Praise for ***Simple Choices for Healthie***

"*Simple Choices for Healthier Eating* is a nutrition fact book disguised as a cookbook—a great tool to help you improve your health. The information is easy to apply, with many tips and recipes that will open you up to new tastes. I found the nutritional facts accurate and understandable—and it's better than many text books for quick reference."
—ADAM INTRONA, DOCTOR OF CHIROPRACTIC

"Creating healthy eating plans and fueling the body's nutritional needs is critical to living well. *Simple Choices for Healthier Eating* is a ready reference guide that simply addresses making good food choices based on scientific facts and personal experience. It's a great time to purchase this cookbook."
—DAN KRAMER, LIFE COACH

"*Simple Choices for Healthier Eating* offers practical resources and specific suggestions without being overwhelming or guilt-inducing. The knowledge and spirit of the authors has inspired me to gradually implement changes into my family's diet. This is no ordinary cookbook!"
—ALLISON JOHNSON, CANCER SURVIVOR, WIFE AND MOTHER

"This book makes a great gift. The information needed to improve health...is presented in a manner to encourage change."
—WINONA L SAATHOFF, R.N., HEALTH EDUCATOR

"At a time when we are being urged by health experts to eat more vegetables and make changes in our diets, it's often hard to know where to begin. *Simple Choices for Healthier Eating* not only provides the nutritional information we need to make healthy food choices, it provides the tools and techniques for preparing the food. Lewis and Fink help us relearn the art of cooking in a manner that is adaptable to our fast-paced lifestyle. This is a wonderful introduction to healthier eating and a wealthy source of information!"
—BOB BRAVERMAN AND SARAH NEARY, FRIENDLY FARM, IOWA CITY, IA

TRANSITIONS TO BETTER LIVING

Simple Choices for Healthier Eating

TRANSITIONS TO BETTER LIVING

Simple Choices for Healthier Eating

Sondra Lewis AND Dorie Fink

Emily
Enjoy healthier
eating.
Blessing
Sondra
9-12-09

Canary Connect Publications
A Division of SOBOLE, Inc.
Coralville, Iowa

DISCLAIMER

This book is not intended to diagnose any illness or disease. Nor is it designed to provide cures and comprehensive solutions. It is not a complete and comprehensive nutritional guide. This information is not intended to replace medical diagnosis or treatment but rather to provide assistance in implementing a healthy approach to eating. Please consult your health care provider for medical advice.

The publisher and authors declare that to the best of their knowledge all material in this book is accurate. We shall have neither liability nor responsibility to any person with respect to any loss or damage alleged to be caused, directly or indirectly, by the information contained in this book.

Cover design by George Foster, Foster & Foster, Inc.
Food photos by Dorie Fink and Sondra Lewis
Illustrations by Rachel Molloy (Pea Patch Graphics) and Christine Hicks

Published in United States of America by
Canary Connect Publications
605 Holiday Road, Coralville, Iowa 52241-1016
For ordering, visit www.SimpleChoices4HealthierEating.com.

ISBN: 978-0-9643462-8-4

Library of Congress Cataloging-in-Publication Data

Lewis, Sondra K.
Simple choices for healthier eating / Sondra Lewis and Dorie Fink.
p. cm. -- (Transitions to better living)
Includes bibliographical references and index.
Summary: "Discusses healthier eating concepts including simple choices for increasing fiber, vegetables, whole grains, and vegetable proteins; lowering fats, sodium, and sugars; choosing healthier fats; and including children. Addresses heart disease and diabetes. Over 80 meal suggestions; over 200 heart healthy, gluten free and/or vegetarian recipes."–Provided by publisher.
ISBN 978-0-9643462-8-4 (pbk. : alk. paper) 1. Nutrition. I. Fink, Dorrit Fryling, 1973- II. Title. III. Series

RA784.L488 2008
613.2--dc22

2008014713

Printed in United States of America

www.Transitions2BetterLiving.com www.SimpleChoices4HealthierLiving.com

Contents

Foreword vii
Preface ix
Acknowledgements xi

Part One: Information Is Key

1 Simple Choices for Healthier Eating: It's a Lifestyle Choice 1
2 Food Labels: Understanding for Healthier Eating 4
3 Fats: A Healthy Balance 8
4 Sodium: How Much Is Too Much? 12
5 Fiber: The Health Difference 14
6 "Sugars": Enjoying in Moderation 16
7 Protein: Quality Counts 18
8 Heart Health: Simple Choices, Big Impact 22
9 Diabetes: Knowledge for Prevention 24
10 Gluten: Understanding Why Some People Need to Avoid It 26
11 Whole Foods: Natural Sources of Goodness 28
12 Maximizing the Benefits of Healthier Eating: Transitions to Better Living 30

Part Two: Recipes – The Heart of It All

13 Tips for Getting Started with the Recipes 32
14 Vegetables 36
15 Condiments 92
16 Making a Meal with Salads 94
17 Breakfast and Brunch Ideas 103
18 Travel Lunches 116
19 Soups, Stews and Casserole Meals 118
20 Quick-Fix Meals 140
21 Cooking for One or Two 159

22 Holiday Dinner Makeover 161
23 Keep Snacking Healthy 166
24 Family Fun Nights 167
25 Beverages 172
26 Breads and Grains 174
27 Desserts 196

Part Three: The Extras

Notes 210
Cook's Glossary 216
Fiber Guide 219
Seasoning Glossary 220
Sweetener Glossary 223
Gadgets, Measuring and More 225
Healthier Choices Shopping Guide 229
Topic and Recipe Index 233
Our Synergism in Action 241
The Making of a Cookbook 241
Contact Us 242
About the Authors 243

Food photos by Dorie Fink and Sondra Lewis

Pumpkin Pancakes with Blueberry Pancake Syrup, page 188
Pepper-Corn Chili, page 130
Fancy Hamburgers, page 146
Confetti Dip, page 42
Wilted Spinach Salad, page 101
Pizza, pages 168–170
Cheese Biscuits, page 183
20-Minute Stir-Fry Dinner, page 61

Foreword

As a doctor, I place a great deal of importance on healthy eating as a critical part of the path to robust health and the prevention of disease. Teaching nutrition and strategies for healthy eating to my patients is a core part of what I do as a physician and is one of the great challenges of my work. We are blessed with an abundance of scientific knowledge about how to eat to support our bodies well. Applying that knowledge meaningfully requires knowing how to extract what is true and important from the enormous amount of information available to us and then to apply it practically in our lives. This can be an overwhelming challenge for the best of us. Many of us have the desire to become healthier but we need guides to teach us what is true in a format that is accessible and practical and easy to integrate into our busy lives.

Sondra Lewis and Dorie Fink are such guides. *Simple Choices for Healthier Eating* is the culmination of years of personal interest, research and experience in the kitchen that has been put in the format of a beautifully written and well-organized manual for how to make healthy food choices and how to prepare good food simply and easily. What you will learn from this book is what constitutes a healthy diet for the majority of people as well as for those with special health issues such as heart disease, diabetes and gluten sensitivity. You will learn how to choose the safest and most environmentally friendly sources of food. Then, most importantly, you will learn how to prepare comprehensive meals for yourself and your family that maximize nutrition while being delicious and easy to incorporate into a busy schedule.

If you are already well versed on the principles of good nutrition, you can skip those chapters and benefit from the marvelous recipes. If you do not have a nutritional background, I believe that you will find the informational chapters to be clear, concise and easy to understand. *Simple Choices for Healthier Eating* is the kind of comprehensive and yet accessible resource that I will make available to all my patients. I know that you will find it enjoyable, informative and, in the end, the road to scrumptious eating and improved health!

Karyn M. Shanks, M.D., F.A.C.P.

Preface

Simple Choices for Healthier Eating is designed to be a resource for those interested in healthier eating. It provides an overview of the nutrients in foods, helpful information about several health issues related to diet and a guide to the selection and usage of various foods. This information is followed by a comprehensive recipe section.

There is a variety of information about "health food" available to us today. It is often hard to sort fact from fiction and know how to prioritize the choices we want to make. In *Simple Choices for Healthier Eating* we start that process for you. Sorting through the hype, we have pulled out the pieces of information that we feel are most critical for making choices that promote healthier eating.

People have a variety of reasons for wanting to eat in a healthier manner. *Simple Choices for Healthier Eating* looks at some key health issues related to diet, including heart disease and diabetes. The book presents simple explanations of the issues, along with evidence that healthier eating is worth the effort because of the disease prevention it promotes.

Once we are motivated to enjoy healthier eating, there is still the element of knowing what to purchase and how to use it. *Simple Choices for Healthier Eating* offers detailed descriptions of various foods, including many vegetables, grains and flours, sweeteners and herbs. It also has a Healthier Choices Shopping Guide, offering suggestions on both ingredients and packaged foods. The recipes are nutrient dense, meaning that they provide a lot of nutrition for the number of calories. Some of them are traditional favorites, while others offer a whole new eating experience.

We believe that healthier eating means eating a variety of foods that provide us with a variety of flavors as well as a host of nutrients. We also believe that it is crucial to have a balanced perspective. For instance, it is important to reduce sodium. But if we reduce it so much that we have to add extra sweeteners to create a satisfying taste, we're being counterproductive.

There is always much discussion about which foods are "healthy foods." While we feel there are many foods that are healthier than others, we also feel it is vital to consume a balanced variety. For all of the knowledge we have about food, there are many things we have yet to find out. Just because one food is described today as a wonder food, that doesn't mean it won't be known tomorrow for its unhealthy properties. Just as important, there is no one food that can meet all of our bodies' needs. In fact, consuming too much of any one food, no matter how healthy it is, can have negative long-term implications. So enjoy a cornucopia of foods, providing your body with a variety of nutrients and taking all things in moderation.

We also believe that healthier eating begins with obtaining information to make smart choices about nutrition and form good habits. Modeling these things to our children is key to investing in their health. Throughout the book, you will find tips for involving children, pleasing finicky eaters, modifying recipes to suit scheduling needs and making recipe preparation easier.

Healthier eating is a lifestyle choice. It is a process that most effectively happens a few choices at a time. We recommend that you read chapters one, two and thirteen before deciding how you will use the rest of the book. If you feel overwhelmed, remember that slow and steady wins the race. We wish you the best in your nutritional journey — it is a transition to better living and is well worth the effort.

Acknowledgments

Everything that has gone into making this book possible
— the knowledge and understanding, the foods, the people, the ideas —
has come from the Holy Spirit, the Lord our God
and His Son, Jesus Christ our Savior.

To Him be all praise and glory!

Sondra and Dorie wish to thank the following people for their help in making this book a reality:

- Our editors, Eric and Elisa, for adding the finishing touches
- Rachel for graphic illustrations that add life and fun to the words
- George for taking our food photos and creating magic with the covers
- The many who read the book at various stages of completion and offered us invaluable comments and endorsements

Sondra wishes to thank:

- My husband, Bob, mother, family and friends for their patience, encouragement and prayers and for being part of the "official tasters"
- My church, First Place group, BSF leaders and my BSF discussion group ladies for their prayerful support and encouragement and also for being part of the "official tasters"
- My dear friend and prayer partner, Carole, whose prayers and encouraging "visits" lighted my path, especially when things seemed to be falling apart
- My friend Dorie, for without her this book would have been only a dream and you would not have the opportunity to enjoy these delicious, healthier recipes

Dorie wishes to thank:

- My husband, Steve, and sons, Nathan and Justin, for encouraging me in my work, tasting and evaluating many recipes and giving me a reason to cook healthy meals
- My extended family, who have supported me all the way and shared with me their discoveries and questions about food
- My small group in Iowa City, who prayed for me and evaluated so many Tuesday evening treats
- My friend Sondra, who gave me the confidence to experiment, the courage to keep trying and who (along with her husband) embraced our family

Part One

Information Is Key

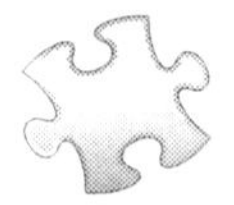

Chapter 1

Simple Choices for Healthier Eating: It's a Lifestyle Choice

Most would agree that the choice to lead a healthier life is a good one to make. But it's a choice that's easy to dismiss or postpone. It involves lifestyle changes — and they can be hard work. However, if we approach the choice to lead a healthier life as a transition, we can allow it to become a process of making simple choices and it becomes much easier to move forward. Nowhere is that more true than with nutrition.

The transition to healthier eating involves making simple choices in a variety of areas.

Simple Choices for Healthier Eating:

- Replace unhealthy fats with healthy fats and, for some, lower fat consumption (chapter three)
- Lower sodium intake (chapter four)
- Increase fiber (chapter five)
- Decrease sugar consumption (chapter six) and use a variety of natural sweeteners (sweetener glossary)
- Increase vegetable proteins (e.g., beans, soy products, nuts/seeds, quinoa, whole grains) (chapter seven)
- Increase vegetables (chapter fourteen) and fruits (p. 196)
- Increase whole grains (chapter twenty-six)

The nutritional choices that we make are also impacted by other lifestyle choices. Choosing to get enough sleep, to be physically active and to reduce the impact of stress on our bodies further enables our bodies to utilize the nutrients we eat and to function properly.

We can look at these nutritional choices as pieces of a large puzzle that fit together to make a complete picture:

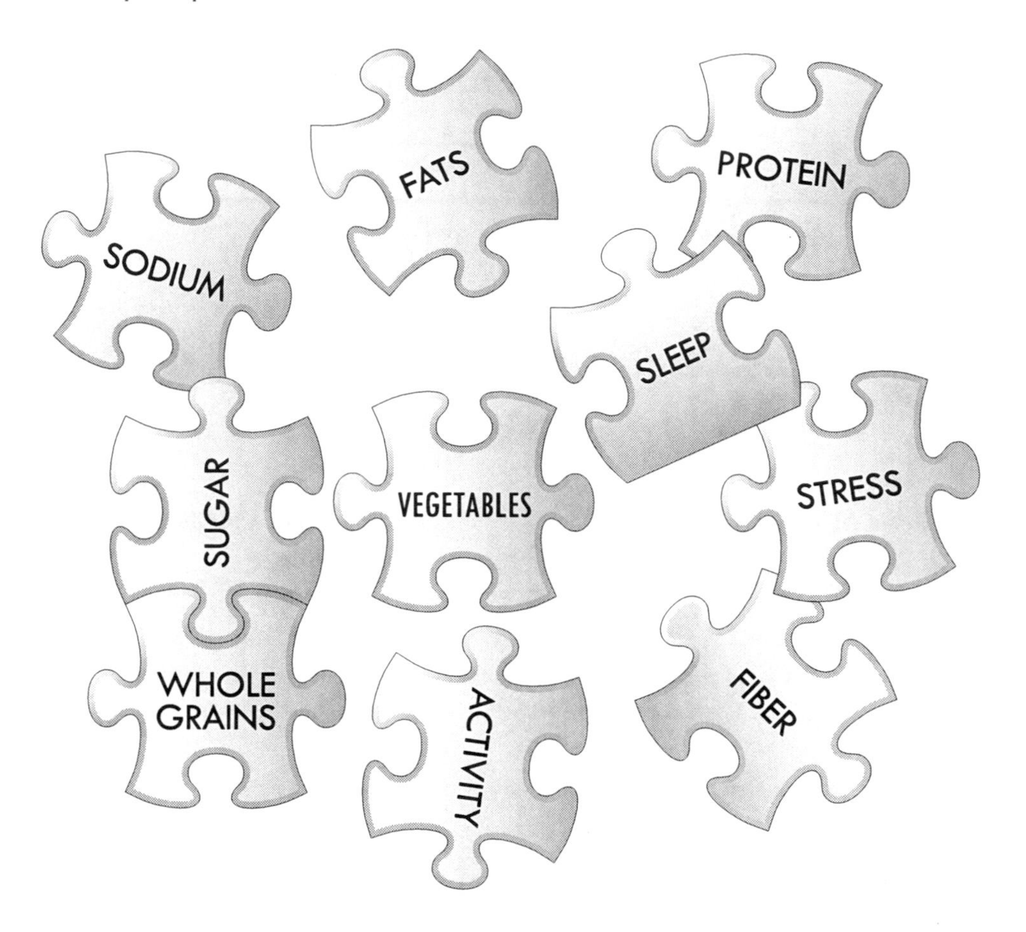

Each choice we make has a nutritional impact on our bodies and gives color and shape to the different puzzle pieces. No piece, by itself, can make a complete picture. But having all of the pieces jumbled together in a box does not make a complete picture either. It is as the pieces are connected in relationship to each other that a picture begins to form. Some pieces will be harder to put in place than others. Completing the puzzle is a process. We will all work at different rates and choose different places of the puzzle on which to work. But the overall picture will be the common framework to which we connect all of our pieces.

Each chapter in part one looks at a different piece of the nutritional puzzle. We recommend that you use the next chapter as a starting point and then read chapters three through twelve in any order, depending on your needs and interests. Ultimately, they all work together to provide support and direction in the transition toward healthier eating.

Likewise, the recipes in part two are designed to be a guide for implementing those choices, providing methods and techniques for adapting them to your own recipes and style of cooking. They are designed to be simple, healthy and appealing. Many of them are also designed to be quick. Most of all, they are designed to be flexible so that you can use them in a manner that enhances your life and moves you and your family toward healthier eating. Before beginning to use the recipes, look through chapter thirteen for tips on getting started with the recipes.

The information and resources in part three expand the ideas introduced in parts one and two. They can be used both as a resource for understanding new ideas and as a catalyst for incorporating those ideas into your daily routine. They also provide ideas for making simple choices about healthier eating beyond the recipes (e.g., Healthier Choices Shopping Guide).

Transitions can be overwhelming. When we try to move too quickly or do everything at once, it becomes too much and the process halts, benefiting no one. Most of us cannot understand, shop for, prepare and enjoy numerous new tastes all at once. We throw up our hands and say, "I can't do it!" Focusing on one or two new things at a time is easier. When we make changes one or two things at a time, we often end up making faster progress in the long run, and the changes we make are more likely to be lifelong changes instead of simply impulsive actions that last only for a short while. Often the small changes can have the biggest long-term impact. Just like putting a few pennies a day into an interest-bearing savings account can yield a large sum of money in the end, so every choice we make toward living healthier lives can increase the impact of each choice before it.

> Andrew Weil, M.D., notes that when a lifestyle change starts slowly and builds over time, the change can "take root and become an ongoing contribution to health."[1]

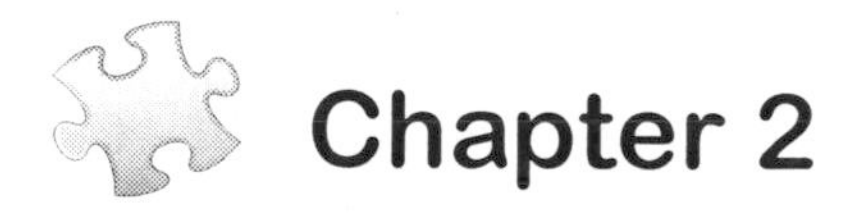

Chapter 2

Food Labels: Understanding for Healthier Eating

Companies often try to make their products sound "healthy" by using catchphrases on their packaging. A bag of jelly beans reads, "A Fat-Free Food!" That sounds good, but most of the reasons for avoiding fat (e.g., weight loss, healthy balance of nutrients) will not be accomplished by eating jelly beans. The trick to understanding the health value of a food goes beyond the marketing phrases. It is important to know what nutrients are present, where they come from and what – if anything – has been added.

Nutrients are the substances our bodies take from food that allow us to function. Nutrients include fats, carbohydrates, protein, water, vitamins and minerals. We need nutrients in varying amounts and for different reasons. Understanding how our bodies use these nutrients and where the nutrients come from is an important part of making informed decisions about the health value of specific foods.

The nutrition facts panel on packages tells us the calories and nutrients per serving.

Calories are a measurement of energy. It is important to balance the calories consumed with the calories burned in physical activity. Extra calories are converted to body fat. The number of calories we need in a given day depends on our age, gender and activity level. For links to Internet programs that help you calculate your ideal caloric need, visit our websites (p. 242).

A sample of recommended calories according to age, gender and activity level.[1]

Men Age	Activity Level (minutes/day)			Women Age	Activity Level (minutes/day)		
	< 30	30–60	> 60		< 30	30–60	> 60
8	1,400	1,600	2,000	8	1,400	1,600	1,800
13	1,600	2,200	2,600	13	1,600	2,000	2,200
18	2,400	2,800	3,200	18	1,600	2,000	2,400
30	2,400	2,600	3,000	30	1,800	2,200	2,400
55	2,200	2,400	2,800	55	1,600	2,000	2,200
70	2,000	2,200	2,600	70	1,600	1,800	2,000

Fat is a nutrient necessary for energy, warmth, the health of skin, hair and cell membranes, the regulation of blood pressure and the absorption of fat-soluble vitamins. It also flavors and moistens food. There is currently a great deal of research about how much fat (or how little fat) we need. High levels of certain fats (saturated and trans fats) are associated with an increased risk of heart disease, diabetes and other health concerns. (See chapter three for more information.) In addition, a high intake of fat can lead to an intake of excess calories. All fat, no matter what type, contains 9 calories per gram, more than any other nutrient. However, there are also some really good fats that are quite beneficial – even essential – to our health.

One study showed that replacing eighty carbohydrate calories with eighty unsaturated fat calories every day lowered the risk of heart disease by 30 to 40 percent. The same study showed that replacing only thirty calories from carbohydrates with thirty calories from trans fats doubled the risk of heart disease.[2] Labels are now required to list trans fats because of their negative impact on health. A growing number of labels are listing the good fats (polyunsaturated and monounsaturated fats) as well.

For many years, it was thought that we should limit fat intake to between 20 and 35 percent of our total calories. Researchers are starting to think that might not be high enough for many people. Some estimate that we need at least 20 percent of our calories to be from healthy fats just in order to absorb the vitamins and essential fatty acids that we need and to maintain healthy levels of HDL cholesterol and triglycerides.[3] (For other benefits of fat, see p. 8). We recommend consuming no trans fats and limited amounts of saturated fats while seeking out good sources of healthy fats.

Cholesterol. Recent research is showing that dietary cholesterol may not impact blood cholesterol levels for most people. Rather, trans fats and saturated fats may be more of the dietary issue.[4] (See chapter eight for more information.)

Sodium should be limited to **2,300 milligrams per day**.[5] (See chapter four.) The recipes within this book were designed to be tasty without high levels of sodium. By nature, some foods will be higher in sodium than others. It is important to keep food consumption throughout the day in mind when looking at sodium intake. (Example: If you enjoyed salsa and chips with lunch, choose a lower-sodium option for dinner.)

Carbohydrates are our bodies' primary source of energy. The quality of energy they provide varies greatly according to their source (see below). On the nutritional panel, the only carbohydrates typically listed are "fiber" and "sugar." However, complex carbohydrates also contain starches.

Fiber is critical for good good health. The average healthy adult should consume a minimum of **35 grams per day**, or 14 grams for every 1,000 calories (see chapter five).

Sugar can be a wonderful enhancement to food, but it can also add a lot of "empty calories" (calories with no nutrition) and can have a negative impact on our health. The nutritional quality of sugar depends on where it came from. Sugar is found in vegetables and fruits (fructose), milk (lactose) and numerous other natural and synthetic sources (see chapter six). It is important that sugars be consumed in moderation. Products of the same type can differ greatly in amounts of added sugars, so checking the quantity on the label is important. In this book, we have tried to make all recipes lower in sugar than common equivalent recipes. We have also attempted to use healthier sugars and to balance the sugar with fiber and protein.

Protein is critical for building and repairing muscle tissue, cells and bones. It also slows the absorption of sugars into the blood and helps us fight disease, produce hormones and digest food. However, too much protein – like too much of anything else – can be harmful (see p. 18). Though scientific studies indicate that more research is needed to determine optimum amounts of protein, it is generally considered accurate to say that the average American adult needs a minimum of 0.8 grams of protein for every kilogram of bodyweight.[6] This is approximately 7 grams for every twenty pounds, or about 10 percent of our total calories (pregnant and breastfeeding women, highly physically active people and chronically ill people need more). Chapter seven shows how easy it is to get adequate amounts of protein.

Vitamins and minerals are powerful substances that can have a great impact on our health. Seeking a variety, from a variety of sources, is a key to good health.

The next five chapters look more specifically at five of the items highlighted above (fats, sodium, fiber, sugars and protein). As above, they are in the same order in which they appear on the nutritional facts panel.

A few other notes about the nutritional panel

Serving Size: When determining the nutrient value of a food, it is important to note the serving size on labels. For example, one can of soup may have 400 milligrams of sodium per serving, while another has only 300. However, if the serving size of the first can is one cup and the serving size of the second can is only a half cup, the first soup is the one with less sodium.

The serving size is also important when considering portions. In the example above, if you require two cups of soup to feel satisfied, you would be consuming either 800 or 1,200 milligrams of sodium – that doesn't sound as good as it looked on the label. The USDA suggests the number of servings per day that we need of each of the following five food groups: grains, vegetables, fruits, dairy and protein. We used these guidelines to design our serving sizes to meet the nutrient needs of the average person. We also took into consideration what the average person would want to eat in order to be full without consuming too much fat, sodium or sugar.

Recipe Nutritional Analysis: We have created our own nutritional facts panel, placing it at the bottom of most recipe pages (see sample at the top of the next page, with explanation of abbreviations used). To do the analysis, we referred to the USDA nutrient

Analysis/Serving:
Calories: 000 (Fat Cal 00) Fat: 00g (00g Sat) Cholesterol: 00mg
Sodium: 000mg Carbs: 00g (00g Fiber 00g Sugar) Protein: 00
Fat Cal = fat calories Sat = saturated Carbs = Carbohydrates
mg = milligrams g = grams

levels and to the actual food labels from brands we used. A few things to note: (1) If a recipe contains a choice of ingredients, the first ingredient listed was used for analysis. (2) If a recipe gives a range in quantity for an ingredient, the lower end of the range was used for analysis, unless otherwise noted. And (3) some ingredients (such as sausage) vary tremendously in their nutrients. For brands we used in testing and analyzing the recipes, please see the Healthier Choices Shopping Guide.

Ingredients: In addition to the quantities of nutrients, it is important to know their source. The ingredient list on a packaged product (listed in order of predominance by weight) or the ingredient list for a recipe provide valuable information. Some key things to look for:

- Is the **fat** from animals or plants? Generally, animal sources will have a higher level of saturated fats.
- Are the **carbohydrates** "smart carbs," providing fiber and long-lasting energy, or do they provide "empty calories" and only short bursts of energy? Generally, carbohydrates found in nature are more nutrient dense than processed carbohydrates. Carbohydrates from starches (e.g., beans and whole grains) produce long-lasting energy, while those from sugars (e.g., fruit, candy, honey) produce short bursts of energy.
- Are the **sources of sugar** natural or artificial? (See chapter six.)
- Is the **protein** from plants or animals? Both are good, but animal proteins should be consumed in moderation since they typically contain more saturated fat.
- Are the **sources of vitamins and minerals** natural sources (such as fruits and vegetables) or synthetic sources? We recommend using natural sources as much as possible (even in supplements).
- Is there added **sodium**? Ingredients with "sodium," "salt" or "soda" in their name (e.g., mono*sodium* glutamate [MSG], garlic *salt*, baking *soda*) contain sodium.

Included in the list of ingredients are various **synthetic products** that are used to alter the taste, appearance or shelf life of a product. While there is great debate about the danger posed by some of these products, it has been shown that many are carcinogenic (can cause cancer over the long term).[7] It has also been shown that, in the short term, people respond to these chemicals in much the same way they respond to drugs and alcohol: some people notice few visible effects, while others notice a marked difference in activity level, concentration, mood swings, depression and/or feelings of illness.[8] The quantity consumed before an effect is noticed varies between people and according to circumstance. We recommend that preservatives, additives and artificial flavorings be limited or avoided as much as possible. For more specifics, as well as further suggestions on what to look for when reading labels, and for recommendations of brands to consider, see the Healthier Choices Shopping Guide.

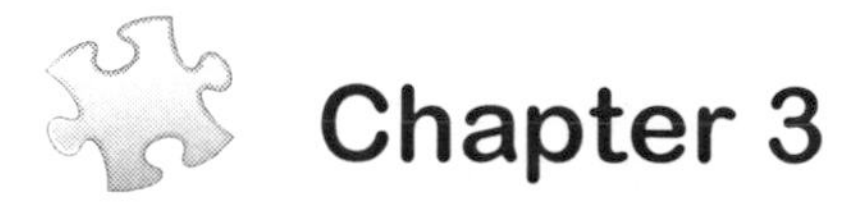

Chapter 3

Fats: A Healthy Balance

Fats are an important aspect of a healthy diet. As with many substances, our bodies need some fats but are harmed by consuming too much. We often hear that "low fat is good," but research is showing that the type of fat we consume is far more important than the quantity.[1]

For many years we were told that eating high-fat foods was directly related to weight gain and that reducing fat intake would lead to weight loss. It is true that fats are high in calories. Since weight gain comes primarily from eating too many calories, reducing extra calories that come from fat can be beneficial. However, fat is not the only source of "extra" calories. Studies are showing that low-fat diets are not any more effective in weight loss than other types of diets; it is lowering caloric intake that is important.[2] Moreover, there is mounting evidence that increasing healthy fats has a beneficial role in moving toward health (see p. 5). So we need to understand the different types of fat and focus on choosing the healthy ones.

Healthy Fats: Polyunsaturated (including omega-3 fatty acids) and Monounsaturated Fats

- Found in fish and many plant foods, including nuts, seeds and nontropical plant oils
- Found in some fruits and vegetables (e.g., avocadoes, olives)
- Typically liquid at room temperature
- Do not raise blood cholesterol levels; may actually lower cholesterol levels if used in place of saturated and trans fats[3] or in place of carbohydrates[4]
- Should make up the bulk of fat in our diet (at least 92% of our total fat intake)[5]

Reasons to Consume Healthy Fats:

- Healthy fats provide us with energy and warmth.
- Healthy fats protect our organs.
- Healthy fats are essential for the function and development of all body cells.
- Healthy fats enable the brain to develop and function properly.
- Healthy fats help with the absorption of nutrients.
- Healthy fats help with the production of hormones.
- Healthy fats slow down digestion, making us feel full longer. (This can be used strategically for weight loss: people who eat breakfast containing some healthy fat usually need less of a snack later in the morning.)

Simple Choices for Consuming Healthy Fats:

- Choose unsaturated over saturated fats.
- Avoid packaged foods with saturated or trans fats.
- Incorporate nuts, seeds and fish into your meals and snacks.
- Blend flaxseed oil with butter to use as a spread (see sidebar on p. 192).
- Use flaxseed oil instead of butter/margarine on popcorn and steamed vegetables.

Two Types of Bad Fats

Saturated Fats:

- Found primarily in tropical oils and in foods we get from animals
- Found in hydrogenated oils
- Typically solid at room temperature
- A dietary cause of high blood cholesterol[6]
- Should be no more than 7 percent of our total daily calories (e.g., a 2,000-calorie diet should contain no more than 16 grams of saturated fat)[7]

Hydrogenated or Trans Fats:

- Oils that have been chemically processed to bind additional hydrogen to the fat molecule
- Used to make many processed goods (including margarine, shortening, chips and baked goods such as bread, crackers and cookies)
- Raise bad cholesterol levels and decrease good cholesterol levels[8]
- Worse than saturated fats[9]
- Increase the risk of vascular disease (disease of the blood vessels)
- Most recommendations are to eliminate them from the diet

Reasons to Consider Lowering Overall Fat Consumption:

- Fats are high in calories (all fat, no matter what type, contains 9 calories per gram of fat) and can lead to unnecessary caloric intake and, consequently, weight gain.
- Being overweight and/or having poor cholesterol levels can lead to heart disease and stroke.[10]
- Being overweight and/or having heart disease increases the risk of diabetes.[11]
- Saturated and trans fats increase blood levels of bad cholesterol.[12]

Simple Choices for Lowering Overall Fat Consumption:

- Reduce quantities of fat in baking and cooking.
  Example 1: Use less fat (pp. 197–199, reducing fat in cookies).
  Example 2: Substitute pureed fruit or vegetables for some of the fat (e.g., applesauce in coffeecakes, pp. 184–185, pumpkin in cookies, p. 85).
- Eat baked or oven-fried foods rather than fried and deep-fat-fried foods (e.g., fish, p. 151; chicken, pp. 98 and 144; potatoes, pp. 21, 39, 76 and 88).
- Choose lower-fat snacks and milk products (check labels since many low-fat products are high in sodium or sugar to make up for lost flavor).
- For stir-fries, use "Water Stir-Fry" method (p. 61).

continue ...

- Use herbs and seasonings to flavor foods instead of using excess oil.
- Use well-seasoned cast-iron cookware since it requires less fat.
- Use condiments, salad dressings and gravies sparingly.

A common source of fat in any kitchen is cooking oil and there are numerous varieties. There are some key differences between oils that allow them to be used for different purposes. While flavor is important, it is also important to use oils that can withstand the temperatures you plan to use. When oils start to smoke, they have reached their smoke point and may produce free radicals. Free radicals can increase the risk of cancer. Since research on this is constantly revealing new information, we encourage you to seek out current scientific studies for updates. We choose to use oils at temperatures below that of their smoke point and have used information from Spectrum Organic Oils as our guide. Safe temperatures for each type of oil will vary depending on whether or not it is refined or unrefined (see next page). Varying the oils we use helps to provide balance to our diets; no oil should be used in exclusion of all others.

<table>
<tr><th>Temperature</th><th>High-Heat Oil to 460°</th><th>Medium-Heat Oil to 375°</th><th>Low-Heat Oil to 320°</th><th>No-Heat Oil</th></tr>
<tr><td>Purpose</td><td>browning
roasting
searing</td><td>baking
stir-frying</td><td>light sautéing
rouxes
sauces</td><td>drizzling on cooked foods
salad dressings</td></tr>
<tr><td>Oils okay to use:</td><td colspan="4">Refined: almond, apricot kernel, avocado, high-heat, organic canola,* grapeseed oil** (to 420°), peanut,* high-heat/high-oleic safflower, high-heat/high-oleic sunflower</td></tr>
<tr><td></td><td></td><td colspan="3">Refined: sesame, walnut
Unrefined: safflower</td></tr>
<tr><td></td><td></td><td></td><td colspan="2">Refined: soy*
Unrefined: corn,* olive, peanut,* sesame</td></tr>
<tr><td></td><td></td><td></td><td></td><td>Unrefined: flaxseed (only for drizzling on cooked foods)</td></tr>
</table>

As we choose oils from a variety of plant sources, we also need to select the type of oil within each variety. The following terms are important to know:

*These oils we recommend avoiding unless you are comfortable with the source: peanut oil (okay if safe from aflatoxins), canola, soy and corn oil unless GMO free. Also we recommend avoiding cottonseed oil because it is exempt from food safety guidelines since it is primarily used for textiles.

**Because of the low oil content of grape seeds, oil cannot be extracted through typical expeller-pressed means. Many companies use chemicals. We recommend finding a company that uses low levels of heat to expeller press their grape seed oil. If solvents are used, alcohol is preferable over hexane.

- **Refined and unrefined:** Refined oils have been treated to increase the time before oxidation occurs. This means that they have a longer shelf life than do their unrefined counterparts and can be safely heated to higher temperatures. However, they generally do not have as much flavor nor as many nutrients as the unrefined oils. In some cases, the refinement involves bleaching or the introduction of other chemicals. Unrefined oils should be used whenever possible for light sautéing and salad dressings
- **Light:** When the term "light" is used with oil (as in "light olive oil"), it means that the oil has been refined; it does *not* mean that it is lower in fat.
- **Cold pressed and expeller pressed:** These are two processes that are used to obtain oils without the use of chemicals.
- **Virgin and extra virgin:** These terms define types of olive oil. Both are judged to have superior taste and neither may contain any refined oil. Extra virgin comes from the first pressing of the olives and is slightly less acidic than virgin olive oil.
- **High oleic:** Oleic acid is a monounsaturated omega acid that is beneficial to health. High oleic oils have large concentrations of oleic acid.
- **Toasted** oils are made from roasted seeds, are generally darker in color and often contain sodium, but they may be a healthier option for flavoring than typical soy sauces.

Whatever oils you use, it is important to store them properly.

- **Slow down oxidation:** Since heat and light increase oxidation, oils should be stored in dark, cool places. Many advocate refrigeration after opening. We choose to refrigerate those oils that we do not use regularly. However, oils that we consume quickly (within two months), we store in a cool, dark cupboard, not near the range. Flaxseed oil should always be refrigerated, even before opening.
- **Keep exposure to air at a minimum:** Purchase oils in small containers so that you use them relatively quickly after opening. Rancid oils not only taste bad but also have high levels of free radicals, which are problematic for health.
- **Avoid exposure to plastics:** We believe it is safest to purchase and keep oils in glass jars so that chemicals from the plastic containers do not leach into the oils.

In addition to a variety of oils, there are a variety of butters and solid fats available.

- **Butter:** We often cut standard recipe amounts in half. Also, use unsalted butter when appropriate.
- **"Margarines":** These products are usually free of cholesterol and lower than butter in saturated fats, but they can contain high levels of trans fats (when they do, they are worse than using butter[13]). Stick margarines are generally higher in trans fats than tub margarines. Margarines are often high in sodium as well.
- **Shortening and lard:** These are usually full of unhealthy fats. Consider using butter or coconut oil instead.
- **Coconut oil:** A tropical oil that is high in saturated fats but that has more nutrients than most saturated fats. Research varies on its benefits and drawbacks.

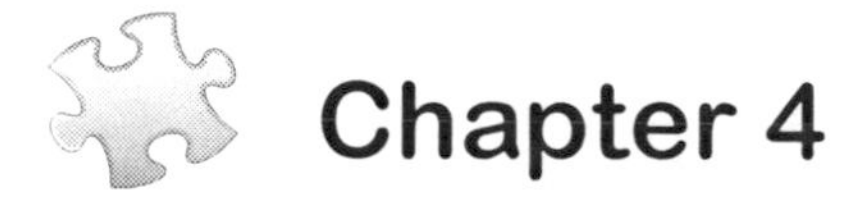

Chapter 4

Sodium: How Much Is Too Much?

Sodium is a mineral that we can't live without, yet living with too much can negatively impact our health. Salt is comprised of sodium and chloride. Sodium naturally occurs in many foods. However, it is also added to many foods in the form of salt.

The **good**:

- Sodium is critical for maintaining an appropriate balance of fluids in our bodies.
- Sodium stimulates the muscles, helps transmit nerve impulses and aids the function of the adrenal glands.
- Sodium keeps minerals (such as calcium) soluble in the blood.
- Sodium adds flavor to food and acts as a preservative.

The **bad**:

- If sodium levels go beyond what our kidneys can regulate, the sodium accumulates in our blood and attracts water, increasing our blood volume.
- High sodium intake is often directly related to high blood pressure.[1] This, in turn, raises the risk for heart disease, stroke and kidney disease.
- Some people, including many older adults, are more sodium sensitive, meaning that they are more likely to experience high blood pressure as a direct result of high intake levels of sodium.
- High levels of sodium intake are also being linked to osteoporosis (because sodium can pull calcium from the bone) and stomach cancer.[2]

The **ugly**:

- We need only 1,200 to 1,500 milligrams of sodium a day[3] but typically consume much more.
- Recommendations are to limit salt intake to less than 2,300 milligrams for healthy individuals;[4] recommendations are lower for high-risk groups.
- Of the sodium we consume, 77% is added during the processing of foods (12% occurs naturally in food, 5% is added during cooking and 6% is added at the table).[5]
- In addition to the obvious (e.g., potato chips and crackers), salt is added in places we might not expect, including salad dressings, poultry, cinnamon rolls and pies.
- In 2007 it was estimated that if the amount of sodium in processed and restaurant foods were reduced by half, 150,000 lives could be saved every year.[6]

- You could meet your sodium quota for the day by consuming half of most frozen pizzas, 2 cups of many canned soups, 2 pieces of many frozen lasagnas, 4 large sourdough pretzels or 10 cookies made from purchased refrigerated dough.

Research is showing that one-third of the people who have high blood pressure can attain normal blood pressure by reducing their salt intake.[7] It also shows that consuming large quantities of sodium early in life might "weaken genetic defenses against developing high blood pressure."[8] So making the choice to lower sodium intake while our blood pressure levels are still normal reduces our risk for heart and kidney disease.[9] The good news is that our taste buds can make the adjustment in just a few weeks.

Simple choices for reducing sodium in our cooking:

- Reduce the salt called for in recipes.
- Add salt only after tasting a dish and determining the true need for flavor.
- Use fresh and dried herbs to add flavor to food.
- When using salty meats, such as sausage, use less meat and cut it into smaller portions so that the flavor comes up in most bites but the quantity is reduced.
- Consider "low sodium" or "no salt added" versions of broth, canned tomatoes and canned beans. Also, compare brands of these products and canned "soup bases" for use in recipes (see pp. 119, 123, 137 and 229–232 for more information).
- Compare brands when using frozen vegetables. Many packages contain no additional salt, while others will have a few hundred additional milligrams.

Simple choices for reducing added sodium at the table:

- Keep the saltshaker away from the table.
- Limit your use of condiments and dressings. When ordering out, ask for these condiments on the side and then use only what you need.
- Use a variety of herbs and spices to liven up your food. Not only will you not need the excess ketchup and mustard, but you will not want to cover up the other great flavors.
- Use lemon as a condiment in place of salad dressings or tartar sauce (on fish).

Simple choices for reducing salt consumed from manufactured products:

- Frequent restaurants that offer oil and vinegar or fresh lemon wedges as alternatives to commercially prepared salad dressings. Or take your own.
- Check the sodium content of cheese products. Many brands are quite high.
- Plan ahead for when you'll want a snack. Choose to have healthy snacks handy (e.g., in your briefcase or in the diaper bag) so you are less tempted to reach for the convenience snacks that are often high in sodium.
- Compare labels; the salt content of similar products varies greatly by brand.
- Consume canned soups and prepared frozen dishes with caution.
- Be aware that products labeled "reduced sodium" may still be high in sodium, though they are reduced from the current norm. "Unsalted" products might not have added salt, but naturally occurring salt may still be present.

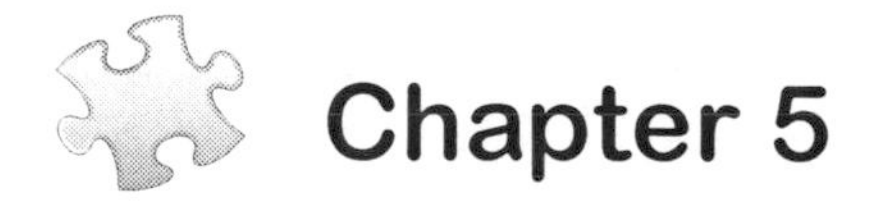

Chapter 5

Fiber: The Health Difference

Fiber is a substance found in plants that is amazingly important to the human body. Fiber plays a crucial role in digestive health, heart health, cancer prevention, weight management and the management of diabetes.

There are two kinds of fiber: soluble and insoluble fiber.

Insoluble fiber:

- Found primarily in whole grains and a variety of vegetables
- Sometimes referred to as "roughage"
- Works much like a street sweeper to help eliminate waste from the digestive track
- Helps to keep bowel function regular
- Regularity and ease of elimination helps to prevent toxins from building up in the body, thus helping in the management of numerous health challenges and in the prevention of diabetes and diverticulitis.[1]

Soluble fiber:

- Found in oats, barley, beans and fruit
- Absorbs water and becomes much like a thick, gummy glue
- Binds with substances such as cholesterol and helps to remove them from the body before they are absorbed into the bloodstream[2]

Other benefits of fiber:

- Fiber slows down digestion, reducing the speed at which sugar passes into the bloodstream and thus helps to regulate blood sugar levels.[3] (This helps anyone wishing to avoid "sugar highs;" it is critical for those with diabetes.)
- Fiber is filling, so it can be used as a weight management tool. Consuming a high-fiber food (such as an apple) shortly before a meal keeps the digestive system busy and signals the body to eat less at the meal. However, there is a reason to use this technique with caution. If we eat too much fiber right before opportunities to eat other nutrient-rich foods, we might deprive our bodies of a complete source of nutrition. This is especially critical for children.
- High-fiber foods are typically low in fat and calories, providing great options for snacks since they keep our stomachs satisfied without filling our bodies with "junk."

- Fiber is not absorbed during digestion but rather helps to move excess fat and chemicals out of the body. For this reason, foods high in fiber often aid digestion.
- Fiber provides food for the friendly flora in our gut. (This flora is important for digestion and is a vital part of our immune system.)

Where do we find fiber? Fiber is found in plant-based foods such as fruits and vegetables, whole grains and beans.

How much fiber do we need? The American Heart Association and the USDA recommended that everyone one year old and above consume **at least fourteen grams of fiber for every 1,000 calories** of food.[4] For someone who consumes 2,500 calories, this works out to 35 grams of fiber a day. We believe this is a minimum at best and that even higher amounts of fiber are beneficial. If your body is not used to consuming this much fiber, it is important to increase fiber amounts slowly, allowing your digestive system to adjust.

It is possible to get our fiber directly from the food we eat, but it is a challenge. Often a fiber supplement is beneficial (see our websites, p. 242). To determine your typical intake of fiber from food, record the foods you eat for three or four days and then use the recipes and Fiber Guide (p. 219) to determine how much fiber you have consumed.

Simple Choices for Including Fiber in a Daily Eating Routine:

- Include lots of fruits and vegetables. Focus on the actual food, not its juice.
- Eat the skins of fruits and vegetables. Use caution with nonorganic fruits and vegetables (p. 37). There is a double reward here in that it also saves time in food preparation. Examples: Use the peel on butternut squash (pp. 128–129 and 209); eat the skins of potatoes (p. 76) and fruits.
- Plan ahead to have high-fiber options available for snacks (e.g., carrot chips and apples). We are more likely to consume these healthier snacks if they are quick and readily available in the refrigerator.
- Use whole grains in cooking such as adding oats to meat loaf patties (pp. 154–155). See page 174 for ideas on how to make the transition to enjoying whole grains in breads and desserts as well as in pasta and rice.
- When possible, choose whole-grain options when eating out. If you do not see a whole-grain option on the menu, ask whether such an option might be available. If enough people ask, things will change.
- Add high-fiber foods such as oats, bran and wheat germ to items like muffins (pp. 186–187), pancakes (p. 188), granola (p. 208), yogurt, salads, applesauce and toppings for ice cream (p. 208) or fruit crisps (pp. 202–203).
- Use flaxseed meal in baking (e.g., granola bars, pp. 112–115; pancakes, p. 189) and as additions to cereal (garnish oatmeal), smoothies (p. 106) and yogurt.
- Find ways to include a variety of beans in your meals and snacks — bean dips (p. 149), adding beans to soups (e.g., 125), casseroles (e.g., pp. 138–139), etc.

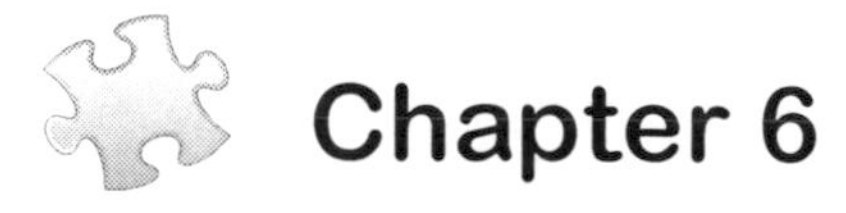

Chapter 6

"Sugars": Enjoying in Moderation

Sugars are a significant part of our diet, and with good reason: they taste good, are found naturally in fruits and vegetables and act as a preservative. However, they can quickly boost our calorie intake and fill us up before we get adequate nutrition. For this reason, the diet and lifestyle recommendations of the American Heart Association include "minimizing the intake of beverages and foods with added sugars."[1]

Understanding why sugars are used can help us make informed choices about how to reduce them. There are a variety of reasons for using sweeteners in foods. Sweeteners:

- Make foods taste sweeter
- Add moisture, creating an appealing texture and a melt-in-your-mouth effect
- Enhance other flavors in foods
- Add flavor and moisture when fats are removed
- Increase the shelf life of many foods
- Save money*

There are also a variety of reasons for limiting sugars. When we limit sugars, we:

- Reduce calories
- Avoid "filling up" before we get adequate nutrition
- Reduce negative effects that are a direct result of sugar consumption (e.g., tooth decay,[2] decreased immunity[3])
- Reduce risk of health conditions that may be influenced by sugar consumption (e.g., diabetes, acid reflux and other digestive issues, difficulty concentrating, heart-related health issues and yeast overgrowth[4])
- Help to promote good blood sugar levels
- Limit the intake of unhealthy fats and sodium since many high-sugar foods are high in these as well

When we find ways to enjoy sugars in moderation, we can maximize the benefits of sugar without experiencing the significant negative consequences.

---

*In some cases, less expensive sweeteners, such as high-fructose corn syrup, are a direct replacement for cane sugar. In other cases, they provide a way of selling a product without needing a large amount of the more expensive whole food (e.g., applesauce with corn syrup requires fewer apples; maple syrup with corn syrup requires less maple syrup – none at all if imitation maple flavoring is used).

The Issue of Corn Syrup

There is much controversy concerning corn syrup and high-fructose corn syrup. Theories are under study for ideas ranging from thinking that corn syrup is hard for the body to absorb,[5] to thoughts that it causes obesity,[6] negatively affects cholesterol[7] and is related to the increase of diabetes.[8] We cannot deny the prevalence of corn syrup in processed foods. According to *The American Journal of Clinical Nutrition*, in 2004 high-fructose corn syrup represented "more than forty percent of caloric sweeteners added to foods and beverages and [was] the sole caloric sweetener in soft drinks in the United States."[9] Whatever the specific health impacts may be, it is a fact that all corn syrups increase calories and decrease the nutritional value of food. For this reason alone, we believe it is worth eliminating or at least limiting consumption.

Simple Choices for Enjoying Sugar in Moderation:

- **Avoid or at least limit corn syrup and high-fructose corn syrup.** Check labels on everything from crackers to canned beans.
- **Avoid or at least limit artificial sweeteners.** Because of compelling evidence of damaging effects with long-term use,[10] our view is that they should be avoided.
- **Limit the quantity of calories that come from sugar.** Check the grams of sugar per serving as well as the serving size.
- **Opt for whole fruit over juice.** Even 100% juice has a high concentration of sugar.
- **Juice consumed should be 100% juice.** Avoid sweeteners and flavorings.
- **Reduce sugars in baking.** Begin in small amounts – even a tablespoon at a time.
- **Use organic cane sugars.** We have found these to be naturally sweeter, allowing less sugar to be used. Dorie's son licked a bit of a common brand of sugar from his finger and liked it, then tried an organic brand and liked it better. He went back to the nonorganic brand and said, "Now this tastes like lemon!"
- **Use a variety of herbs and spices to enhance flavor.** See Seasoning Glossary.
- **Use a variety of sweeteners.** See Sweetener Glossary.
- **Taste before topping.** Sometimes we add toppings to food out of habit rather than necessity (e.g., syrup, dressing, sauce). There may be enough flavor already, so adding a lot on top hides those good flavors and "wastes" the use of great ingredients!
- **Add sugar strategically, allowing the sugar quantity to be reduced elsewhere.**
  Example 1: When Dorie added a bit of sugar and some chocolate chips to her pancake batter, her son stopped using syrup and reduced his overall sugar intake.
  Example 2: Sprinkle sugar on the top of muffins and coffee cake. This provides an initial sweet taste so the sugar inside the batter can be reduced.
- **Watch ingredients in "low-fat foods."** When companies cut fats, they often find flavor elsewhere by increasing the sugars (e.g., low- or no-fat salad dressings).
- **Discriminate among brands.** Some companies use less sugar or find better sources. Foods that commonly have discrepancies between brands include cereals, bread, crackers, condiments, applesauce and canned foods (e.g., soups, beans, fruit).

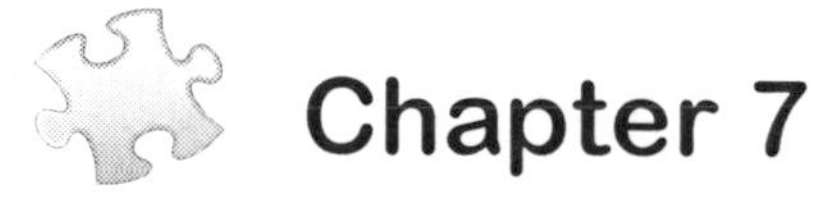

Chapter 7

Protein: Quality Counts

Protein is an important part of any diet. Our bodies need protein in order to grow, repair cells, fight disease, produce hormones and digest food. However, we usually do not need large amounts. The average adult needs a minimum of about 7 grams of protein for every 20 pounds,[1] (only about 10 percent of our total calories). This need varies depending on health and activity level.*

Proteins are constructed of combinations of amino acids. There are twenty known amino acids, but our bodies can produce only half of them. The others, "essential amino acids," need to be obtained from food. Proteins from animal sources typically contain all essential aminos and are known as "complete proteins." However, they often come packaged with saturated fat. Proteins from vegetable, or plant, sources often lack one or more essential amino acids but provide much more nutrition per calorie. Some people make the choice to eat mostly or only vegetable proteins.** These diets are referred to as "vegetarian" (includes egg and dairy products) and "vegan" (contains no animal products). We support those who choose vegan or vegetarian diets. An edmame symbol indicates recipes that are vegetarian or have a vegetarian option.

We believe that everyone can benefit from eating more vegetable proteins. They are consistently lower in saturated fats and typically more nutrient dense than animal proteins. People who consume higher amounts of vegetable protein have greater health advantages, including lower blood pressure.[3] However, we also promote the consumption of a variety of foods and believe that animal proteins can be part of a healthy diet. Therefore, we recommend lean portions of meat and poultry from grass-fed and free-range animals (p. 29) and small but regular amounts of wild-caught fish (p. 97).

---

*Researchers are still trying to determine optimum protein levels. Since the digestion of protein requires calcium, consuming high levels of protein can cause the body to take calcium from the bone. One study showed that "women who ate more than 95 grams of protein a day were 20% more likely to have broken a wrist over a 12-year period" than those who ate less than 68 grams a day.[2] Consequently, long-term high protein diets should be evaluated carefully.

**It used to be common belief that sources of vegetable proteins should be combined properly at each meal to get the right balance of aminos. "Protein combining" was thought to be especially important for vegetarians. Research is now showing that this is not as critical as once thought. What's important is to simply eat a variety of vegetable proteins throughout the day.

Some healthier animal proteins with their saturated (sat) fat and protein content.

Animal Proteins (4 oz. raw)	Sat Fat (grams)	Protein (grams)	Animal Proteins (4 oz. raw)	Sat Fat (grams)	Protein (grams)
Beef, 90% ground	4.6*	22.7	Venison, ground	3.8	24.7
Chicken, white/dark (skinless, boneless)	0.8/1.2	23/22	Pork, lean (boneless loin chops)	2.5	24.7
Turkey, ground breast/dark	0.5/3	23/21	Cheese (hard) 1 oz.	3.6–4.2	7.4–7.9
Egg, 1 whole	5	6.3	Low-fat Milk (1 cup)	1.5	8
Salmon, wild coho	1.4	24.5	Cod/Halibut/Tilapia	0.1–0.7	avg. 21

*Cattle that are allowed to get exercise and forage for their own food (e.g., grass-fed) produce meat with 47% less saturated fat and 133% more omega-3 fatty acids than cattle fed from a trough (e.g., grain-fed).[4]

Vegetable proteins are found in many foods, including vegetables, fruits, legumes, grains, nuts and seeds.

Below is a partial list of fruits and vegetables with their protein content. For simple choices on how to increase vegetable consumption, see pages 40–41.

Vegetable (1 cup)	Protein (grams)	Vegetable (1 cup)	Protein (grams)
Acorn Squash (cooked)	1.6	Kale (raw)	2.2
Artichoke (medium)	4	Leeks (raw, sliced)	1.3
Asparagus (raw)	3	Onions (raw, diced)	1.8
Avocado (pureed)	4.5	Peas (frozen)	6
Beets (raw)	2.2	Peppers, bell (diced)	1.4
Broccoli (raw)	2.1	Potatoes (diced)	3
Butternut Squash (raw, cubes)	1.4	Pumpkin (canned)	2.7
Cabbage (raw)	1.2	Spaghetti Squash (cooked)	1
Carrots (raw, sliced)	1.1	Spinach/Collards (raw)	0.9
Corn (frozen kernels)	4.5	Summer Squash (raw, sliced)	1.4
Fennel (raw, diced)	1.1	Sweet Potatoes (raw, diced)	2.1
Green Beans (frozen cuts)	2.2	Tomatoes (raw, diced)	1.6

Fruit —1 cup (unless otherwise indicated)	Protein (grams)	Fruit —1 cup (unless otherwise indicated)	Protein (grams)
Banana (med., 7-inch)	1.3	Cherries, sweet fresh w/ pits	1.2
Blackberries, fresh	2	Grapefruit, CA white ½ (~4")	1
Blueberries, fresh	1.1	Peach/Nectarine, fresh slices	1.4/1.5
Cantaloupe/Watermelon	1.5/0.9	Raspberries, fresh	1.5

Legumes are another excellent source of protein. (See pp. 48–49 for more information on the nutrition of beans.)

Beans — 1/2 cup cooked	Protein (grams)	Beans — 1/2 cup cooked + Soy Products	Protein (grams)
Adzuki	5.6	Pinto	5.8
Black	7	Red	6
Black-eyed Peas	6	Split Peas	8.2
Cannellini (white kidney)	6	**Soy Products**	
Garbanzo (chickpeas)	7	Black Soybeans	9
Great Northern	5	Edamame (green soybeans)	10
Kidney	6.7	Soy Protein Isolate, 2 Tbsp. (unsweetened; p. 89)	16
Lentils	8		
Lima	5.9	Soymilk (1 cup)	7
Navy	9.8	Tofu (3 oz.)	7

It is easy to increase the consumption of beans. Unlike many foods, beans do not lose nutrients in the canning process, so there is nothing wrong with grabbing a can of beans to use warm or cold. (Just make sure they are packed only in water; some are packed in corn syrup.) Try adding them to any of the following:

- Soups, stews and chilies (e.g., pp. 118, 122, 123, 125, 129, 130 and 132)
- Tacos (e.g., p. 100). Special Note: If you have people eating the tacos who do not like the appearance or texture of beans, try pureeing some black beans and stirring them into the taco meat. Large quantities will change the texture, but small amounts will hide nicely behind the meat and seasonings.
- Dips and spreads (e.g., Bean Dip, Hummus)
- Salads (e.g., pp. 94 and 101)
- Casseroles (e.g., pp. 138–139)

Soy is one of the few plant sources of a complete protein. Coming in many forms (see chart above and p. 89), it can be used in a variety of ways. Consider the following:

- Use soy protein isolate in smoothies (p. 106 for ideas).
- Add soy protein isolate to baked goods (e.g., Pumpkin Cookies, Protein Bars).
- Use soy protein isolate as a binder (e.g., Sweet Potato Cakes, Veggie Burgers).
- Consider tofu (e.g., Seared Tofu, Pepper-Corn Chili – tofu version).
- Use edamame beans in soups and salads (e.g., Basic Soup, Wilted Spinach Salad).

Grains (pp. 174–180) and meals (e.g., flaxseed meal) can also be a great place to find protein. Quinoa is another plant source of a complete protein (p. 178).

Grains	Protein (grams)	Flours — 1/4 cup	Protein (grams)
Barley, 1/2 cup cooked	1.8	All-Purpose Flour	3
Flaxseed Meal, 2 Tbsp.	3	Cornmeal	5
Oat/Wheat Bran, 1/4 cup dry	3.8/2	Spelt, Whole-Grain & White Flour	4
Oats, quick/reg., 1/2 cup dry	7/5	Wheat Germ	8
Quinoa, 1/4 cup dry	5	Whole-Wheat Pastry Flour	3
Rice, brown, 1/2 cup cooked	2.7	Whole-Wheat Flours	4

One way to increase the amount of protein we get from grains is to use whole-grain flours as much as possible. (See p. 181 for ideas on introducing this taste.) We can also add whole grains where they might not normally be, including in soups and baked goods. One of the perks of adding protein to sweet treats is that protein helps to reduce sugar highs and lows. (For simple choices for increasing whole grains, see p. 174.)

We can also get protein from nuts and seeds. Though a great source of unsaturated (healthier) fats, they are high in calories and should be consumed in moderation. Adding small amounts to foods can enhance flavor, texture and nutrition. Consider using nuts and seeds to enhance:

- Salads
- Muffins, pancakes, baked goods
- Snacks
- Granola and Protein Bars
- As a topping for yogurt/ice cream
- Mixed with cereal (hot or cold)

Here is nutritional information for a sampling of nuts used in recipes in this book:

Nut (1/4 cup raw)	Calories	Fat Calories	Saturated Fat (grams)	Protein (grams)
Almonds	207	163	1.4	7.6
English Walnuts	191	172	1.8	4.5
Pecans	171	160	1.5	2.3

Meal Idea ~ Topped Baked Potato

Preheat oven—400°. Scrub and dry potato. Rub High-Heat oil on the skin. Pierce several times with a fork. Bake 45–50 minutes, or until tender. Split open. Enjoy creating your own topping or use one of the following to increase the nutrition and make it a complete meal. Many of these utilize vegetable proteins:

- Roasted asparagus and cheese*
- Steamed broccoli, onions and cheese*
- Sautéed spinach or chard, red onions and cheese*
- Corn-bean salsa (p. 91)
- Meat/bean taco mixture (p. 100)
- Sautéed fennel and leeks
- A dollop of Confetti Dip (p. 42) with your favorite vegetable

*We recommend only one ounce of cheese per potato.

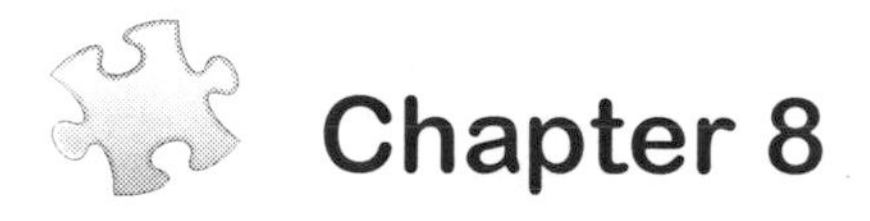

Chapter 8

Heart Health: Simple Choices, Big Impact

Every day, scientists are learning more about heart disease and how to prevent it. As it has been for almost a century, heart disease is still the number-one killer in the United States, accounting for one out of every 2.8 deaths.[1] Yet it is a disease that can be significantly impacted by choices we make in our eating and lifestyle habits. In fact, healthy eating and lifestyle changes can reduce the risk of heart disease more than drug therapy.[2] And the 2006 guidelines of the American Heart Association for "diet and lifestyle goals for cardiovascular disease reduction" begin with the consumption of an "overall healthy diet."[3]

When the risk factors of heart disease are examined, the above statements make sense. Certainly some risk factors, such as age, gender and family history, cannot be changed. However, many of the risk factors can be reduced or eliminated by simple lifestyle choices. These areas of focus include the following:

- The prevention and control of diabetes
- The maintenance of low blood cholesterol levels
- The reduction of high blood pressure

  and
- The maintenance of a healthy body weight

This knowledge provides good motivation for making healthier eating choices. Unfortunately, the task often appears too large. Overwhelmed, we fail to make any changes at all. By making a few simple eating choices at a time, we can have a positive impact on heart health without feeling so overwhelmed.

As you prepare and consume foods, **make the choice** to do the following:

- **Increase fiber** (fiber helps remove cholesterol from your body and can help you lose weight[4]). See chapter five.
- **Increase essential fatty acids** (varieties include EPA, DHA and omegas). Found in fish oils and many nut and seed oils, fatty acids have been proven to lower blood pressure and reduce the risk of heart disease.[5] See chapter three.
- **Reduce saturated fats and trans fats** (helps avoid weight gain and lower cholesterol[6]). See chapter five.

- **Reduce sodium intake**. See chapter four.
- **Reduce high-calorie foods**, especially if weight loss is important.
- **Balance calorie consumption with physical activity** (reduces weight gain).
- Increase consumption of a variety of **vitamins and minerals** (this can come from both food and food-based nutritional supplements). See our website (p. 242) for more information.

These things can be accomplished, in part, by **choosing** to:

- Include a variety of **whole-grain** products. See page 174.
- Eat **baked** rather than fried (reduces intake of saturated and trans fats as well as calories).
- Increase consumption of **beans** (increases fiber and intake of vitamins and minerals). See page 48.
- Include more **vegetables and fruits** (increases fiber, increases consumption of vitamins and minerals and gives you more food for less calories). See pages 40–41.

To locate recipes in this book that make use of several of the choices listed above, look for a heart symbol at the bottom of a page. (If a recipe has a choice of ingredients and not all are heart healthy, a "c" by the heart symbol c indicates that an appropriate choice is to be made in order for the recipe to be heart healthy. There are also times when a recipe is at the upper end of an appropriate limit on fat or sodium content. It can be part of a heart-healthy diet so long as other foods paired with it are not excessively high in fat or sodium. In these cases, we have marked the heart symbol with a "c" and then written the words "paired with" below.)

Studies have shown that people who eat at least a single serving of whole grains each day reduce their risk of heart disease by as much as one-third compared to those who eat only refined grains.[7]

The American Dietetic Association now recommends eating from five to nine servings of fruits and vegetables per day. They cite research that shows:

- Stroke rates decline with each additional serving of fruits and vegetables.
- An increase in fruits and vegetables can lower blood pressure within a month.[8]

About Cholesterol

For years it was thought that lowering dietary cholesterol would lower blood cholesterol levels. Researchers now believe dietary cholesterol may not have a significant impact on blood cholesterol for most people. However, saturated fats have been shown to increase bad levels of blood cholesterol and trans fats have been shown to both increase bad cholesterol levels and decrease good cholesterol levels.[9]

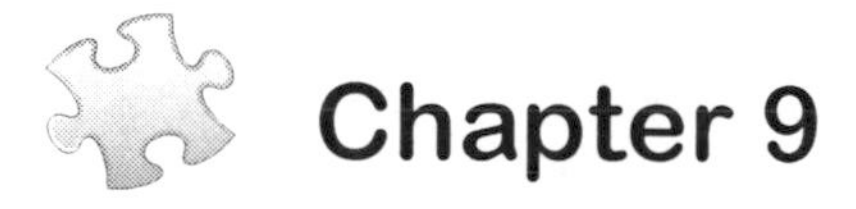

Chapter 9

Diabetes: Knowledge for Prevention

Diabetes is becoming an increasing concern. Particularly alarming is evidence that the increased incidence of diabetes is directly related to our lifestyle. Research is proving that diabetes can be prevented and/or delayed.[1] We are also learning that many of the life-threatening complications that accompany diabetes can be avoided if diabetes is diagnosed early and managed well.[2] It is important that we become aware of the eating habits that can help lower our risks and maintain our health.

Insulin is a hormone that is needed to allow sugar from the bloodstream to move into cells where it can either be converted to energy or stored as fat. People with diabetes have difficulty regulating their blood sugar levels because their bodies either do not produce enough insulin or do not respond to the insulin effectively. Elevated blood sugar levels are damaging to the body, causing the complications of diabetes, such as kidney and heart disease.

Type 1 Diabetes

- Involves the body failing to produce insulin because the insulin-producing cells are destroyed by the immune system
- Affects about 5 to 10 percent of Americans with diabetes[3]

Type 2 Diabetes

- Involves the body not responding to insulin normally, leaving sugar in the blood
- Is the more common form of diabetes

About 20.8 million Americans have diabetes, but only about 14.6 million are aware of it.[4] In addition, approximately 54 million Americans have pre-diabetes, a condition in which "blood glucose levels are higher than normal, but not high enough for a diagnosis of Type 2 diabetes."[5]

It is not the intent of this book to diagnose or provide treatment plans for people with diabetes. Information on symptoms and how to seek professional care can be found from the American Diabetes Association and your physician.

It is prudent, however, that we seek to understand lifestyle habits that can help to prevent diabetes and lessen its impact. Studies show exercise and diet to be more effective in delaying and managing Type 2 diabetes than medication; in one study, thirty minutes of moderate exercise each day along with a 5 to 10 percent reduction in weight reduced the effects and development of diabetes by 58 percent.[6] Treating and controlling conditions such as obesity, high cholesterol, high blood glucose and high blood pressure can go a long way toward preventing or delaying diabetes. Therefore, it is critical that we pay attention to what we eat.

To help prevent or delay the onset of diabetes, we need to **make the choice** to:

- Manage our weight (involves watching calorie intake).
- Use heart-healthy eating strategies (see chapter eight).
- Manage blood glucose (sugar) levels.

We all benefit from avoiding sugar highs (see chapter six). Some of the ways we can keep our blood glucose levels in check involve **making the choice** to:

- Reduce sugar consumption.
- Consume sugar with protein, fiber and/or fats (to slow down sugar absorption and avoid sugar spikes).
- Reduce consumption of refined carbohydrates (easily digested into sugar).
- Be aware of total carb intake during the course of the day (all carbs are converted into sugar by our bodies).

Choose to center meals on vegetables and whole grains since these foods quite naturally meet the above criteria, provided they are prepared in a suitable manner (few added sugars and saturated fats). It is also important to consider **total carbohydrate intake**. Starchy vegetables such as potatoes, yams, peas and corn, whole-grain breads, cereals, pasta and rice can be beneficial in preventing and managing diabetes because they are rich in fiber. However, they are high in carbohydrates and need to be consumed in moderation, especially for those with diabetes. Thus, **portion size** is critical.

Making the effort to prevent diabetes is well worth it. **Diabetes increases the risk of several major illnesses**, including cardiovascular disease (heart attack, stroke, high blood pressure), blindness, dental disease, kidney disease, nervous system disease, complications in pregnancy, amputations and sexual dysfunction.[7] The **financial cost** of diabetes is significant as well. In 2002, people with diabetes had more than five times the annual health care costs per capita of people without diabetes.[8] In 2002, diabetes resulted in a loss of almost 88 million disability days and accounted for 176,000 cases of permanent disability, at an estimated cost of $7.5 billion.[9]

Perhaps nowhere do these preventative strategies pay off as much as they do in children. The earlier diabetes starts, the more years a person has to develop complications. The National Institutes of Health states that a "lack of physical activity and unhealthy eating patterns ... play important roles in determining a child's weight [and] the risk for Type 2 diabetes."[10] Dr. Francine Kaufman, pediatric endocrinologist and former president of the ADA, says "What was once a disease of our grandparents is now a disease of young adults and teenagers. And it's pretty much due to the life we all live."[11]

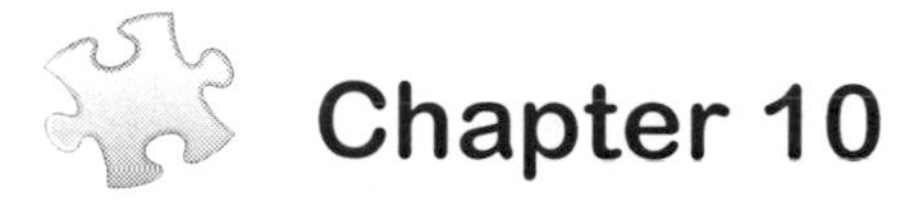

Chapter 10

Gluten: Understanding Why Some People Need to Avoid It

Gluten is a protein that provides structure to bread so that when it rises, it doesn't collapse. It is found in many grains, including wheat, rye and barley. It is also found in some medications, some vitamins and things like envelope adhesives. Many people add gluten (often sold as "vital wheat gluten") to whole-grain bread recipes to cause them to rise more and have a lighter taste.

However, some people cannot tolerate gluten. The most common type of intolerance is an immune system response in which the body responds to the presence of gluten by causing damage to the intestinal villi (lining of the intestinal wall). This damage prevents nutrients from being absorbed into the bloodstream, which means that they are malnourished no matter how much good food they eat.

People who have this response to gluten have a condition known as celiac disease, or celiac sprue. It is a common disease (affecting 1 in every 133 people)[1] but widely unrecognized (only about 3 percent of people with celiac disease have been diagnosed with it).[2] Celiac disease is different from a food allergy/sensitivity in that it does not cause a histamine reaction. Nor is it a response to IgE (a type of antibody) in the bloodstream. It is a genetic, inheritable condition. People with celiac disease can reverse the effects of intestinal damage and malnutrition and live a symptom-free life if they avoid foods containing gluten.[3]

Symptoms of celiac disease vary tremendously and often intensify the longer the disease goes undetected. Amazingly, some people with celiac disease do not display any symptoms at all.[4] Symptoms can include, but are not limited to, abdominal cramping, bloating, immense appetite, diarrhea, muscle cramping in hands and legs, constipation, fatigue, weight loss, iron-deficiency anemia, depression, mood swings and an inability to concentrate.

Some individuals do not have celiac disease but do have a sensitivity to gluten and feel better if they avoid it. Damage does not occur to their small intestine when they ingest gluten, but they still may have systemic (whole-body) responses that can include fatigue, muscle and joint pain, headaches and inflammation.

Grains and grain-like products that are gluten free and considered safe for people who need to avoid gluten include amaranth, buckwheat, corn, millet, oat (see * below chart), quinoa, rice, sorghum, teff and wild rice. It is important for people who need to avoid gluten – and the people who cook for them – to become familiar with products that contain gluten. Many sauces (such as Worcestershire sauce), condiments and processed foods contain traces of gluten that can be harmful.

The recipes in this book that are made with all gluten-free ingredients are marked with this symbol. In some recipes with a choice of ingredients, this requires choosing a gluten-free ingredient. Such cases are indicated with a "c" following the gluten-free symbol. c (Sometimes the variable ingredient is indicated just below the symbols [e.g., omit Worcestershire sauce for a gluten-free recipe or choose a gluten-free brand].) Please note that when we suggest using "whole-grain" breads or pastas, this does not need to be a product made from wheat or other gluten-containing grains. (See chart below for non-gluten-containing grains.)

Gluten Containing Grains	Gluten-Free Grains and Grain-like Products	
Barley	Amaranth	Quinoa
Kamut®	Buckwheat	Rice
Rye	Corn	Sorghum
Spelt	Millet	Teff
Wheat	Oat*	Wild Rice

*Oat must be certified gluten free (see our website, p. 242, for more information).

Gluten-Free Flour Mix

Mix: 5 minutes

2 1/4 cups brown rice flour
1 cup tapioca starch
3/4 cup cornstarch
1/2 cup potato starch
2 teaspoons xanthan gum

Measure ingredients into a storage jar. To mix, rock jar back and forth several times.

Yield: 4 3/4 cups

Gluten-Free (GF) Mixes

To the left is our Gluten-Free (GF) Flour Mix that is used in some of our recipes. Some recipes were developed using Bob's Red Mill brand mixes. Each recipe will either refer you to this page or list the brand label.

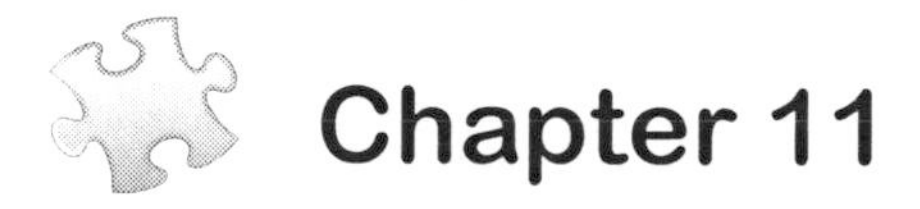

Chapter 11

Whole Foods: Natural Sources of Goodness

In our desire to eat healthier foods, one of the things to focus on is using whole foods. "Whole foods" are foods that have been unaltered by humans, so that they retain their natural sources of nutrients. This chapter offers guidelines for finding and purchasing a variety of whole foods.

What Is "Organic"? The term "organic" generally refers to farming practices that avoid synthetic materials and emphasize land conservation and the use of renewable resources. Organic produce is grown without the use of synthetic or petroleum-based pesticides or herbicides. It is generally more nutrient dense since farmers give the soil time to be naturally enriched. In addition, organic plants experience more stress than nonorganic plants. This stress prompts the plants to produce defense molecules. These defense molecules are strong antioxidants (e.g., resveratrol in red grapes) and detoxicants (e.g., sulfurophan in broccoli) and provide important nutrition for us.

Organic animal products come from animals that were raised without antibiotics or growth hormones and were fed food that was organically grown.

Some organic farmers go beyond organic definitions and/or choose not to apply for certification but still use organic practices. If you talk to farmers at local farmers' markets, you can get to know which farmers utilize farming practices with which you feel comfortable.

Why Local? It is estimated that the typical food on the American table travels an average of 1,500 miles.[1] This increases pollution *and* decreases the nutrient level and the taste of food. Local farmers are more likely to use sustainable farming practices and are more likely to grow a variety of crops. Locally grown food is usually fresher because it can be purchased soon after it is harvested. Shopping locally supports local farmers, and quite frankly, the food tastes much better!

Why in Season? Food that is in season is more likely to be local and fresh and has a much better taste. It also provides us with variety at our tables. Since it is so easy to get foods from all over the globe at almost any time of year, we tend to use the same foods repeatedly. Choosing to eat many of our foods in season helps vary our diets.

What Is Non-GMO? "Non-GMO" is a term that refers to foods that have not been genetically modified. There is a lot of controversy over GMO; we choose to avoid GMO foods whenever possible (corn and soy are key ones to watch for).

Which Is Best — Canned, Frozen or Fresh?

- **Canned** fruits and vegetables often have added ingredients (e.g., salt, sugar) and typically lose nutrients in the processing (except beans, tomatoes and pumpkin).
- **Frozen** produce is a great option if it is frozen soon after picking (when the nutrient value is highest and before molds have a chance to grow). Sometimes it is actually fresher than "fresh" produce that has sat on trucks and in storerooms. However, some vegetables have sodium added. Packages sold with seasonings or sauces often contain high levels of sodium, sugar, fat and/or preservatives.
- **Fresh** fruits and vegetables are the ideal option if truly fresh and cared for well.

Finding a good source of whole fruits and vegetables can take a bit of time and exploration. Many grocery stores are selling more and more local and organic foods. Another wonderful source of local organic foods is a CSA (Community Supported Agriculture). Members buy a share in a farm and in return receive a weekly box of fresh, local produce during the growing season. (See our websites, p. 242, for more information.)

Whole Grains: There are many grains available to us today. Often they have been processed to alter their appearance, texture, shelf life and response to baking. This alteration takes away many of the nutrients in the natural grain. Using grains that have been left "whole" means that more nutrients are consumed. For ideas on making this transition from refined grains to whole grains, see pages 174 and 181.

Meat, Poultry and Dairy Products: Finding meat and poultry from a local farmer is ideal but not always possible. Besides the distance your meat has traveled, some things to consider when reading labels are the following:

- Were the animals raised free of steroids, antibiotics and growth hormones?
- Were the animals fed food grown free of pesticides?
- Are the poultry and processed meats packed free of chemicals such as nitrates and nitrites and with minimal sugar and only natural preservatives?
- Were the animals allowed to get exercise and forage for their food instead of being fed from a trough? Meat from grass-fed animals is lower in saturated fats (p. 19).

Some of the terms used to answer the questions above include "all natural," "free range," "grass fed" and "organic." However, there is not yet an industry standard to define these terms, so look closely at the label for the company's definitions, check out their website or write to the company or farmer and ask some questions.

As we bake and cook, we pull many ingredients from our shelves beyond produce and grains. Making simple choices in the grocery store to purchase brands that use whole ingredients can also impact our health. (See Healthier Choices Shopping Guide.)

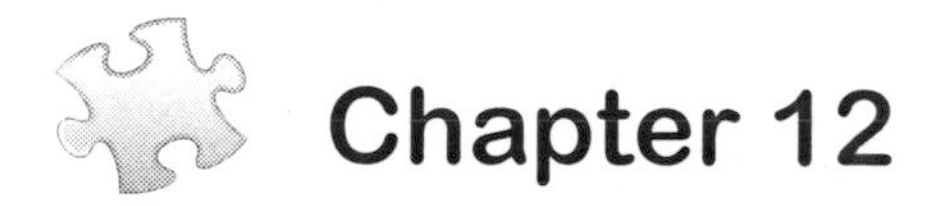

Chapter 12

Maximizing the Benefits of Healthier Eating: Transitions to Better Living

While there are many things we can do to make it simpler, no one can deny that eating in a healthy manner takes intentionality and resources. It only makes sense, then, to maximize our efforts by taking care of our bodies in as many ways as possible. This will help our bodies to best use the nutrients in our food.

Exercise: Medical studies show that exercise is beneficial in many facets of life. Regular exercise:

- Improves energy
- Aids digestion
- Increases circulation
- Boosts our mood (by raising serotonin levels in the brain)
- Reduces stress
- Helps to maintain optimal bodyweight
- Helps to maintain healthy blood pressure levels
- Helps to control blood sugar
- Increases bone and joint health (can even increase bone mass)
- Increases balance and flexibility
- Strengthens muscles
- Helps the body to get rid of toxins
- Improves lung function

Stress Reduction: *Stress* is a modern-day buzzword when it comes to health issues, and for very good reasons. It can cause havoc throughout our bodies, depleting important stores of nutrients and interfering with our ability to function in a variety of ways. Consider the following stress-reducing techniques:

- Exercise (even just a few minutes a day)
- Breathing exercises
- Sleep
- Prayer and reflection
- Talks with an understanding friend
- Balancing time indoors and outdoors, getting plenty of sunlight

Sleep: Few of us get the full restorative sleep that we need each night. Our bodies were designed to rest; when we sleep, our bodies are hard at work doing things they cannot fully do when we are busy. Nutrients are utilized, hormones are regulated and cells are built and repaired while we rest.

Bodywork Therapies: There are many different bodywork therapies, including chiropractic care, acupuncture, yoga and massage.

Proper **chiropractic** care naturally restores proper nervous system function, which in turn controls all body functions.

Acupuncture is a facet of Eastern medicine that addresses a wide range of ailments by harmonizing the various systems of the body, striving to treat the root of the problem and not just the symptom.

Yoga is a practice of postures, breathing practices and meditative control.

Massage therapy uses soft tissue techniques (e.g., myofacial release, shiatsu, Swedish massage) to increase blood circulation. This brings oxygen to the cells of the muscles, tendons and ligaments, reviving their elasticity and range of motion.

All of these therapies – and many others – can benefit our bodies in many ways, including, but not limited to improving digestion, managing pain, strengthening the immune system and increasing circulation. As we experience these benefits, our sleep improves, our stress is reduced, our energy increases and the nutrients we consume are more easily absorbed and utilized.

Food-based Supplements: For many years it was a commonly held belief that all the nutrients we need can be obtained by eating the right foods in the right quantities. In recent years, that belief has been challenged, partly because the nutritional value of food is not as high as it used to be.* A basic supplemental program does not take the place of a healthy diet, but rather enhances it, allowing the healthy food we eat to be used more effectively by our bodies.

In June 2002, the *Journal of the American Medical Association* stated their official belief that vitamin supplementation should be part of a healthy American's diet.[1]

The best supplements are food-based, meaning they are derived from food sources, not synthetic (man-made) sources. They are easily absorbed by our bodies and are processed in such a way as to retain their nutritional value. Recent tests have reveled that some supplements contain substances not on the label. Often, this is occurs because raw materials are not tested for their purity or because machinery is not properly cleaned. It is critical that supplements be purchased from a company of high integrity with excellent quality control. (See our websites [p. 242] for tips on choosing a company as well as for suggestions on starting a supplemental program.)

---

*One study showed that farming practices have lowered the nutritional value of food sometimes by as much as 38 percent compared to produce grown in 1950.[2] In addition, long periods of storage, shipping conditions, processing and some cooking methods deplete foods of many nutrients.

Part Two

Recipes – The Heart of It All

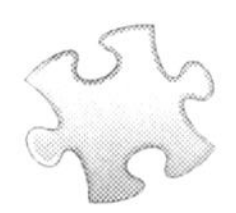

Chapter 13

Tips for Getting Started with the Recipes

Before beginning the recipes, we encourage you to read the next few pages for a guide to the symbols, helpful hints and sanitation tips.

Symbols to Guide You

Symbols Used in the Recipe:

Preparation Time* (symbols below recipe title):

S→T: From Start to Table. Inactive or semi-inactive time is occasionally indicated to help you with the timing of other meal preparation or tasks.

S→O: From Start to Oven.

*The **estimated time** assumes that (1) you are familiar with the recipe (it always takes longer the first time) and (2) you use some helpful equipment/gadgets (e.g., food processor to chop/slice large quantities of onions.)

 **Timing:** offers advice on timing so the preparation goes more smoothly; sometimes located in the sidebar.

Bolded Words Within Recipe Directions: highlights key parts of each step.

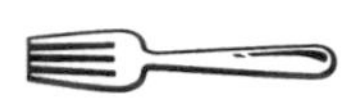 **Serving Suggestion:** highlights serving ideas, garnishes and meal complements; sometimes located in the sidebar.

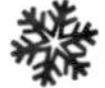 **Storage:** offers information about freezing, chilling and/or storage.

Symbols Used in the Sidebar:

Healthy Bites: bits of nutritional information

Little Chef: ideas on what children can do in the kitchen. Some involve helping with the preparation, while others are simply fun learning activities.

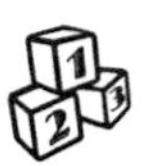

Variations: tested or suggested ingredients to make the recipe your own

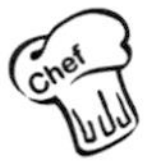

Helpful Hint

Equipment Tip

Symbols located at the bottom of the page opposite the nutritional information:

Heart Healthy recipe if appropriate portions are consumed. (See chapter eight for more information).

Recipe made with **Gluten-Free** ingredients so they are safe for those with celiac disease. (See chapter ten for more information.)

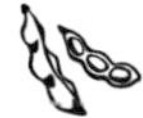

Recipe is **vegetarian** or has a vegetarian option.

c c c A "c" following the heart, gluten-free or vegetarian symbol stands for "choice." This means that here are ingredient choices that can make the recipe heart healthy, gluten free or vegetarian. Sometimes the variable ingredient is indicated just below the symbols.

Ingredients

- If an ingredient is listed that comes from a variety of sources (e.g., "milk" can be from a cow, soybeans, rice, nuts), the ones listed in parenthesis are the ones we tested. The first one listed is our favorite.
- "High-Heat oil," "Medium-Heat oil," etc., refers to an oil that will not reach its smoke point at the temperatures required by the recipe. For a list of appropriate choices, please see page 10.

Nutritional Analysis

A description of the nutritional analysis and how it was calculated is on pages 6–7. Certain brands we used for the analysis are listed in the Healthier Choices Shopping Guide.

Helpful Hints in Preparing to Use the Recipes

- **Oven temperatures** are listed just below the ingredients.
- **Baking dish sizes** are listed just before the recipe directions with an indication if the dish is to be prepared (e.g., oiled, lined with parchment paper).
- **Begin with a clear and clean counter.** Especially with recipes that involve mixing batters and/or chopping.
- **Handling distractions and interruptions.** Before you begin, set out all ingredients and equipment to make the process faster and calmer. (They are listed in the order in which they will be used.) Use a table knife or other straight edge to mark your place in the recipe.
- **Measurements** are provided as a guide. It is a good rule of thumb to use the quantities suggested until you get to know a recipe. Then adjust the quantities according to your tastes and preferences. However, close to accurate measuring is the best guarantee of success with baked goods (see p. 230 for measuring guidelines).
- **Abbreviations** used:

  tsp. = teaspoon(s)
  Tbsp. = tablespoon(s)
  lb. = pound(s)
  oz. = ounce(s)
  g. = grams
  mg. = milligrams
  mcg. = micrograms
  ~ *or* approx. = approximately
  sm. = small
  med. = medium
  lg. = large
  min. = minute(s)
  pkg. = package
  GF = gluten free

- **Cooking definitions** can be found in the Cook's Glossary (pp. 216-218). Please note that many recipes follow the **"Chop & Drop"** method for sautéing vegetables. It consists of slicing/dicing/chopping vegetables, beginning with the vegetable that takes the longest to cook. Begin sautéing the first vegetable while you dice the next vegetable in the order listed on the recipe. Occasionally the "Chop & Drop" method is applied to only one or two vegetables with ground meat or chunks of meat (e.g., Tacos, p. 100).

Sanitation Tips[1]

- **Wash your hands** with warm, soapy water before, after and during food preparation (especially after handling raw meat, eggs, poultry or seafood).
- **Wash countertop** surfaces before and after food preparation. Disinfect with a natural product (see our websites, p. 242) after handling raw meats.
- **Cutting boards.** Have one cutting board for raw meats and poultry and another for other foods (especially vegetables) so that foods do not get contaminated by the juices of raw meat and poultry. Any cutting board surface with cuts can harbor bacteria, so a dishwasher-safe, nonporous surface is a good style to use.
- **Cook foods to a safe temperature.** Contaminated food may look and smell normal. Use a food thermometer to know that you have cooked meat and poultry to a safe temperature that will destroy bacteria (see chart below).
- **Refrigerate or freeze foods promptly.** Since harmful bacteria can rapidly reproduce, refrigerate or freeze perishable foods soon after purchasing or preparing them. Keep hot food hot and refrigerate leftovers after the meal.
- **Defrost food safely.** Bacteria can reproduce rapidly on raw meats at room temperature, so defrost in the refrigerator (see chart below). While thawing, keep meats wrapped and refrigerated below cooked or ready-to-eat foods. For meats in sealed packages, you can immerse in cold water, changing water every 15 minutes.
- **Store food safely.** Store food away from cleaning supplies and chemicals. Use or freeze foods within an appropriate amount of time (see chart below). If there is any question about a product's storage or expiration, discard it.

Safe Internal Temperature of Cooked Foods[2]	
Beef, Veal, Lamb	145–170°
Chicken*	180°
Pork	160–170°
Turkey	180–185°
Venison	160°
Patties: Beef, Lamb, Pork, Veal, Venison	160°
Patties: Poultry	165°
Eggs: until yolk, whites are firm	
Egg dishes	160°
Casseroles/Left-overs/Stuffing	165°

*no longer pink; juices run clear

Raw Food Cooked Food	Safe Refrigerated Storage Time[3]
Beef Roasts/Steaks	3–5 days
Fish	1–2 days
Ground/Stew Meat	1–2 days
Pork Chops/Roasts	2–3 days
Poultry, pieces/whole	1–2 days
Whole Turkey	3–4 days
Sausage	1–2 days
Venison (all cuts)	1–2 days
Eggs, raw in shell Hard-Cooked Eggs	3 weeks 1 week
Leftover meat/poultry** Leftover gravy/broth	3–4 days 1–2 days

**only 1–2 days for chicken nuggets/patties

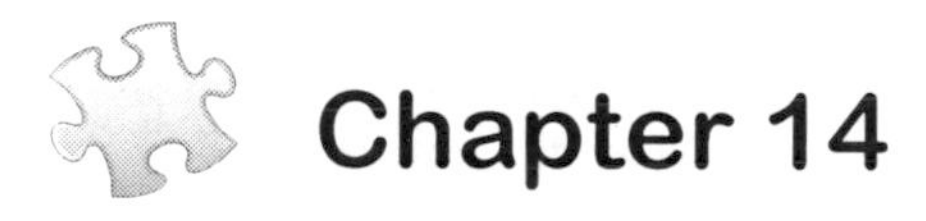

Chapter 14

Vegetables

Children's books are full of stories about kids who don't want to eat their vegetables and parents who insist that they must. How did vegetables get such a bad name? Well, in part, it's because we buy them in cans or from the produce section long after they were harvested, so much of the good flavor is gone (to say nothing of the nutrients!). Then we cook them so long that they lose much of their color, and the flavor and nutrients are further depleted. To top it off, we cook the same ones in the same manner over and over again. It's no wonder we get tired of them!

But there's a bright side: the variety of vegetables available to us is enormous and there are unlimited possibilities for consuming them. They can be colorful, flavorful and fun. They make good finger food and healthy snacks. They can perk up any meal and are probably the easiest way to add variety to your favorite casseroles and soups. Furthermore, vegetables are some of the most nutritionally dense foods around. They have an enormous quantity of vitamins and minerals per calorie (along with less sugar and fat). The maxim that we "ought to eat our vegetables" is correct, but it's the way in which we do it that can turn that concept into a delightful experience instead of a dreaded necessity.

This chapter highlights many vegetables in alphabetical order. There are tips for selection and storage as well as ideas for serving the vegetable. Most pages have a recipe that features that particular vegetable. The material on the next six pages is information that pertains to vegetables as a whole.

We often overlook a great variety of vegetables because they are unfamiliar and we do not know what to do with them or if we will like them. Make the exploration of vegetables a game: choose a new one each week, perhaps choosing vegetables that start with the same letter as the names of family members. Try one of the suggestions listed for that vegetable in this book. If you buy it from a farmer, ask her how she likes to prepare it. CSAs (p.29) are a great way to explore new vegetables; someone else selects them for you, choosing ones that are fresh and ready to eat – and you get a new variety each week. Remember, vegetables taste differently depending on how they are prepared. If you try something and don't like it, wait a little while and then try it again in a different way. Taste buds change over time, so you never know when an old dislike might become a new favorite.

Washing Vegetables

It is important to wash vegetables well before using them. This helps to remove dirt and sand that have accumulated as well as bacteria and residues. There are some specific washing techniques that are good for certain vegetables. These are highlighted on the individual vegetable pages. If nothing unique is noted, here are some general guidelines to follow:

- **Leafy Vegetables:** Swish leaves in water to loosen sand and dirt. Pour out wash water and repeat until water remains clean. (For heading leaf vegetables – e.g., cabbage – remove and discard the outer leaves.)
- **Vegetables with Skins:** Scrub skins well with a rough sponge or soft vegetable brush. Even if you choose not to use the skins, scrub them well before peeling or cutting to avoid spreading mold and bacteria, which may have accumulated on the surface during the growth or storage process.

Vegetable Peels

The outer peel, or skin, of a vegetable is the primary source of fiber in a vegetable and is often where we find the greatest concentration of nutrients. Sometimes there are nutrients present in the peel that are not present in any other part of the vegetable. For this reason (and the fact that it saves time), we try to use the peel as much as possible. Some skins are tough and not edible; some are edible only when cooked. The recipes in this book all use the peel (butternut squash included), unless otherwise noted.

Special Note: There is a greater risk to using the peel of vegetables that are not organic since these peels likely contain chemical residues. Therefore, we do not recommend using the peel of nonorganic vegetables.

Healthy Bites

Prostate Cancer: In a study of 1,200 men, those who ate four or more servings of vegetables a day had reduced their risk of prostate cancer by 35%. Those men reduced their risk by 44% when they consumed at least three servings of cruciferous vegetables (vegetables belonging to the mustard family, including cabbage, broccoli and kale) every week.[1]

Cholesterol: Several substances in vegetables can help reduce cholesterol. One of the more surprising ones is vitamin C, which neutralizes free radicals. This, in turn, means that the free radicals are not able to oxidize cholesterol, which is the process that allows cholesterol to stick to the artery walls. Four strips of yellow bell peppers have 48 mg. of vitamin C!

Immune System: Inulin is a particular kind of carbohydrate found in foods such as asparagus. Though we don't digest it, it provides food for the friendly bacteria in our large intestine.[2]

Equipment Tips

Steamer Pan: A double-boiler-style pan that has holes in the top pan which allow steam from the bottom to cook vegetables in the top without water touching the vegetable.

Steamer Basket: A collapsible basket that fits inside a saucepan can also be handy for cooking vegetables.

Healthy Bites

Best Tasting Corn: Even corn on the cob tastes better when steamed (instead of boiled in a full pan of water) — and you save the nutrients (p. 58)!

Benefits of Vitamin C: Many vegetables contain large amounts of vitamin C, which may help people lose weight because it increases the body's ability to burn off fat.

Steamed Vegetables

When vegetables sit in water to simmer, flavor and nutrients are drained from the vegetables into the water. In order to minimize the loss, consider steaming instead of simmering. Use very small amounts of water in the saucepan or use a steamer basket. Here's a good method to use:

1. Pour small amount of water in saucepan. The trick is to have essentially no or very little water (e.g., 1 or 2 teaspoons) remaining after cooking. The amount of water used depends upon:
   a. the vegetable
   b. the length of cooking time
   c. the simmering temperature
   d. the tightness of the pan lid
2. Add vegetable(s); sprinkle with salt, pepper and/or other seasonings. Bring to boil, reduce heat, cover and steam until desired tenderness (check water level occasionally so it does not cook dry). Most vegetables are best when slightly crunchy (similar to al dente cooked pasta). Many of the vegetables in the next fifty-three pages indicate ideal cooking durations.

Serve immediately with a drizzle of flaxseed oil if desired.

Carryover Cooking

If the steamed vegetables are cooking faster than the rest of a meal, remove them from the heat source, drain liquid off and allow them to "carryover-cook" from the steam in the covered saucepan.

Stir-Fry Vegetables

Stir-fry does not need to mean a big Chinese dinner. Stir-fry almost any individual vegetable (or a mixture of them) to make a tasty side. Or add meat, poultry and/or tofu for an attractive entrée. Vegetables such as broccoli, asparagus and cauliflower are best if used blanched or frozen. Spinach, chard, tomatoes, nuts and seeds are best to add during the last minutes of cooking. We recommend using our "Water Stir-Fry" method (see p. 61). Add garlic, herbs and seasonings to replace some of the salt. If you desire an Asian flavor, use liquid aminos (p. 230), which are lower in sodium than most soy sauces.

Roasted Vegetables

S→T: 35 minutes (25 minutes is inactive)

Since roasting vegetables infuses their flavor while maintaining their nutritional content, it is a wonderful method for preparing easy, rich and flavorful side dishes. We have also found that many people who do not generally care for plain vegetables will devour the roasted ones – and ask for more!

Vegetables that lend themselves well to roasting:

- **Asparagus** (p. 46)
- **Beets** (p. 50)
- **Bell peppers**
- **Carrots**
- **Onions**
- **Potatoes**
- **Winter squashes** (pp. 82–87)

Authors' favorite combo: diced red or Yukon gold potatoes (unpeeled), sliced onions and carrots, frozen tri-color pepper slices, frozen asparagus cuts and freshly minced garlic. Our method is:

Preheat oven—450–500°. Cast-iron skillet.

1. Preheat oven while preheating cast-iron skillet on stovetop. **"Chop & Drop"** carrots, potatoes and onions in small amount of High-Heat oil. **Season** with salt, pepper and dried thyme. Place skillet in preheating oven. **Roast** 15 minutes. (If using stainless steel, do not preheat pan.)
2. Remove briefly, **stir** in asparagus and pepper slices (lightly oiled and seasoned) and some minced garlic. **Roast** 15 minutes, or until vegetables are tender, stirring in more fresh garlic during the last few minutes.

Roasting Winter Squash Whole:

1. Place the whole squash (do not prick or cut) in baking pan, place in oven, turn oven to 400–500° and roast for about an hour (depending on size), or until skin gives slightly when pushed gently with thumb.
2. Cut in half. Scoop out seeds and remove flesh. Serve as a side, use for casseroles or soups, or use in baked goods (e.g., pumpkin).

Roasting Vegetables Equipment Tip

We prefer a cast-iron skillet to roast vegetables (clean up is so much easier). But since cast iron should not be placed in a preheated oven, we offer the following solutions:

- Preheat skillet inside preheating oven. Add veggies to warm skillet.
- Do not preheat oven. Allow approximately ten extra minutes for roasting (excellent method for asparagus).
- Preheat oven and cast-iron skillet as described in "Authors' favorite . . ." to left.

Hints for Roasting Frozen Vegetables

- Frozen pepper slices and asparagus spears can be roasted from a frozen state or thawed. If frozen, allow five extra minutes.
- Brush off ice crystals before roasting so the melting ice does not prolong cooking time or make the vegetables soggy.

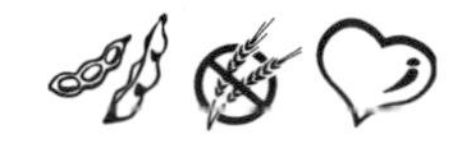

Increasing Vegetable Consumption

Increasing vegetables can sound overwhelming, if not impossible – especially to the cook who is preparing food for people who claim to not like vegetables. However, there are several things that can be done to add vegetables to favorite foods in appetizing ways – sometimes even disguising the vegetables for times when you need to "sneak" them in!

Simple Choices for Increasing Vegetable Consumption:

- **Use vegetables as sweeteners.** Carrots, bell peppers, beets and sweet potatoes can all be good choices for sweetening sauces (e.g., p. 136), baked goods (e.g., p. 200), casseroles (e.g., p. 150) and soups and stews (several pages).
- **Use vegetables to add moisture and flavor to baked goods.** Pumpkin is a good one for this task (e.g., pp. 85 and 206).
- **Make veggies fun.** Kids love to dip, and small amounts of healthy dips are a great way to increase vegetable consumption (p. 42). Many veggies can also be cut into shapes and used to make faces or other designs on a plate.
- **Use variety.** We often get tired of the same thing all the time. Or we assume that we don't like something because it looks like something we didn't like before. In addition to varying the types of vegetable offered, vary the way in which they are offered. For example, carrots can be served cooked or raw, in soup or salad, as a side dish or a snack. They can be sliced, diced, grated, cut into matchsticks or purchased as chips. Here's a fun thing to try: Use a vegetable peeler to shave a carrot. Place the shaved pieces on a plate in the fridge. In an hour or so, they will curl, making fun shapes to eat and a decorative garnish to boot!
- **Be strategic about hunger.** Right before dinner is a prime time for snacking in most households; the smells of food cooking only accentuate the hunger pangs and desire to eat. Instead of fighting it, make use of it – put out a plate of cut veggies or a handful of those snow peas you're stir-frying and let everyone munch away!
- **Make vegetables accessible.** Veggies are much more likely to be used for snacks if they are easy to get to and don't require much effort to eat. When you use a vegetable to prepare a meal, consider whether there are ways it could make a good snack the next day. Cut a few celery sticks; slice an extra cucumber; or wash a few extra cherry tomatoes. Then they will be ready and easy to grab when snack time comes around. (You might even put handfuls of cut veggies in plastic bags so that they are an easy on-the-go snack to grab for the trip to the park or to slip into a lunch box.)
- **Puree vegetables.** Pureeing vegetables, such as carrots or onions, allows you to slip them into a variety of dishes without causing a big difference in texture. Be aware, however, that using large amounts of pureed vegetables can change the texture of some foods. See our recipes using pureed vegetables in baked goods (p. 200), sauces (p. 136) and even hamburgers (p. 146).

- **Utilize casseroles.** Casseroles are known for being a combination of several ingredients. It is usually easy to throw in an extra handful of vegetables (e.g., if the recipe calls for one cup of green beans, try a cup and a half) or to throw in a couple of additional vegetables. Spinach often "disappears" in meat dishes, and diced peppers rarely fail to enhance a dish's color and taste. Chances are, you will increase the number of servings you get out of the casserole as well, thus being economical with both time and money.
- **Capitalize on taste.** It is often amazing to taste fresh produce side by side with produce that has spent time in packaging crates on a delivery truck. Choose fresh, local produce as often as possible, or look for frozen varieties that were packed soon after picking to incorporate quickly in soups and casseroles. The taste is much more appealing and your efforts will be worthwhile.
- **Involve everyone in the effort.** When we're involved with the process, we are usually more motivated to enjoy (or try) the result. Let everyone in the family chime in on what vegetables to put on the grocery list. Kids can help select the produce. (Dorie's kids like the challenge of looking for unblemished produce and have great fun weighing it.) Everyone can help to wash, prepare and cook the vegetables, even the frozen ones. (Dorie's kids used to think it was great fun to dump out a bag of frozen vegetables, especially if there were ice crystals! Take time to enjoy these little curiosities in life ... they can do a lot more than just get dinner on the table.)
- **Grow your own vegetables.** It will likely increase the flavor, increase the accessibility, involve everyone in the family and lower the cost.

Healthy Bites

Taste: It often takes 20 or 30 times of tasting something to develop a taste for it (especially in kids), so keep offering a variety!

Weight Loss: Vegetables (prepared properly) offer few calories per ounce, allowing you to eat a much larger amount of food without consuming an excessive amount of calories.

Cognitive Ability: A study found that "consuming an average of 2.8 servings of vegetables a day was associated with a 40% decrease in cognitive decline compared with those who ate an average of less than one (0.9) serving a day."[3]

Little Chefs

Eating "5 Colors a Day" is a great way to make sure you are getting a variety of nutrients. Help your child to create a color chart and cover it with clear contact paper. Allow your child to use a dry-erase marker to check off the colors he or she eats each day — it can even double as a place mat.

Make an extra color chart for grocery shopping.

Consider making a family outing out of a trip to a farmer's market.

Maximizing the Benefit of Dips

Kids, like most of us, love to dip.
Take advantage of that and give them good quality foods to dip!

- Serve with vegetables — many people who are not likely to eat raw vegetables will pick them up for the chance to enjoy a good dip.
- Before dinner, when everyone has the munchies and reaches for something "quick" that is often unhealthy, pull out the dip and set it on the table with a few raw vegetables. People can satisfy that urge to munch and get quality food inside at the same time.
- Use whole-grain crackers or wafers as another way to increase fiber.

Healthy Bites

Processed Dips: Many processed dips contain an array of unhealthy ingredients. A popular brand of green onion dip includes corn syrup, partially hydrogenated oils, MSG, many preservatives and artificial colors and flavors. By preparing simple dips at home, the great taste can be enjoyed without the negative impact of potentially harmful ingredients.

Neufchâtel Cheese: This is one of many varieties of cream cheese to choose from. Typically it has fewer calories, one-third less fat, 20% less cholesterol and a bit more protein than conventional cream cheese.

Confetti Dip

Photo on Front Cover with Raw Vegetable Tray

Mix: 10 minutes + chilling time

1 green onion (scallion)
OR small wedge of red/yellow onion
1–2 thin slices each: yellow, red and green bell peppers
1 small radish
2 small carrot sticks
2 sprigs parsley
1 small clove garlic, crushed
1/8 tsp. celery salt
8 oz. Neufchâtel cheese (see sidebar)
OR 1 cup low-fat sour cream

Dice onion, peppers, radish and carrot (approximately ½ cup). In small food processor, finely **chop** vegetables, parsley and garlic. **Blend** in celery salt and Neufchâtel cheese (or sour cream) until creamy.

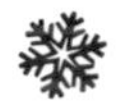
Chill several hours or overnight to blend flavors.

Yield: 20 (1 Tbsp.) servings ~1 1/4 cups

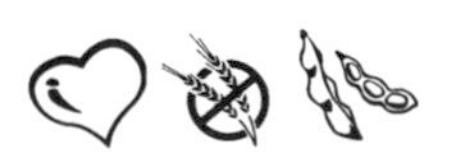

Analysis/Tablespoon:
Calories: 32 (Fat Cal 24) Fat: 2.7g (1.7g Sat) Cholesterol: 8mg
Sodium: 54mg Carbs: 0.8g (0.1g Fiber 0.2g Sugar) Protein: 1.2g

Artichoke (Globe)

Prep: ~5 minutes Cook: 30–40 minutes

Artichokes are low in calories yet abundantly rich in nutrients (e.g., fiber, vitamin C, calcium, iodine, folate, magnesium, chromium, manganese, potassium).

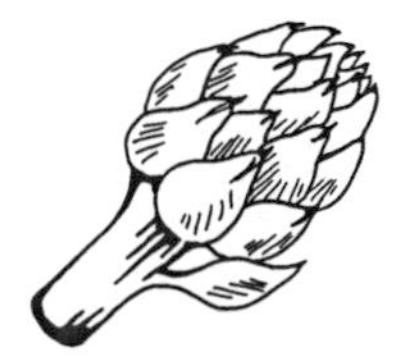

Globe Artichoke

1. **Prepare** artichoke:
   (a) Wash thoroughly under running water.
   (b) Cut off stem to be even with base.
   (c) Cut off top about 1 inch down.
   (d) Pull off loose leaves from bottom.
   (e) With scissors, snip off leaf tips, if desired.
   (f) Brush all cut edges with lemon juice.
2. In saucepan, place bottom side up in approximately 1 inch of simmering water. Season with salt. Cover and **steam** for 30–45 minutes, depending upon the size. To test for doneness, tug on a leaf; it should release with just a little resistance.
3. *Meanwhile,* **prepare** sauce (recipe below).

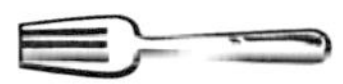

See sidebar for serving

Lemon-Butter Sauce

2 Tbsp. unsalted butter, melted
2 Tbsp. flaxseed oil
1 Tbsp. freshly squeezed lemon juice
1 Tbsp. minced fresh parsley
Freshly ground black pepper

Combine ingredients. Serve as dipping sauce with artichokes. Extra is great drizzled over steamed broccoli. For a sauce for fish, use one part butter/oil and one part lemon juice with a sprinkle of pepper and little fresh parsley. Yield: 4 servings

Artichoke

Shopping Tips:

Select tight and heavy artichokes.

Serving Suggestions:

Enjoy steamed artichokes with baked fish and potatoes.

To eat artichokes, remove leaves, starting with outermost leaves. Dip each leaf base in Lemon-Butter Sauce. Scrape the vegetable "meat" off with your teeth.

When you come to the center (the heart), remove the "fuzz" with sharp knife and savor the "heart" with a drizzle of Lemon-Butter Sauce. The "heart" is simply the best!

Uses for canned hearts:

- Hummus
- Meal-in-a-Salad
- Pilafs

More Facts:

Easy to digest, artichokes also improve liver function and help lower cholesterol.

Analysis for Lemon-Butter Sauce/Serving:
Calories: 111 (Fat Cal 108) Fat: 12g (4.1g Sat) Cholesterol: 15mg
Sodium: 0mg Carbs: 0.4g (0g Fiber 0.1g Sugar) Protein: 0g

C
sauce - portions; frequency

Arugula

Shopping Tips:

Leaves should be firm and green. Small, young leaves are more tender and do not have such a strong flavor.

Storage Tips:

Store leaves in plastic bag in crisper drawer. Best if used within 2 days.

Serving Suggestions:

- Use the young, tender leaves to perk up a salad of leafy greens.
- Ribbon-cut or mince and stir into warm or cold pasta dishes.
- Use as a garnish on sandwiches – you'll likely find you don't need as much mayo or mustard!

Recipes Using:

- Fancy Scrambled Eggs
- Pea & Celery Salad
- Meal-in-a-Salad

Salad Dressing Storage Guidelines

Store covered in refrigerator for 7–10 days. Freeze extra in ice cube trays.

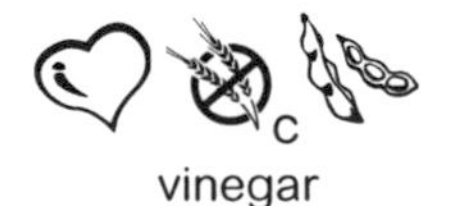

Arugula

A vegetable with a peppery, almost mustard-like taste, arugula adds a nice kick to salads and pesto. It is also a healthy way to add flavor to sandwiches and eggs.

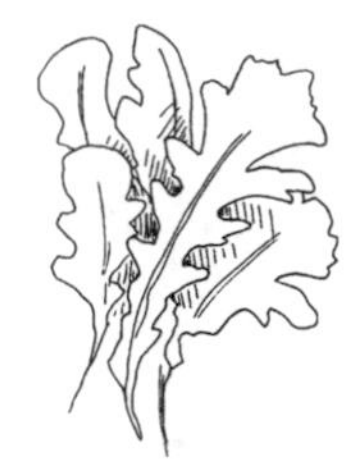

Arugula Leaves

Arugula Pesto Salad Dressing

Mix: 10 minutes

This recipe was inspired by the Friendly Farm farm stand newsletter (Iowa City, Iowa). Arugula and spinach are Sondra's favorite combination, but you can use any vegetable-herb combination desired (see Pesto recipe on p. 93 for ideas).

1 cup fresh arugula (loosely packed)
1 cup fresh spinach (loosely packed)
2 cloves garlic, cracked
2 Tbsp. raw apple cider vinegar
1/4 cup water
1 1/2 tsp. freshly squeezed lemon juice
1/4 cup olive oil
Freshly grated nutmeg

1. **Rinse** arugula and spinach and **spin-dry**.
2. Add arugula, spinach and garlic to food processor with chopper blade (or blender jar). **Process** until finely chopped. Add vinegar, water (for a thicker consistency, use less water) and lemon juice to processor. **Process** while **streaming** in oil. Season with nutmeg and salt to taste.

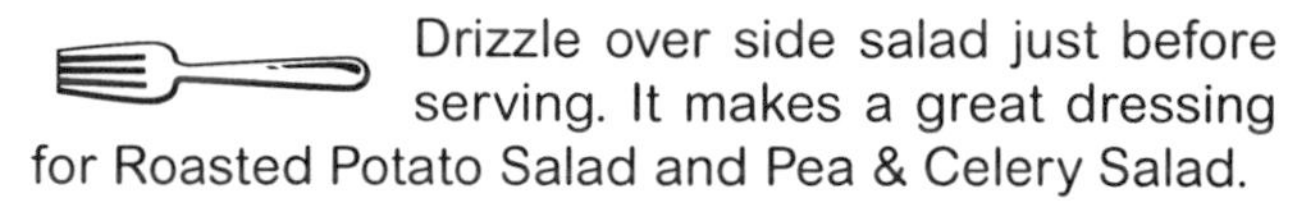

Drizzle over side salad just before serving. It makes a great dressing for Roasted Potato Salad and Pea & Celery Salad.

Yield: 16 (1 Tbsp.) servings 1 cup

Analysis/Tablespoon:
Calories: 32 (Fat Cal 30) Fat: 3.3g (0.5g Sat) Cholesterol: 0mg
Sodium: 10mg Carbs: 0.3g (0.1g Fiber 0g Sugar) Protein: 0.1g

Roasted Potato Salad with Arugula Pesto Salad Dressing

Inspired by the Food Network, this salad is delicious and safe for potlucks or picnics!

Make it quick and easy: Allow the below recipe to serve only as a guide. Sondra likes to dice a handful of leftover oven fries, grate a little red onion with a microplane, dice a carrot or rib of celery, and stir in a dab of Dijon-style mustard with Arugula dressing. If desired, eggs may be added to the salad. It's a great addition to a simple lunch!

2 lb. red potatoes, chunked
1 Tbsp. High-Heat oil
1/2 tsp. each: salt, garlic powder, paprika
Freshly ground black pepper, as desired
1 med. red onion, chopped (1 cup)
1/2 tsp. Dijon-style mustard
1/2 cup Arugula Pesto Salad Dressing (p. 44)
Vegetable Combos:
2 cups diced red pepper
2 cups diced green pepper
OR
3 cups green beans (blanched 3 minutes)
1 cup diced red peppers
1 cup diced green peppers

Preheat oven—450°.
Baking pan (stainless steel or preheated cast iron).

1. **Drizzle** oil over potatoes and sprinkle with seasonings. **Toss** to coat potatoes. Place in oven and **roast** 7–10 minutes.
2. **Stir** in onions and continue roasting until potatoes are tender (about 20–25 minutes total time). **Chill**.
3. **Stir** mustard into dressing. Add dressing and vegetable combo to potatoes. **Stir. Chill**.

Yield: 8 servings 8 cups

Arugula (continued)

More Facts:

Arugula is a green that's easy to grow at home, in your yard or in a pot on your kitchen counter. As long as you harvest the leaves, they will continue replenishing themselves for months.

The ancient Romans used arugula frequently in their salads. They also used the seeds to flavor oil.

Paprika Facts:

Paprika is made by grinding dried red sweet bell peppers. It has different names throughout the world and is made from more than one kind of pepper. Interestingly, the paler the color, the hotter the flavor.

Nutritional Comparison

Compared to a traditional potato salad, our salad increases fiber by 142% and at the same time reduces:

Calories by 31%
Fat by 40%
Saturated fat by 57%
Sodium by 32%.

Analysis/Serving:
Calories: 167 (Fat Cal 48) Fat: 5.3g (0.8g Sat) Cholesterol: 0mg
Sodium: 156mg Carbs: 26.2g (3.4g Fiber 4.2g Sugar) Protein: 3.3g

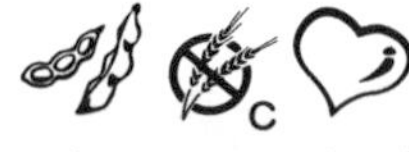

vinegar, mustard

Asparagus

Shopping Tips:

Look for tight buds and bright green color.

Serving Suggestions:

- Blanched asparagus spears add an elegant and flavorful touch to a tray of veggies and dip.
- Fantastic in soups! (Even the woody part of the stalk can be peeled and added to soup stock.)
- A treat in stir-fries.
- Roasted is our personal favorite. There are never any leftovers.

Recipes Using:

- Roasted Vegetables
- Basic Soup
- Hearty Chicken Noodle Soup

More Facts:

Since asparagus tastes best right after being picked, frozen asparagus (frozen soon after picking) often has a richer flavor than fresh asparagus found in the produce section of the store.

---

1 lb. raw asparagus = ~14 spears = ~3 cups

Asparagus

Prep: ~5 minutes   Cook: see below

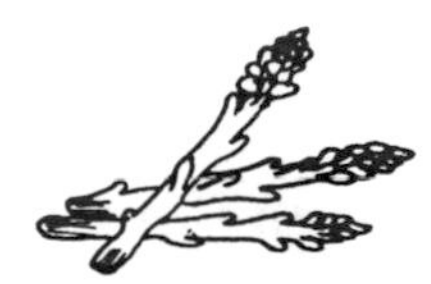

Asparagus Spears with Tips

Whether you are savoring the rich flavor of roasted asparagus or enjoying the delicate taste it adds to soups, asparagus is one vegetable you do not want to miss … and it is good for you! Asparagus has a rich source of nutrients, providing ample amounts of vitamin A, B-complex, C, E, K, potassium, iron, zinc, rutin, glutathione (an important anticarcinogen) and fiber.

1. Remove woody end by gently bending spears and snapping where they naturally break.
2. If desired, cut tender portion into 1-inch lengths for cuts/tips, or leave as spears.
3. Soak in cold water to remove sand and dirt.
4. **Steaming Asparagus:** Arrange in top of steamer pan or in a steamer basket. Sprinkle with salt and/or other seasonings (e.g., seasoned garlic salt). Cover. Steam until tender (spears 10–15 minutes; cuts/tips 5 minutes). If desired, drizzle with flaxseed oil or Butter-Lemon Sauce (p. 43).

Roasted Aspargus

Preheat oven: 425°/450° (convection/conventional). Baking pan (stainless steel or preheated cast iron).

1. Using your hands, lightly coat asparagus spears with High-Heat oil. Sprinkle with seasonings (e.g., seasoned garlic salt or garlic 'n' herb; see p. 222).
2. Place single layer in pan/skillet. Roast until tender (fresh about 5–7 minutes; frozen about 10–12 minutes), turning asparagus halfway through cooking time. Serve immediately.

Avocado

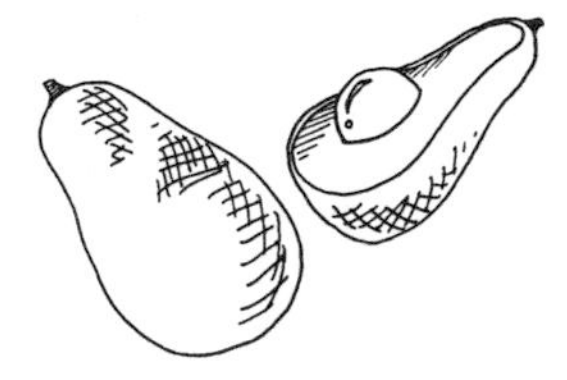

The smooth and creamy avocado is best known as an ingredient in guacamole, but it can be served many ways. Rich in a variety of nutrients, it has many health benefits. Research shows that the carotenoids (such as lutein) found in avocados are more easily absorbed by our body because of the healthy fats that are also present. In addition, the carotenoids found in other vegetables are easier to absorb if consumed with avocado.[4] Only a small amount of avocado is necessary to greatly multiply the health benefits of numerous other foods.

Because the avocado is high in calories (88 percent comes from unsaturated fat), it should be enjoyed in moderation.

Avocado

Shopping Tips:

Choose avocados that are heavy for their size and just ripe or almost ripe. (When ripe, they give a little when gently pushed in at the stem.) Smooth-skinned avocadoes stay green when ripe; rough-skinned ones get darker.

Ripening & Storage Tips:

Ripen avocados on the kitchen counter. To speed up the process, wrap them in a brown paper bag. Once they are ripe, store them in the refrigerator until ready to use.

Serving Suggestions:

See ideas below Easy Guacamole recipe.

Heart Health

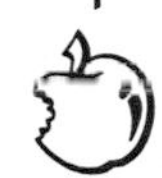

When eaten in moderation, the avocado is a great food for heart health. The rich oleic acid reduces cholesterol; the potassium helps to regulate blood pressure; and the folate lowers the risk of heart attack.[5]

Easy Guacamole

1 avocado
Seasoned garlic salt (p. 222)
Freshly squeezed lemon juice
Diced tomatoes (optional)

Slice avocado lengthwise, circling knife around large seed in center. **Remove seed** with spoon. Scoop out flesh, place in bowl and gently **mash** with a fork until smooth. **Season** with garlic salt and lemon juice (also helps to retain color) as desired. **Stir** in tomatoes. Serve immediately.

Serving ideas for guacamole and avocado slices.

- Use as a dip or spread.
- Use as a replacement for cream cheese (e.g., on bagels).
- Use as a replacement for mayonnaise on sandwiches.
- Use as a replacement for sour cream (e.g., soups, tacos).
- Dice and add to salads.
- **Salad Dressing:** Omit tomatoes. Stir olive oil and additional lemon juice into guacamole.

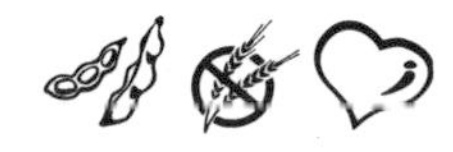

Beans

While they might provide a rustic and down-to-earth tone to meals, beans have nothing to be humble about. A versatile food, beans are an excellent source of nutrients. Unlike most foods, beans lose few nutrients when they are canned, so using canned beans can be healthy and convenient. (For instructions on how to prepare dried beans, see Black Bean Soup on p. 122.)

Nutrition of Beans

Beans have a lot to offer. They are high in **fiber** (helps to lower cholesterol, aids intestinal health and helps with blood sugar levels) and make a good source of **protein**, especially when combined with grains. Beans also have many **antioxidants**. Generally, the darker the bean, the higher the level of antioxidants (black beans have ten times the amount of antioxidants as oranges and comparable amounts to cranberries).[6] Beans also contain several vitamins and minerals that we need for good health. The minerals they contain are of key importance because our bodies cannot manufacture them – we have to get them from dietary sources. Beans are particularly rich in potassium, folate, magnesium and iron.

Potassium works with sodium and chloride to help our muscles contract and expand and to help our nerves function properly. It helps to slow the excretion of calcium and thus is influential in the accumulation and maintenance of bone mass.

Folate can be difficult for the body to absorb, but it is a key nutrient for heart health, red blood cell formation, circulation and the development of the fetus. It has been linked to the prevention of neurological diseases such as Parkinson's and to slowing dementia in patients with Alzheimer's.[7] It is also beneficial in preventing osteoporosis-related fractures.

Magnesium is critical for bone health and muscle relaxation. It is required for the function of over three hundred enzymes and is used in so many ways that it affects almost every system in our bodies.

Iron helps to give us energy and is involved with the transportation of oxygen throughout our bodies.

Bean (½ cup)	Fiber	Protein	Potassium	Magnesium	Folate	Iron
Edamame	2.3g	7.5g	345mg	50mg	241mcg	1.8mg
Black	6g	7g	280mg	60mg	128mcg	1.8mg
Garbanzo	5g	7g	250mg	35mg	80mcg	1.6mg
Kidney	8.2g	6.7g	329mg	36mg	65mcg	1.6mg
Pinto	5.5g	5.8g	292mg	32mg	72mcg	1.8mg
Tofu (3 oz.)	0.8g	7g	126mg	31mg	16mcg	1.2mg

Beans come packaged with or without added salt. Sometimes, as in the hummus recipe below, salted beans add more flavor and no additional salt is necessary. In other cases, such as stews, unsalted beans are fine because the beans simmer and absorb the other flavors of the stew.

Here is an example of the sodium content in salted and unsalted beans. The range of salt reflects variances by brand — another reason to read the labels.

Bean (½ cup)	**Beans** with salt	**Beans** without salt
Black	85–200mg	15mg
Garbanzo	100–350mg	30mg
Red	140–200mg	25mg

*Note: We suggest caution when purchasing canned baked beans; they often are loaded with sodium and sugar.

Quick & Easy Hummus

S→T: 10 minutes

1 (15 oz.) can garbanzo beans (with added salt) (drained, reserve some liquid)
2 tsp. lightly minced fresh garlic (~2 cloves)
1 Tbsp. tahini
Seasonings (see sidebar for some ideas)
1 Tbsp. freshly squeezed lemon juice
1 tsp. olive oil
1–3 Tbsp. bean liquid

Add beans, garlic, tahini and seasonings to food processor (with chopper blade). **Process** until finely chopped. Process while **streaming** in lemon juice, followed by oil and then bean liquid, until hummus is a smooth, spreadable consistency.

Serve with raw or blanched vegetables. Use as a spread on crackers, sandwiches or toast.

Yield: 20 (1 Tbsp.) servings $1\frac{1}{4}$ cups

Analysis/Tablespoon:
Calories: 23 (Fat Cal 8) Fat: 0.9g (0.1g Sat) Cholesterol: 0mg
Sodium: 21mg Carbs: 3g (0.8g Fiber 0.5g Sugar) Protein: 1.1g

Beans

Purchasing Tips:

For canned beans, note the sodium content and make sure the beans are packed in water, not syrup.

Storage Tips:

Dry beans can last for years. However, they fade and take longer to cook as the beans get older. Store beans in glass away from heat and light.

Seasoning Ideas for Hummus

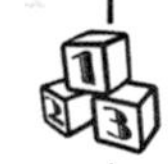

Most any spice can be added to hummus. Sondra likes onion powder with dried basil and paprika *or* with dried parsley, ground cumin and coriander.

Vegetables can also be included, such as canned artichokes (drained) and raw carrots. Finely chop them with the beans.

Magnesium for the Heart

Magnesium helps prevent heart attacks and can prevent free-radical damage after a heart attack.[8]

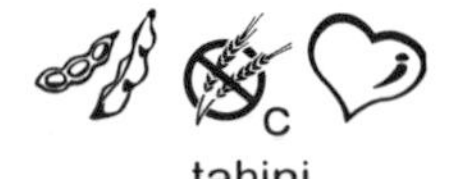

Beet & Beet Greens

Shopping Tips:

Beets sold with greens intact are fresher. Smaller beets are more tender and offer more flavor.

Storing Tips:

Remove greens 2 inches from bulb and store separately for 2–3 days. The bulb will keep for a few weeks stored in an open bag in the crisper drawer.

Serving Suggestions:

Traditionally, beets are served cooked. They are, however, delicious served roasted or raw as a garnish to lettuce salad or on raw vegetable platters.

Recipes Using:

- Beet Salad
- Meal-in-a-Salad

Other Facts:

There are many varieties of beets, offering a subtle range of flavors and colors. Involve the family in the fun with a test for the most popular.

---

10 oz. = 1 1/2 cups unpeeled

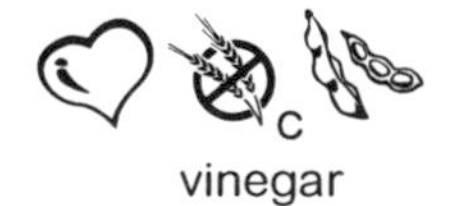

vinegar

Beets

Though high in natural sugars, beets are healthy for the liver and aid both circulation and the relief of constipation. The leaves contain calcium, iron, magnesium, phosphorous and vitamins A, B and C.

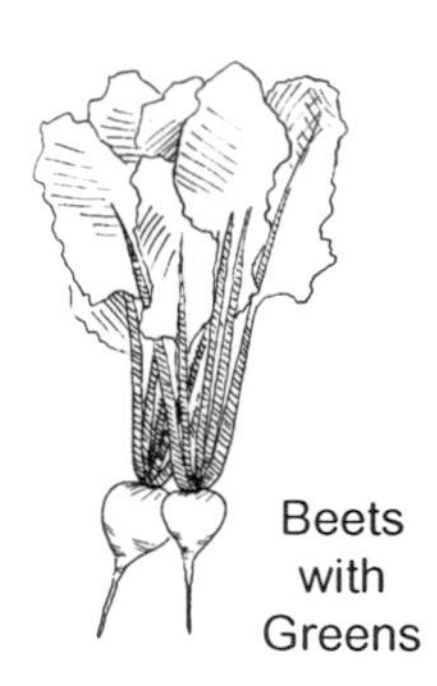
Beets with Greens

Roasted Beets with Greens

S→T: ~30 minutes (12 minutes inactive)

Beets
Onion, diced (use ~1/2 cup/1 cup beets)
Ground coriander (use 1/4 tsp./1 cup beets)
Medium-Heat oil, salt and pepper
Balsamic vinegar

Preheat oven—375°.
Baking pan (stainless steel or preheated cast iron).

1. Cut off stems and greens, reserving greens for Step 3. Scrub bulbs thoroughly. Dice (¼ inch).
2. **Roasting**:
   - Drizzle diced beets with oil, seasonings (salt, pepper and coriander). Toss to coat. Roast 10 minutes.
   - Stir in onions and more oil, if needed. Roast another 10–15 minutes until al dente.
3. *Meanwhile,* wash greens. Leave whole or tear into pieces. **Sauté** 3–5 minutes or **simmer** covered 5–7 minutes, seasoning with salt and coriander and balsamic vinegar as described on page 64. Serve immediately with beets.

Simmered Beets and Greens

Simmer sliced/diced beets as with any simmered vegetable (see p. 38), allowing 20 minutes, or until beets are tender. If desired, add greens and simmer for 5 additional minutes. Season as described above.

Bok Choy

Sometimes referred to as "white cabbage," bok choy looks like a cross between celery and collards. It has broad white or greenish-white stems with loose, dark green leaves and is an excellent source of calcium and vitamins A and C.

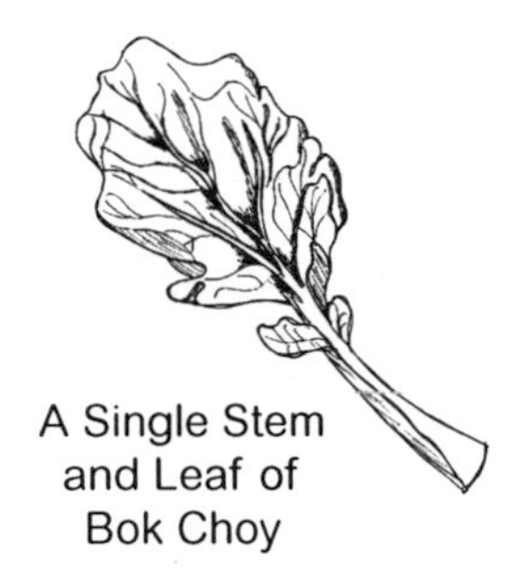
A Single Stem and Leaf of Bok Choy

Bok choy has a pungent fragrance and taste, especially when eaten raw, but becomes milder when cooked. Baby varieties are much more tender and less pungent.

To Prepare:

Wash stems and leaves. Chop stems into small pieces. Cut leaves with scissors or tear into small pieces.

Baby Bok Choy & Leeks

Medium-Heat oil
Matchstick carrots
Sliced leeks
Baby bok choy, chopped
Seasoned garlic salt (p. 222)

"Chop & Drop" vegetables in oil, sautéing until the colors pop.

 Serve immediately as a side dish.

For an easy stir-fry and pasta meal:

1. In saucepan, bring water to boil for pasta. After adding leeks to stir fry (Step 3), begin cooking whole-grain fettuccini without salt until al dente.
2. In a large skillet, sauté raw chicken chunks or strips in small amount of High-Heat oil.
3. When chicken is halfway done, "Chop & Drop" vegetables and seasoning. When done, remove pan from burner, add drained pasta and sprinkle of seasoning. Stir and serve immediately.

Bok Choy

Shopping Tips:

Bok choy stalks should be firm and leaves green and crisp. Chop off the core of the stem and wash stalks individually.

Serving Suggestions:

While bok choy can be served as salad greens, many prefer the more gentle taste of sautéed bok choy. It's a tasty addition to stir-fries, pilafs, casseroles and eggs.

Recipes Using:

- Fancy Scrambled Eggs
- Breakfast Squares
- Breakfast Pizza
- Stir-fry

More Facts:

There are over twenty varieties of bok choy. If you are new to bok choy or prefer mild greens to pungent ones, look for baby bok choy that is fresh from the farm. Its delicate flavor is a wonderful summer treat.

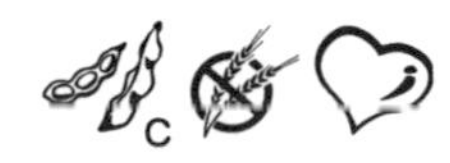

Broccoli

When broccoli is fresh and cooked correctly, it is a tender, flavorful treat. Even if you have resisted broccoli before, give farm-fresh broccoli (lightly steamed) a try. The nutrition of broccoli abounds, with cancer-preventing compounds, antioxidants, fiber and calcium.

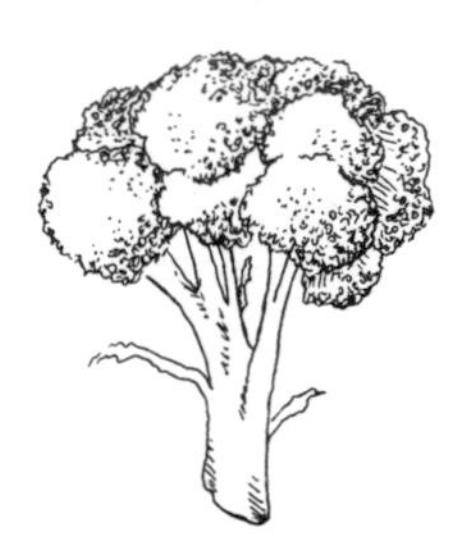

Broccoli Florets with Stem

Method to prepare fresh broccoli for casseroles, stir-fries or as a steamed side dish.

1. Cut off florets. **Peel** stalk portion with vegetable peeler or paring knife to remove fibrous outer bark.
2. **Cuts:** Cut stalk into medallion (disk) pieces and floret portion into bite-size pieces.
   Spears: Cut both stalk and floret portion into strips.
3. If necessary, **soak** pieces in salted water for 5 minutes to kill hidden pests. Drain. Rinse.
4. **Steam** (3–5 minutes) or blanch (1–2 minutes) as desired.

Broccoli

Shopping Tips:

- Choose stems that are narrow (less woody).
- Look for florets with a purple or blue tone. A yellowish tinge indicates that broccoli is old and likely to be bitter.

Serving Suggestions:

- Blanched with dip
- Blanched in salad
- Steamed on potatoes
- Blanched in stir-fry

Recipes Using:

- Meal-in-a Salad
- Slow Cooker Chowder
- Chicken-Broccoli Mac 'n' Cheese
- Salmon & Pasta

More Facts:

When cooking broccoli, include the leaves -- they contain the greatest concentration of nutrients.

~9 oz. stalk = ~2 cups

Broccoli & Red Pepper

Broccoli spears
Sliced red pepper
(~1/4 of a pepper for 2 servings of broccoli)
Salt, pepper and/or
seasoned garlic salt (p. 222)

In saucepan, **steam** seasoned vegetables with small amount of water for 3–5 minutes. Serve immediately since overcooked/mushy broccoli is bitter. If needed, use the carryover cooking technique (p. 38). If desired, drizzle with flaxseed oil or Butter-Lemon Sauce (p. 43).

Cabbage

Cabbage varies in color as well as flavor, but all varieties are rich in antioxidants and folate and contain cancer-preventing compounds. Bok choy and collards are discussed independently. Here we focus on the green and purple head varieties of cabbage, as well as napa cabbage, a delightful mild cabbage sometimes referred to as Chinese cabbage.

Sautéed Cabbage

S→T: 10 minutes

Sautéed cabbage is a colorful, nutritious, tasty and easy side dish for almost any meal. It can also be used in place of rice for serving with chicken.

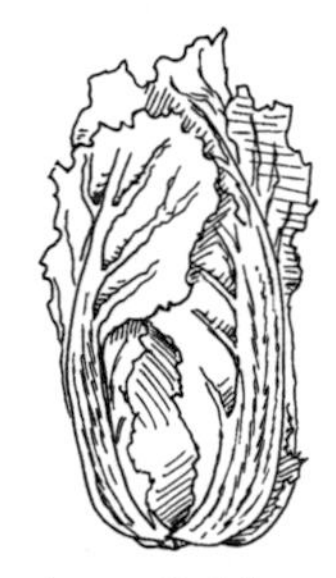

Napa Cabbage

Medium-Heat oil
1/2 small head or napa cabbage, chopped
1 small leek, chopped (optional)
Seasoned garlic salt (p. 222)

In skillet, **season** and **sauté** cabbage and leeks in oil until color is a vibrant green and vegetables are just tender.

Cabbage

Shopping Tips:

Choose heads of cabbage that have bright colors and are tight and heavy for their size.

Storage Tips:

Loosely sealed, fresh cabbage heads will last 1–2 weeks in the refrigerator, and cut cabbage will last 5–6 days.

Serving Suggestions:

- Shred for use in salads or coleslaw.
- Chop/shred and add to casseroles or stir-fries.

Recipes Using:

- Cabbage-Fish Bake
- Cabbage Patch Soup
- Chicken-Cabbage Delight

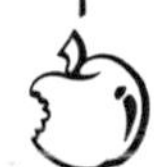

Lower Cancer Risk

A six-year study in the Netherlands looked at dietary data for over 100,000 people. Those eating the most vegetables had a 25% lower risk of colorectal cancers. Those who ate a lot of crucifers (e.g., cabbage, broccoli, kale) reduced their risk by 49%.[9]

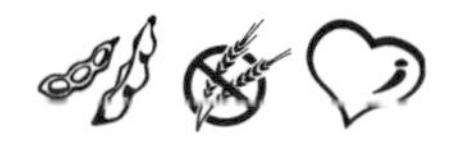

Carrot

Shopping Tips:

Choose small to medium carrots that are crisp and firm.

Storage Tips:

Remove green tops before storing.

Serving Suggestions:

- Roasted – yum!
- Shredded for salads, stir-fries and garnishes
- Raw as snacks, with dip or in a salad

Recipes Featuring Carrots for Sweetness:

- Chunky Garden Spaghetti Sauce
- Spice "Muffin" Cake/ Cupcakes

More Facts:

Darker varieties have more vitamin K.

Carrot Tops

Carrot tops (fresh or dried) are full of nutrients. Mince the fresh tops and use as garnish (like parsley) for any recipe.

Carrot

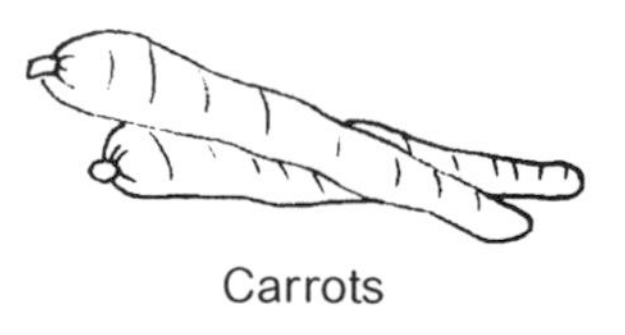

Carrots

A versatile vegetable, carrots can be enjoyed raw, cooked in casseroles, soups and stir-fries or served as a side dish. If eaten with the peel, they are a great source of carotenoids, including vitamin A. Their fiber helps to prevent constipation and alleviate indigestion. Carrots are a great natural sweetener for a variety of foods.

Glazed Carrots

S→T: 15 minutes (mostly inactive time)

Carrots are naturally sweet, so taste buds can be retrained to enjoy them without sweeteners. But sometimes even the most "all natural" taster desires something a little sweeter.

2 cups sliced/julienned carrots
Salt and pepper

Glaze Ingredients:

1/4 cup water and/or cooking liquid
1 tsp. cornstarch
1/2 tsp. honey or agave nectar, if necessary

In saucepan, **simmer** seasoned carrots in small amount of water until al dente (approx. 10 min.). **Drain** cooking liquid into measuring cup, leaving carrots in pan. Add water to measure ¼ cup. **Whisk** in cornstarch and sweetener, if using. Pour over carrots and heat to **thicken**, stirring often. Taste. If needed, add more seasonings. **Garnish** with carrot tops (see Healthy Bite in sidebar).

Yield: 4 vegetable servings

Analysis/Serving:
Calories: 30 (Fat Cal 1) Fat: 0.2g (0g Sat) Cholesterol: 0mg
Sodium: 108mg Carbs: 7.1g (1.7g Fiber 3.6g Sugar) Protein: 0.6g

Celery

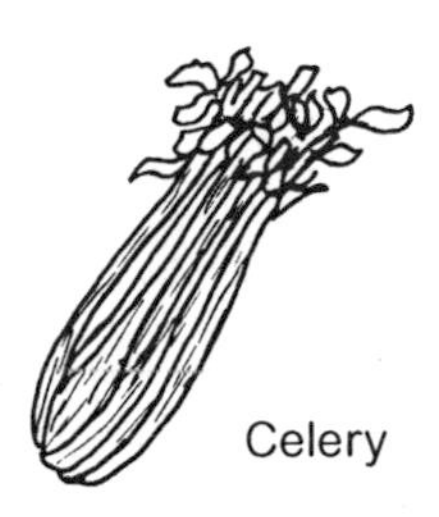
Celery

Easily forgotten, celery is a great source of nutrients and a wonderful way to subtly enhance the flavors of soups, salads and casseroles. Rich in vitamins and bioflavanoid antioxidants, celery also contains allicin, the healthy nutrient in garlic. Leaves may be saved for use in soups, casseroles or stir-fries

Serving Suggestions:

Great for Snacks – good finger food!

- Cut into pieces to have ready for a snack on the run.
- Fill celery ribs with a small amount of healthier-choice fillings (e.g., nut butter, cream cheese, dip, salsa, hummus).
- Serve with Confetti Dip (p. 42), Spinach Dip (p. 79), Hummus (p. 49) or Black Bean Dip (p. 149).
- Dice or slice and eat by the handful.

Other Serving Ideas:

- Add to salads, casseroles, soups and stir-fries.
- Sauté and use to top a baked potato.
- Put in lunch boxes.

Celery

Shopping Tips:

Choose celery with firm, crisp ribs and dark leaves. Avoid celery with browning stalks or yellowed leaves.

Important Purchasing Tip:

Since most of the celery available in grocery stores has been blanched in ethylene gas, it is one of the most chemically altered whole foods in North America.[10] We recommend organic celery with dark, unbleached leaves.

Crave the Crunch

Often the craving for chips or salted nuts can be satisfied with another crunchy food. Celery offers a great crunch while also providing fiber to give the "full" feeling that stifles the tendency to keep munching.

Wilted Celery

Place in ice water to recrisp.

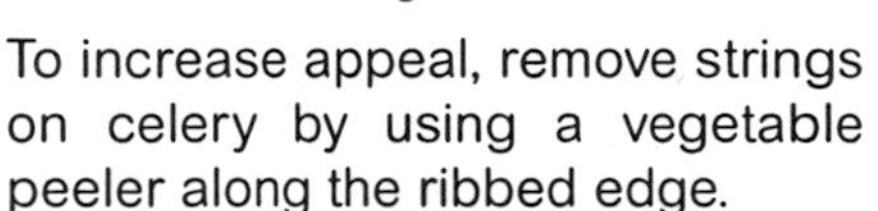

Finicky Eaters

To increase appeal, remove strings on celery by using a vegetable peeler along the ribbed edge.

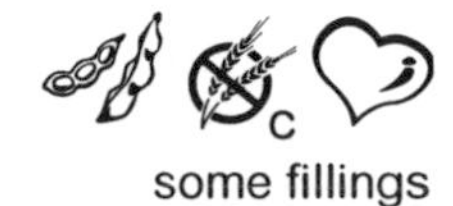

some fillings

Chard

Shopping Tips:

Select chard with crisp, vibrant-colored leaves.

Storage Tips:

Store unwashed chard in a plastic bag in the refrigerator. It can also be blanched and frozen.

Serving Suggestions:

- Use stalks and leaves in cooking (sauté, steam or add to soups).
- Use stems of white chard in salads.

Recipes Using:

- Greens & Onions
- Stir-fry

Healthy Bites

Sodium and Chard: Since chard is high in sodium, use less salt in recipes with chard.

Good Nutrients: With higher levels of more nutrients than almost any other vegetable, Swiss chard is excellent for your health. It is especially good for bone, eye and heart health.

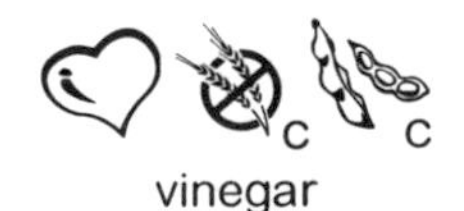

vinegar

Chard

A quick-cooking green, chard provides an alternative to spinach. It comes in red and white varieties, with both flat and crinkly leaves. Chard is a good source of vitamins, fiber and several minerals, including zinc and magnesium.

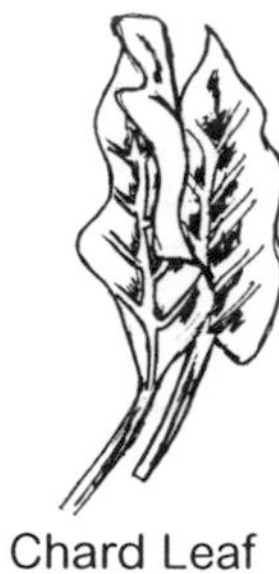
Chard Leaf with Stem

Sautéed Chard with Balsamic Grilled Chicken

Red onion slices
Medium-Heat oil
Boneless, skinless chicken breast (butterfly cut)
Balsamic vinegar
Salt, pepper, garlic powder and/or nutmeg
Swiss chard

1. **Sauté** onions in oil until almost tender.
2. *Meanwhile,* place chicken on platter. **Coat** with vinegar (approx. 2 tablespoons per pound of chicken). Lightly season with salt and garlic powder. Slide onions to side of skillet and lay chicken in skillet. **Cook** chicken approximately 3–4 minutes on each side.
3. *Meanwhile,* wash, spin-dry, remove rib and chop (or tear) chard. Slide chicken and onions to side. (If skillet is not large enough, remove fully cooked chicken and keep warm.) Add chard and seasonings (nutmeg, especially freshly grated, is delicious). **Sauté** approximately 3 minutes, stirring often. **Add** a splash of balsamic vinegar about halfway through to deglaze pan. Serve with raw vegetables.

Chard & Potato Bake

Follow Kale & Potato Bake (p. 65), using 4 medium chard leaves (~2½ cups ribbon-cut) and sautéing chard with onions instead of simmering.

Collards

Collards — nonheading cabbages with broad, smooth, dark-green leaves and fairly long stems — are a good source of dietary fiber and omega-3 fatty acids as well as an excellent source of vitamins and minerals.

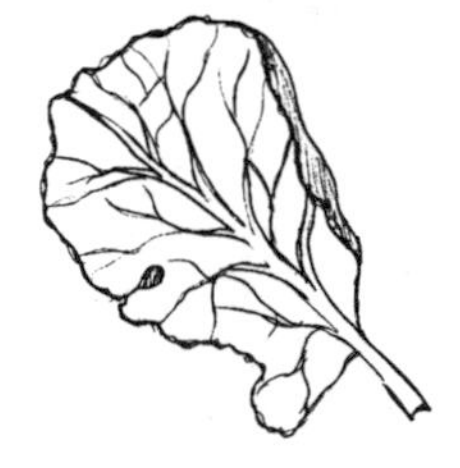
Collard Leaf

Collard Wraps

S→T: ~22 minutes

2 collard leaves, per wrap
1/2 cup chopped onions, per wrap, (divided)
Splash balsamic vinegar
Seasoned garlic salt (p. 222)
Grilled chicken chunks (4 oz./wrap)
Cooked brown rice (~1/2 cup/wrap)
Dijon-style mustard, as desired

1. Remove center rib from collards.
2. In large skillet, bring a thin layer of water to boil. Lay collards flat (or with as few folds as possible) into boiling water. Add half the onions (between layers of collards), vinegar and a light sprinkle of seasoning. Cover and **simmer** 15 minutes, or until tender.
3. *Meanwhile,* **sauté** chicken, remaining onions and a sprinkle of seasoning in Medium-Heat oil, stirring occasionally; add rice near end.
4. Using two large slotted spoons/spatulas for support, **transfer** collards onto a large platter. Unfold. **Spread** mustard on collard. **Spoon** on chicken mixture. Pick up edge of 2 leaves and **roll** leaves around filling, moving carefully and quickly so as not to get burned. Transfer wrap to serving plate.

 Serve immediately.

Collards

Shopping Tips:

Choose collard leaves that are firm and vivid in color, with no browning or yellowing. Smaller leaves are tender and less bitter.

Use collards soon after purchasing since they increase in bitterness the longer they are kept.

Storage Tips:

See Greens on page 64.

Recipes Using:

- Southern-Style Shepherd's Pie
- Greens & Onions

More Facts:

Collards contain almost as much calcium as milk.

While eaten from the wild since the earliest of times, collards have been cultivated since the times of the ancient Greek and Roman civilizations.

Other Filling Ideas 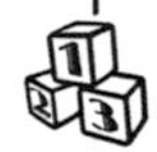

- Brown rice, cheese, onions
- Salmon, brown rice

Analysis/Serving:
Calories: 314 (Fat Cal 76) Fat: 8.4g (1.6g Sat) Cholesterol: 63mg
Sodium: 411mg Carbs: 32.6g (3.7g Fiber 4.2g Sugar) Protein: 27.1g

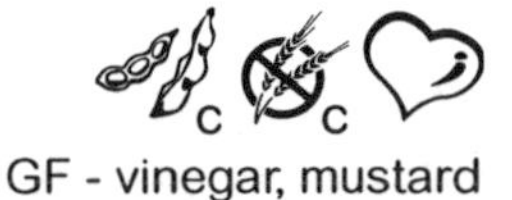

GF - vinegar, mustard

Corn

Shopping Tips:

Choose corn that is still in the husk because the husk retains moisture. The husk should be supple, not dry, and the kernels should be firm and in even rows. Since heat causes some of the sugars to convert to starch, look for corn that is kept near some refrigeration in the store; at the farmer's market, it should be kept in the shade.

Storage Tips:

Store corn in the husk until ready to use. Once blanched, whole ears of corn may be frozen and kept for up to a year.

Corn on the Cob

Boiling corn drains away both nutrients and flavor. So instead of boiling, try steaming it. We place a stainless steel slotted disc in the bottom of a large skillet or kettle, add just enough water to cover the disc, place the corn on the disc, cover the pan and simmer, allowing the steam to cook the corn until fork tender. The taste is fantastic!

Corn

There are five different types of corn: dent corn (used to make many corn products, including corn syrup), flint corn, flour corn, popcorn and sweet corn. While most corn is considered a grain, the sugars in sweet corn do not easily convert to starch, making it a vegetable and not a grain. Corn contains a variety of nutrients, the most notable being fiber and folate. The darker the corn is, the stronger the flavor and the higher the nutrient level. Blue corn, an increasingly popular form of flint corn, is superior in nutritional value. Flint corn and popcorn are less allergenic than other varieties.

Scalloped Corn

S→O: 15 minutes Bake: 15–20 minutes

1 (10 oz.) pkg. frozen corn
3/4 cup finely chopped onions
1 cup diced red/green bell peppers
(*or* use tri-color frozen peppers)
1/4 cup water
1/4 tsp. each: salt, paprika
Freshly ground black pepper (optional)
1 egg, slightly beaten
1/2 cup milk (unsweetened soy or low-fat cow)
1 Tbsp. brown rice flour
1 Tbsp. Medium-Heat oil (divided)
1/4 cup dry bread crumbs* (p. 98)

Preheat oven—350°. Prefer ovenproof saucepan.

In saucepan, bring corn, onions, peppers, water and seasonings to boil, reduce heat and **simmer** for 3 minutes. In small bowl, **whisk** egg, milk, flour and half of the oil together. In separate bowl, **stir** the remaining oil into bread crumbs. **Stir** egg mixture into cooked corn mixture. **Sprinkle** oiled crumbs on top. **Bake** 15–20 minutes.

Yield: 4 servings

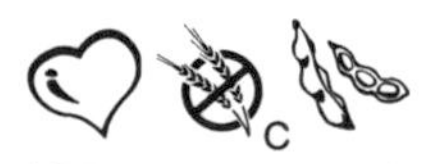

Analysis/Serving:
Calories: 182 (Fat Cal 56) Fat: 6.2g (1g Sat) Cholesterol: 53mg
Sodium: 181mg Carbs: 26.8g (2.7g Fiber 8.3g Sugar) Protein: 6.5g

*GF - use coarsely chopped puffed brown rice; add 1/8 teaspoon more salt in corn mixture.

Fennel

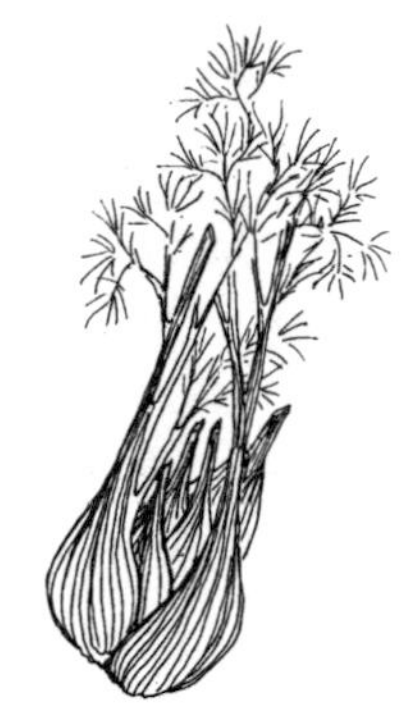
Fennel with Fern-Like Top

Fennel has been an important part of Mediterranean cooking for centuries. Closely related to parsley, carrots and dill, fennel is available fall through early spring. Its texture and crunch resemble those of celery, but its licorice flavor is distinctive. Fennel has an unusual combination of antioxidant properties, which makes it a vegetable of high health value. Its high levels of fiber, folate and potassium make it excellent for heart health.

Fennel leaves can be used as a garnish or a seasoning, and the stalks and bulbs can be enjoyed in a variety of soups, salads, casseroles and side dishes. Cooking softens the flavor.

Preparing Fennel: Cut off stalks. Cut globe portion into fourths, remove core and slice or dice. Slice or dice the stalks as well, saving the feathery leaves for a garnish or extra flavor.

Fennel & Mashed Potatoes

S→T: 40 minutes

2 lbs. new potatoes, diced
1 cup diced fennel
1/2 cup chopped onion
1 clove garlic, finely minced

1. Place potatoes, fennel and onions in saucepan. Sprinkle with salt and pepper and add ½ cup water. Bring to a boil, reduce heat, cover and **simmer** approximately 30 minutes, or until vegetables are fork tender.
2. **Add** garlic and **mash** with electric mixer to blend flavors evenly (do not overmix).

Yield: 6 servings ~4 1/2 cups

Fennel

Shopping Tips:

Choose fennel with green leaves and stalks that are fairly close together. The bulb should be firm and white or pale green, with few blemishes. The sweet fragrance should be noticeable and there should be no signs of flowering.

Storage Tips:

Fennel loses its flavor as it is stored, so use fennel shortly after purchasing.

Serving Suggestions:

- Use where you would normally use celery.
- Leaves make a beautiful garnish on mashed potatoes, steamed carrots and salad.

Recipes Using:

- Cabbage-Fish Bake
- Slow Cooker Chicken & Veggies
- Salmon & Pasta

More Facts:

Wild fennel is harvested for its seeds and used as a spice in foods such as sausage, breads and pickles. Sweet fennel is cultivated as a vegetable.

Analysis/Serving:
Calories: 457 (Fat Cal 2) Fat: 0.2g (0g Sat) Cholesterol: 0mg
Sodium: 17mg + varies Carbs: 26.6g (3.2g Fiber 2.1g Sugar) Protein: 3.2g

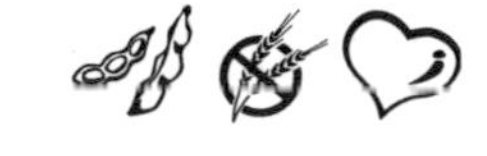

Garlic

Shopping Tips:

Choose firm, dry, rounded garlic heads with little or no unbroken skin.

Storage Tips:

Whole garlic heads can last for weeks, especially when kept away from direct heat and light. Once the head of garlic is broken, the cloves lose flavor and nutrient value after just a few days.

Reduce Cancer Risk

There is strong evidence that regular consumption of garlic and onions may lower your risk of cancer. In one study, participants reduced their risks for certain cancers by as much as 88% for esophageal cancer, 73% for ovarian cancer and 71% for prostate cancer.[11]

A chef's knife is perfect for mincing garlic!

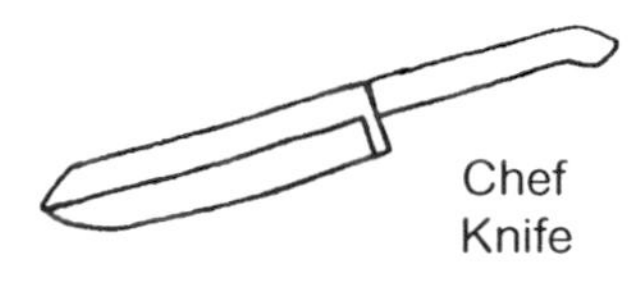

Garlic

One of the most ancient foods, garlic has been praised throughout history for both its flavor and its healthful properties. Though native to Central Asia, it is now used all over the world.

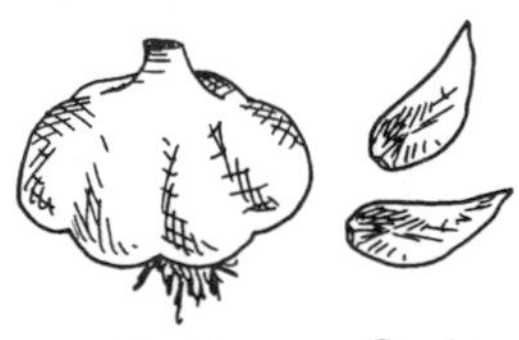

Scientists are conducting an increasing number of studies proving what people have believed for centuries – that garlic is highly beneficial for promoting heart health, reducing inflammation (thus helping arthritis), fighting bacterial and viral infection and aiding gastritis. It is beginning to be understood as an agent in reducing cancer risk and even in preventing weight gain.

Since it is most healthful when fresh, add garlic to dishes (such as stir-fries) during the final stages of cooking, and choose fresh over flaked and powdered versions whenever possible.

Mincing Fresh Garlic:

1. **Separate** cloves from bud (head) and lay on cutting board. Place blade of large knife flat on clove, with sharp edge facing away from you. Pound blade hard with "heel" of hand to **crush** garlic and loosen the peel. Remove **peel**.
2. Rock sharp edge of a chef's knife back and forth to finely **mince**. To rock, use fingers of left hand to hold tip of blade firmly on cutting board. With right hand, lift blade from board to rock up and down across the garlic. Occasionally remove garlic from blade; gather garlic into pile and repeat rocking procedure. (If left-handed, use reverse hands.)
3. To release more flavor, gather garlic into pile and gently smash with flat side of knife blade.

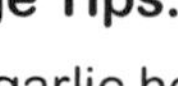

Estimated Analysis/Serving for 20-Minute Dinner on next page:
Calories: 318 (Fat Cal 85) Fat: 9.4g (1.6g Sat) Cholesterol: 42mg
Sodium: 313 Carbs: 30g (6.4g Fiber 7g Sugar) Protein: 28.7g

20-Minute Stir-Fry Dinner

Photo on Front Cover

This recipe incorporates the **"Water Stir-Fry"** *method to cut the fat and offer an opportunity to use flavorful oil that should not be used at high stir-fry temperatures. Start sautéing with a small amount of High-Heat oil (approximately one-half teaspoon for every two servings). Throughout the sautéing process, add water a teaspoon or so at a time to prevent food from sticking to pan. (For ease, place small container of water by range.) Garnish with a drizzle of flavored Low- or No-Heat oil (e.g., olive, toasted sesame, flaxseed). See pages 10-11 for more info on these oils.*

2 oz. whole-grain or gluten-free pasta
(linguine, fettuccine, spaghetti)
1/2 tsp. Medium-Heat oil
8 oz. raw skinless chicken breast strips
1–2 cups red onion slices
Garlic 'n' Herb seasoning (p. 222)
2–3 cups bell pepper strips (fresh or frozen)
1 small yellow or pattypan squash, sliced
1–2 cloves garlic, minced
Flavored oil (olive, toasted sesame, flaxseed)

1. In saucepan, bring water to **boil** for pasta. Just before adding peppers to stir-fry, cook pasta without salt until al dente.
2. *Meanwhile,* in skillet, **sauté** chicken in Medium-Heat oil, stirring often and adding water as needed (see "Water Stir-Fry" method above). While chicken is cooking, **stir** in onions, sprinkle of salt, pepper and Garlic 'n' Herb seasoning. Stir in peppers when meat is almost done; add squash a little later. Stir in minced garlic during the last minute.
3. When stir-fry is done, remove pan from burner and **add** drained pasta, sprinkle of salt and pepper and a drizzle of flavored oil to skillet. **Stir** to toss. Taste and add more oil and seasonings as needed. Serve immediately.

Yield: 2 servings (can be doubled or cut in half).

Garlic
(continued)

More Facts:

Chopping and crushing garlic is what begins the reaction that allows the allicin (the source of most of garlic's health benefits) to form and be digested by the body. Exposure to air aids this process, so chop or crush your garlic a few minutes before using, allowing time for the allicin to reach its full benefit.

Research has shown that light cooking does not reduce the health benefits of garlic, though cooking for several minutes does.[12] For this reason, we recommend adding garlic at the end of your cooking time. (In some recipes, we add half the garlic early on for flavor and the other half at the end for health.)

Research has shown that microwaving garlic removes much of its healthful properties.[13]

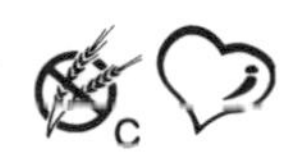

Green Beans

Shopping Tips:

Choose beans that are firm, smooth and vibrant in color, free of brown spots and bruising.

Storage Tips:

Green beans age quickly and should be used soon after purchasing. The shelf life can be extended somewhat if they are stored, unwashed, in a plastic bag or sealed container in the refrigerator, keeping their exposure to air at a minimum.

Serving Suggestions:

- Dice for salads (Roasted Potato Pesto Salad on p. 45), soups, stews or casseroles
- Steam for stir-fries
- Sauté for side dishes
- Pair with pork and fall squashes

More Facts:

All forms of beans probably originated in Peru. Taken back to Europe by Spanish explorers, they then spread around the globe as traders carried them on trade routes.

Green Beans

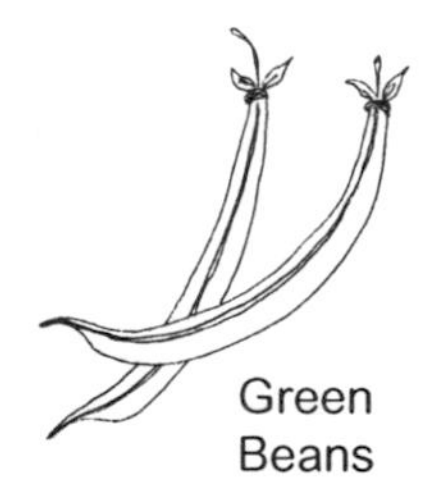

The term green beans can refer to any number of bean varieties eaten before reaching maturity – when they are still "green" in their pod. Often referred to as snap beans or string beans, the green bean family includes yellow or wax beans and French beans.

A low-cal food, green beans have an extensive list of nutrients; few vegetables can match the green bean for the variety and richness of the nutrients it provides, including vitamins K, C and A, manganese, fiber and iron. It is a fantastic food for both bone and heart health.

Sautéed Green Beans with Almonds

S→T: ~10–12 minutes

In skillet with lid, **steam** frozen (or fresh stemmed) green beans (seasoned with salt and black pepper) in small amount of water* for 4 minutes (frozen) or 6 minutes (fresh). (The trick is to have no or very little water remaining.) Remove lid; **drizzle** freshly squeezed lemon juice and Medium-Heat oil over beans. Add a tablespoon or so of minced or sliced red onion and **sauté** to desired doneness, stirring often (best served slightly crunchy). Toward the end, taste for seasoning and stir in a handful of slivered almonds.

Notes: When pattypan squash is in season, we add some slices when sautéing. To cut the fat, use the "Water Stir-Fry" method (p. 61).

*Often, when using frozen green beans in this recipe, water is not needed at all. Simply pour frozen green beans into skillet, turn burner on medium and slowly bring to a simmer.

Estimated Analysis/Serving: (using 5 oz. frozen green beans/serving)
Calories: 86 (Fat Cal 37) Fat: 4.1g (0.9g Sat) Cholesterol: 0mg
Sodium: 138 Carbs: 11.5g (1.9g Fiber 2.2g Sugar) Protein: 1g

Tired of Green Beans? *Green beans are often taken from a can, where the processing and extra sodium have zapped them of good flavor. Or they are overcooked, draining away their color, flavor and nutrients. Plopped down next to a serving of meat, they look sad and tired and don't taste much better. Try rejuvenating your image of green beans! Feature them in a salad (as in the recipe below) or steam them just until the color "pops." You'll be amazed at how much this "mundane" vegetable can appeal to your senses of sight, smell and taste.*

Green Bean Basil Salad

Prep: ~20 minute + chilling

1 lb. fresh green beans, stemmed (5 cups)
1 Tbsp. olive oil
4 cloves garlic, minced
2 handfuls fresh basil, ribbon-cut
2 medium fresh tomatoes, diced (3 cups)

1. **Steam** green beans 3–5 minutes, lightly seasoned with salt. Immediately transfer to ice-cold water to stop the cooking process and **chill**. Drain and spin-dry in salad spinner.
2. To fuse flavors, **heat** oil, garlic and basil on low for 2 minutes, stirring often. Add 1 tablespoon of water to oil mixture. (This helps to spread the flavored oil more evenly without needing more oil and calories.)
3. **Drizzle** oil mixture over green beans. **Toss**. Gently **stir** in tomatoes and **chill**.

Best served within 24 hours.

Yield: 7 (~1-cup servings)

Green Beans
(continued)

Recipes Using:

- Hearty Meat & Veggie Chili
- Fall Harvest Stews
- Beef Barley Soup
- Salmon & Pasta
- Barley Casserole
- Southern-Style Shepherd's Pie

Healthy Bites

Quick Cooking: Vegetables such as green beans and broccoli require little time to cook, so less water is required for steaming (approximately 1–2 teaspoons of water per cup of vegetables).

Health Benefits: The high levels of vitamins A and C in green beans help to prevent the build-up of cholesterol, act as anti-inflammatory agents (good for arthritis), boost immune health and protect against several cancers.

Analysis/Serving:
Calories: 58 (Fat Cal 20) Fat: 2.2g (.3g Sat) Cholesterol: 0mg
Sodium: 7mg+ varies Carbs: 8g (3.6g Fiber 2g Sugar) Protein: 2.2g

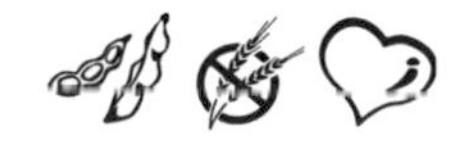

Greens

Purchasing Tips:

Choose greens that are firm and vibrant in color with crisp edges. They should be free of brown or slimy spots.

Storage Tips:

Greens keep best if wrapped in a damp paper towel and placed in a plastic bag in the crisper drawer.

Serving Suggestions:

- Sauté or simmer for side dishes (recipes to right).
- Ribbon-cut and add to almost any dish (see collards, chard, kale and spinach pages).
- Stir-fry fast cooking greens (e.g., chard, spinach).

For ideas on using a variety of salad greens, see pages 68–69.

More Facts:

Before scientists had determined what makes greens "healthy," commanders of armies were telling their soldiers to eat greens for strength.

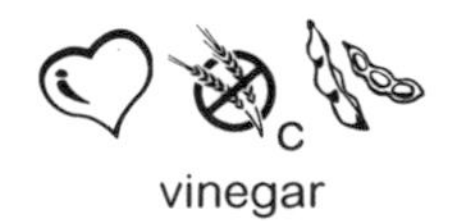

Greens

For centuries, people have used greens as an inexpensive way to increase the quality of their diet. Some greens come attached to edible roots (e.g., beet greens). Others are eaten primarily for their leaves (e.g., spinach). All leafy greens are packed with nutrition and are wonderful contributors to the prevention of heart disease, eye disease and cancer. They have multiple phytonutrients as well as a generally high amount of fiber. This page features a recipe for using the hardier, bolder greens. For discussion on some of the more delicate salad greens, see pages 68–69.

Greens & Onions

1. Wash and spin-dry greens. Remove tough center rib (often stronger, more pungent) from large leaves (e.g., collards, kale). Tear, chop or ribbon-cut.
2. **Sauté method** (works for the quick-cooking greens, such as beet, chard or spinach): In skillet, sauté red onion slices in oil until tender. Add greens, lightly season with salt, pepper and freshly grated nutmeg (or coriander for beet greens). Sauté for 3–5 minutes, stirring often. Add a splash of balsamic vinegar or freshly squeezed lemon juice about halfway through.

   Simmer method (works for all greens): In saucepan, place greens and diced red onions. Season as described in sauté method. Add a small amount of water. Bring to boil, reduce heat, cover and simmer (see chart below). If desired, drizzle with balsamic vinegar, freshly squeezed lemon juice and/or flaxseed oil.

Greens	Minutes to Simmer	Green	Minutes to Simmer
Beet	5 min.	Kale	15–20 min.
Chard	3–5 min.	Kohlrabi	20 min.
Collards	15 min.	Spinach	3–5 min.

Kale

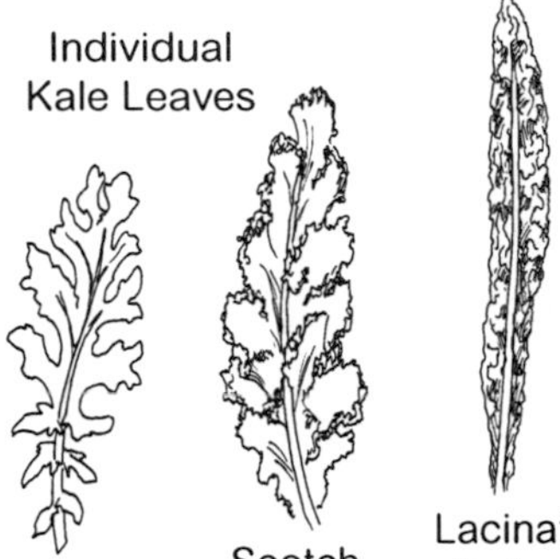

An ancient member of the cabbage family, kale has few calories and huge nutrition. With high levels of vitamins K and A, kale is wonderful for eye health and reduces the risk of several cancers. Steaming is the preferred method for cooking kale; not only does it soften the flavor, but it actually makes the nutrients more available to the body than when kale is eaten raw.

Kale

Shopping Tips:

Choose leaves that are deep green and fresh with strong, not cracked or dry, stems. Small leaves are more tender than large ones. The sweetest kale is harvested after a frost or after it has "wintered over."

Storage Tips:

Unwashed leaves may be wrapped in a damp paper towel, placed in a plastic bag and stored in the crisper drawer of your refrigerator. The longer kale is kept, the more bitter it becomes.

Serving Suggestions:

Because kale has a strong flavor, start with small amounts as you and your family are developing a taste for it. Kale may be substituted for cabbage or spinach in most soups and casseroles.

Recipes Using:

- Beef Barley Soup
- Pepper-Corn Chili
- Grilled Chicken Kale-Carrot Soup

Kale & Potato Bake

S→T: 30 minutes (~15 minutes inactive)

2 cups ribbon-cut kale (loosely packed)
3/4 cup finely chopped onions (divided)
3 cups diced red potatoes (~1 lb.)
Salt, pepper, freshly grated nutmeg (as desired)
1 clove garlic, minced

Preheat oven—375°. **Oil** baking dish.

1. In saucepan, **simmer** kale, half of the onions and seasonings in about ½ cup water until tender and water is absorbed (about 20 min).
2. In another saucepan, **simmer** potatoes, remaining onions and seasonings in about ¼ cup of water for about 15 minutes, or until tender and water is absorbed. Coarsely **mash**.
3. **Stir** in kale and garlic. Transfer to baking dish. **Bake** for about 5 minute to heat through.

Yield: 4 servings

Optional Versions:

- Stir in 2 oz. low-fat shredded cheese (Monterey Jack, mild cheddar) with kale.
- Omit salt. Add diced nitrate-free ham and low-fat cheese with kale. Serve with a side salad.

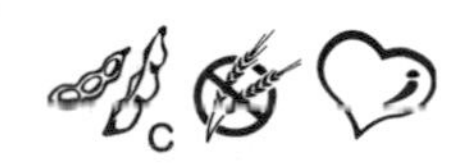

Kohlrabi

Shopping Tips:

Choose firm, small plants (tennis ball size) because they will be the most tender and flavorful. The leaves should be attached to the bulb and vibrant in color.

Storage Tips:

Kohlrabi can be stored for several weeks in the refrigerator and will be good as long as its leaves stay green.

Preparation Tips:

The tough outer edge of kohlrabi should be removed with a paring knife.

Fun Fact:

The name *kohlrabi* comes from the German words *kohl*, meaning "cabbage," and *rabi*, meaning "turnip." Indeed, kohlrabi looks a bit like a "cabbage turnip," though the taste is much closer to that of a "radish cucumber."

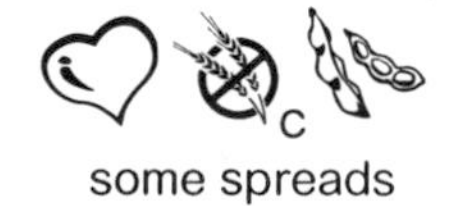

some spreads

Kohlrabi

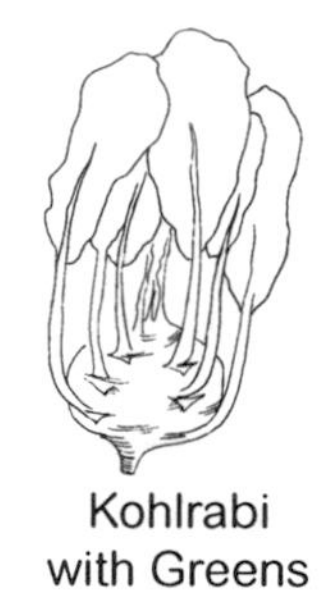
Kohlrabi with Greens

Another member of the cabbage family, kohlrabi comes in several varieties. There are both green and purple varieties. Much like a cross between a radish and a cucumber in taste, the young kohlrabi has a mildly sweet flavor and can be as juicy and crunchy as an apple.

Because of its ability to stabilize blood sugar, it is a good choice for those with hypoglycemia or diabetes. High in potassium and fiber, kohlrabi is a good low-cal choice for those afternoon munchies.

Serving Suggestions:

- Shred, grate or dice for salads (it absorbs flavors of dressings well, allowing you to use little salad dressing and still have the taste spread throughout the salad).
- Slice or julienne for munching or relish tray.
- Slice and spread with healthier choices of peanut butter (or other nut butters), dip (pp. 42, 79 and 149) or Hummus (p. 49) or top with a thin slice of low-fat cheese.
- Julienne and add a small amount to a stir-fry.
- Enjoy leaves steamed with onions (p. 64). Kohlrabi greens are a stronger, more pungent green so they are an acquired taste. Remove the center rib and ribbon-cut the leaves. Simmer the greens of one kohlrabi with a cup of onions and seasonings (salt, pepper and freshly grated nutmeg). Add a drizzle of balsamic vinegar about 15 minutes into simmer time and drizzle with flaxseed oil before serving.
- Some people lightly steam diced kohlrabi or add the diced vegetable to soups and stews. We recommend starting with small amounts in soups and stews and finding the balance that works best for you.

Leeks

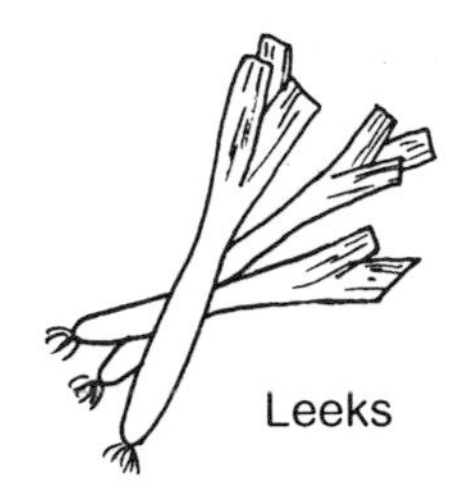

Related to garlic and onions, leeks contain many of the healthful properties of these two vegetables, though in lesser amounts. Leeks have a unique combination of nutrients that work together to stabilize blood sugar and can be influential in lowering cholesterol and easing the pain of arthritis.

Leeks have a milder, sweeter taste than onions, with a slight hint of garlic. They are perfect for dishes that have more delicate flavors because they are not overwhelming. At the same time, they are a great complement for stronger flavors, such as cabbage. Leeks are excellent when paired with potatoes or eggs and make a great addition to many soups.

Preparing Leeks:

Because leeks collect sand between their leaves, getting them clean can be a bit tricky. Here are some tips:

1. Remove wilted, dried or spongy portions. Rinse to remove surface dirt and sand.
2. Slice stalk down the middle lengthwise, stopping just short of the roots. Fanning the leaves apart with your fingers, run under cool water to remove dirt and sand.
3. Remove the roots. (Generally these are not used, though they are edible. If you choose to use the roots, wash them thoroughly in a bowl of water.)
4. Lay cut side down on cutting board. Slice at desired thickness, working from root end toward open end, using as much of the darker leaves as desired.
5. If desired, place slices in bowl of water. Any remaining sand will fall to the bottom. Drain.

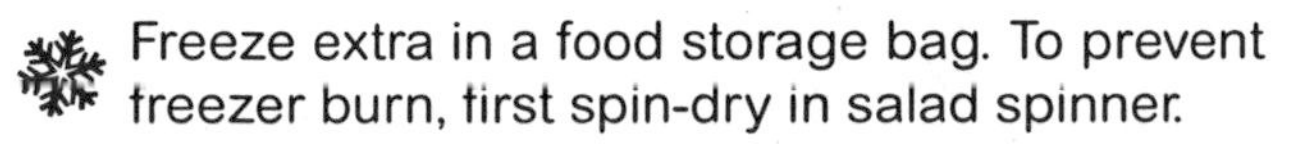
Freeze extra in a food storage bag. To prevent freezer burn, first spin-dry in salad spinner.

Leeks

Shopping Tips:

Look for green leaves and white stalks, firm and without blemish.

Storage Tips:

Leeks can be stored for up to two weeks in the refrigerator. Once chopped, they can also be frozen, ready to add to soups, casseroles and hot side dishes. (Frozen leeks do not work in salads.)

Recipes Using:

- Cabbage Patch Soup
- Breakfast Squares
- Sautéed Cabbage
- Breakfast Pizza

Just for Fun:

What is the one vegetable that you do not want in your boat? Answer: Leeks!

Many Uses

The entire stalk and all of the leaves can be chopped and used as you would onions or garlic.

---

1 medium leek =
~1 cup sliced leeks

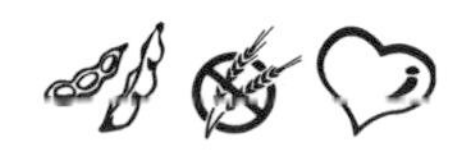

Lettuce and Salad Greens

Shopping Tips:

Choose lettuce and salad greens that are crisp and free of brown or slimy spots. Torn greens should be well sealed because they lose their nutritional value when exposed to air.

Serving Suggestions:

- Use as a garnish on hot and cold sandwiches.
- Consider a variety of salads (pp. 94–102).
- Add torn tender greens to scrambled eggs.
- Fill large leaves with any combination of foods to make a breadless wrap.

Fun Facts:

California is the "lettuce capital of the world."

Although lettuce is usually served cold in the United States, it is cooked in many Asian countries.

Salad Spinner

A salad spinner is helpful to wash and dry salad greens. One with a small basket inside is great for delicate foods (e.g., fresh herbs, berries).

Lettuce and Salad Greens

Hundreds of varieties of lettuce and salad greens are used in numerous ways the world over. They add flavorful nutrition to any side salad. Usually high in fiber, these low-cal leafy greens are chock-full of nutrients. The various shades and pigments of leafy greens indicate a variety of phytonutrients and other vitamins and minerals — generally the darker the color, the more the nutrients. These leafy greens aid digestion and increase liver health, and they lower the risk of heart and eye disease, cancer and stroke. For a delightful variety of texture, color and flavor, as well as a spectrum of nutrients, select a variety of salad greens for your table.

There are three basic types of lettuce:

- **Head** lettuce includes crisphead (e.g., iceberg) and butterhead (e.g., Boston and Bibb) varieties
- **Leaf** lettuce includes red and green leaf varieties
- **Romaine** or "cos" lettuce (full of nutrition; commonly used in Caesar salads)

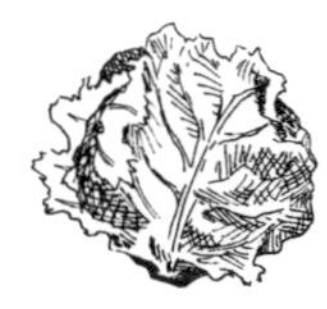

Iceberg Lettuce

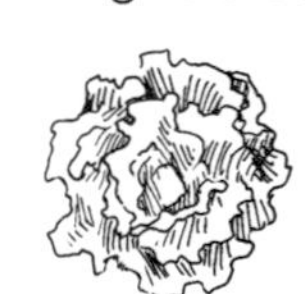

Leaf Lettuce

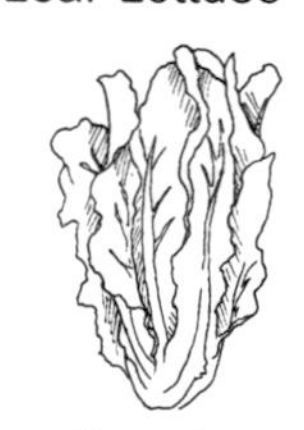

Romaine

In addition to lettuce, there are a variety of other salad greens to enjoy. In fact, many are packaged along with lettuce in the bagged salads available in most grocery stores. Some of the more common greens include:

- **Arugula** (p. 44)
- **Endive, Radiccio and Escarole** – all varieties of chicory. Since they have a rather sharp taste (slightly bitter, almost spicy), these greens are most often enjoyed when mixed with other, lighter greens and/or combined with fruit such as pear or apple.
- **Herbs** – several herbs, such as parsley and basil, make a nice accent to side salads.

- **Mustard greens** – taken from the same plant that produces the seeds used to make Dijon mustard, these leaves are bursting with nutrients and add a delightfully subtle kick to many dishes, hot and cold. Consider them for side salads or as a garnish for sandwiches. They are also great added to scrambled eggs.
- **Spinach** (p. 79)
- **Watercress** – the somewhat peppery taste of this ancient leaf vegetable complements strong flavors such as onion, ginger, garlic and chili in both hot and cold dishes. It perks up mild dishes such as rice and pasta, is great in pesto (p. 93) and is a nice, crunchy accent to any side salad. Amazingly, this simple leaf, gram for gram, has more vitamin C than an orange, more calcium than milk and more iron than spinach.

Europeans mix greens so regularly that they have special words to describe different types of mixtures. From the French word *mesclumo*, we derive the popular mesclun mix. This mix can be made in a variety of ways but generally combines four basic flavors:

- Mild (e.g., leaf lettuce)
- Bitter/tart (e.g., radicchio, escarole, endive)
- Piquant (e.g., mustard greens)
- Peppery/spicy (e.g., arugula, watercress)

Side Salad

For a simple side salad, take a mixture of greens and serve with a drizzle of flavorful dressing (pp. 44, 47, 70, 97 and 99). For variety, add a vegetable (e.g., sliced avocado, matchstick carrots, diced pepper), a fruit (e.g., apple, blueberries) or a sprinkle of nuts or seeds. This provides varying textures and tastes and increases the nutritional value of your meal — an opportunity too good to pass up!

Lettuce and Salad Greens
(continued)

Storage Tips:

Romaine and leaf lettuces can be washed and dried before storing.

Greens and lettuce varieties do best if stored in a plastic bag or container, preferably in the crisper drawer.

For greens that are sold with their roots (e.g., watercress, mustard greens), wrap the roots in a damp paper towel and place in a plastic bag or container.

Greens and lettuce should be stored away from fruits, such as bananas, apples and pears, that give off ethylene gas as they ripen (this causes brown spots on the leaves).

Finding Greens

Though many salad greens may sound "exotic," they are found in almost any grocery store, often bagged with a variety inside. Choose a new one each week.

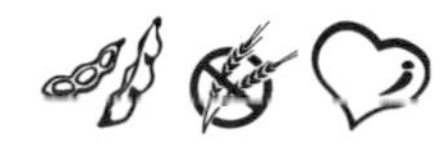

5-Minute, Full-of-Flavor, Healthy Salad Dressings

Never the need to buy a bottled version again!

In an effort to reduce fat in bottled salad dressings, many manufacturers add corn syrup, artificial flavorings and an abundance of salt in an attempt to increase the flavor lost when removing the fat. We choose to find flavor in the olive oil along with the combination of natural ingredients and seasonings, using only a light sprinkle of salt, if any. While this increases the fat content (the better monounsaturated fat), the robust flavor allows for the use of less salad dressing. So how about taking five minutes and whip up a delicious, low-sodium, healthy salad dressing. *(See pp. 44, 47, 97 and 99 for more recipes.)*

Portions

Most salad dressing bottles list two tablespoons for a serving. If this much dressing is used, the primary taste that comes through is the dressing. Drizzling dressings on your salad (instead of pouring) enhances the flavor of the salad without masking it and keeps the fat intake to a minimum. We recommend trying only two teaspoons of our low-sodium, full-of-flavor salad dressing on a side salad (about 1½ cups of salad).

Xanthan Gum

Xanthan gum is a fermented sugar derived from corn that is used to give body to a liquid without affecting taste. It is also used to add volume and viscosity to gluten-free baked goods.

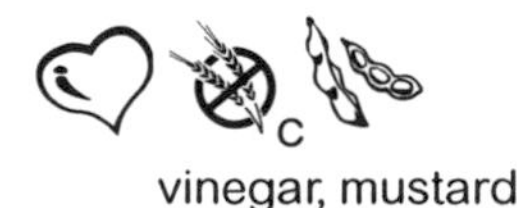

vinegar, mustard

Balsamic Vinaigrette Dressing

Mix: 5 minutes

1 Tbsp. balsamic vinegar
1 Tbsp. raw apple cider vinegar
1 Tbsp. sweetener—agave nectar or honey
1/4 cup water
1 tsp. garlic powder
1/4 tsp. onion powder
1/2 tsp. dried basil (optional)
1/2 tsp. dried oregano (optional)
1 tsp. Dijon-style mustard
3–4 pinches xanthan gum (optional, see sidebar)
1/4 cup olive oil

In bowl, **combine** all ingredients except oil, crushing basil and oregano with your fingers. **Whisk** while streaming in oil. Continue to whisk until opaque. Lightly **season** with salt and pepper.

Drizzle over mixed salad greens just before serving.

Store in refrigerator for 2–3 weeks. Empty glass jars/bottles (e.g., purchased salad dressing bottles, spice jars) make excellent containers. Allow leftover to come to room temperature before serving.

Yield: ~15 (2 tsp.) servings

Analysis/Serving (2 tsp.):
Calories: 37 (Fat Cal 32) Fat: 3.7g (0.5g Sat) Cholesterol: 0mg
Sodium: 13mg Carbs: 1.4g (0g Fiber 1.9g Sugar) Protein: 0g

Okra

Commonly used in the southern United States for gumbos and soups, okra is not well known in the North. A native of northern Africa, okra contains a surprising amount of fiber (two grams per half cup cooked) as well as good amounts of potassium, calcium and several vitamins.

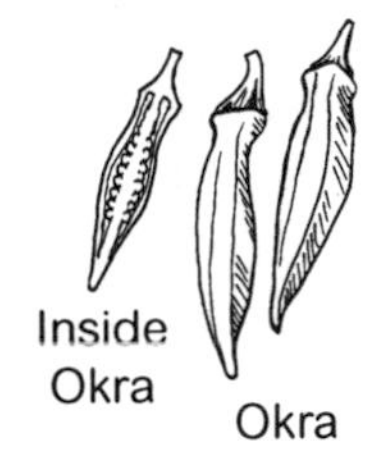

Pan-Fried Okra

S→T: 15 minutes

Because of its slimy texture, many people do not think they like okra unless it is deep-fat fried. Well, no more! This recipe adds great flavor without the slime. It also reduces the empty calories found in deep-fat fried foods.

~ 20 (3 inch) okra
1 Tbsp. High-Heat oil
1 Tbsp. butter

1. If using electric range, **preheat burner** on medium for about 8 minutes.
2. *Meanwhile*, remove ends; **slice** okra ¼ inch.
3. Place noncoated stainless steel skillet on hot burner. **Add** oil and butter and heat to melt butter. Add okra, lightly season with salt and pepper and **sauté** for about 5–8 minutes, or until golden brown and slightly crispy, stirring occasionally.

Transfer to a paper-towel-lined bowl to drain excess oil.
Serve immediately.

Yield: 2 servings

Okra

Shopping Tips:

Quality taste starts with tender fresh-picked okra, so we recommend purchasing okra at your local farmer's market or ask your CSA (see p. 29) to offer okra. Choose bright-green, two- to three-inch-long okra without black spots (a sign of spoiling).

Storage Tips:

Store okra in the refrigerator and use within a few days of harvesting. Whole okra (stem removed but cap intact) can be blanched and frozen.

Serving Suggestions:

The slime from okra provides a natural thickener for soups and stews. If the texture is unappealing, puree cooked okra before adding to soups.

Steam, sauté, bake or eat okra raw.

More Facts:

As okra spread around the world, it became known as gumbo in the southern states and West Indies. In some places it is known as *Lady Fingers*.

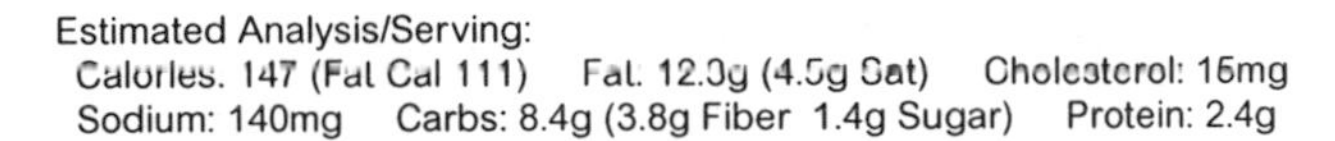
Estimated Analysis/Serving:
Calories: 147 (Fat Cal 111) Fat: 12.3g (4.5g Sat) Cholesterol: 15mg
Sodium: 140mg Carbs: 8.4g (3.8g Fiber 1.4g Sugar) Protein: 2.4g

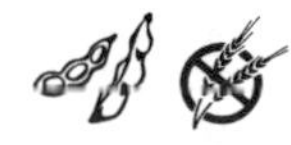

Onions, Scallions and Shallots

Shopping Tips:

Onions and shallots should be clean and firm, with no soft spots or indication of mold. The skins should be dry and crisp and the necks should be closed, not broken or open.

Scallions should be crisp and firm, with a white bulb and deep, green leaves.

Storage Tips:

Onions do best when stored at room temperature with good ventilation (such as in a wire basket). Do not store with potatoes since they absorb the moisture from potatoes and spoil more quickly.

Once cut, onions should be kept in the refrigerator. The nutritional value of a cut onion deteriorates quickly after a day or two.

Some Recipes Using Onions:

- Caramelized Soups
- Venison Teriyaki
- Black Bean Soup
- Slow Cooker Pork

Caramelized Onions

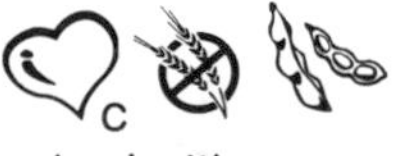

paired with

Onions, Green Onions (Scallions) and Shallots

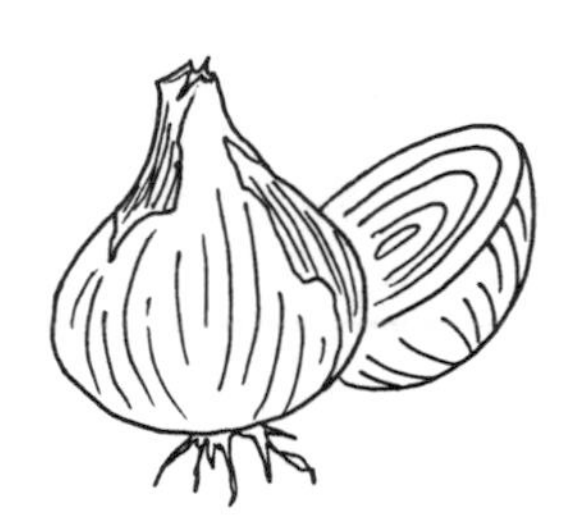

Onion (whole/cut)

Onions *are a low-calorie, tasty and healthy way to add flavor to almost any dish. There are many varieties of onions; the sweeter ones have a higher sugar content.*

The onion is an antibiotic, antifungal and antiviral agent. It also has anti-inflammatory and anticancer properties, and because of its high sulfur content, it is useful in eliminating heavy metals and parasites. It also lowers cholesterol.

Caramelized Onions

S→T: ~30 minutes (20–25 minutes mostly inactive)

1 Tbsp. Medium-Heat oil
2 lg. onions, thinly sliced (~4 cups)
Salt and freshly ground black pepper, to taste

In skillet, **sauté** onions in oil for 25 minutes, or until golden brown. **Season**. **Stir** occasionally, adding water to prevent onions from sticking to pan or burning (see "Water Stir-Fry" on p. 61.)

Yield: 4 servings 1 cup

Caramelized Onion Dinner

S→T: ~35 minutes (if Marinara Sauce is prepared in advance)

1 Tbsp. Medium-Heat oil (divided)
1 lg. onion, thinly sliced (~2 cups)
Salt and freshly ground black pepper, to taste
8 oz. boneless, skinless chicken/turkey breast/tenders (cut into strips)
2 cloves garlic, minced (divided)
2 lg. bell peppers (green/red or yellow)
or 1 (10 oz.) pkg. tri-color frozen peppers
1 cup Marinara Sauce (p. 90)
2 oz. whole-grain pasta (cooked al dente)

continue ...

Preheat cast-iron skillet (can use stainless steel but may require more oil).

1. In large skillet, season and **sauté** onions in half the amount of oil over medium heat for about 20 minutes. Stir occasionally, adding water as needed to prevent onions from sticking to pan or burning (see "Water Stir-Fry", p. 61).
2. Slide onions to side of skillet. Drizzle remaining oil on empty side. Add poultry strips and half of the garlic; season. **Sauté** poultry (continuing to caramelize onions) for 5 minutes. Stir often and add water as needed. Add and **sauté** peppers, stirring all food together when meat is done and onions are golden. Add rest of garlic during last 30 seconds. If desired, drizzle with olive or flavored oil.

Layer pasta (lightly seasoned with salt), stir-fry and Marinara Sauce.

Yield: 2 meal servings

Green Onions *(also called scallions) are the immature onion and have most of the same nutritional benefits, though they are richer in some vitamins and minerals. They are a great digestive aid and make foods with a high fat content more digestible. Use from green tip to root.*

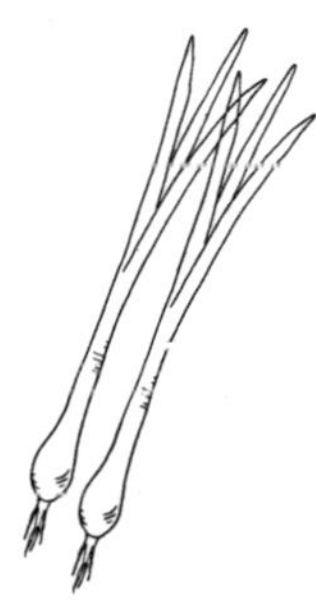
2 Scallions

Shallots *are a milder, sweeter member of the onion family. When cooked, they become thick and creamy. They flavor oil well and are a nice addition to salad dressings. One shallot bulb has two halves.*

Shallots with and without stem

Onions, Scallions and Shallots (continued)

Serving Suggestions:

- Use raw as a garnish on spicy soups or tacos.
- Chunk and place under meat in slow cooker to provide flavor and a natural place for fat to drain away from meat.
- Thinly slice (especially red) for salads, sandwiches and on pizza

Powerful Onions

The more pungent the onion, the more nutrients.

Sweet Onions

Sweeter onions are best when used raw or lightly cooked. (Their sugars often mask the flavors you want to feature in "hearty" soups and casseroles.)

Recipes Using Green Onions:

- Confetti Dip
- Spinach Dip

Recipes Using Shallots:

- Fancy Scrambled Eggs
- Meal-in-a-Salad
- Salmon & Pasta

Analysis/Serving: Caramelized Onions/Estimate for Dinner
Calories: 76/417 (Fat Cal 31/111) Fat: 3.4/12.3g (0.6/2g Sat) Cholesterol: 0/42mg
Sodium: 77/521 Carbs: 11/46g (2/9g Fiber 5/12g Sugar) Protein: 1/30g

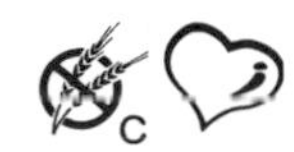

Peas

Shopping Tips:

Purchase peas in pods that are firm and crisp. The garden pea should not have much "rattling room" inside.

While both canned and frozen peas have added sodium, the nutrients and flavor of frozen peas are superior.

Storage Tips:

Peas are best enjoyed the day they are picked, before the sugars convert to starch. They should be refrigerated even in the store. Peas protected by a pod stay sweet longer.

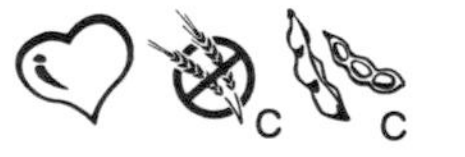

GF - vinegar, mustard

Peas

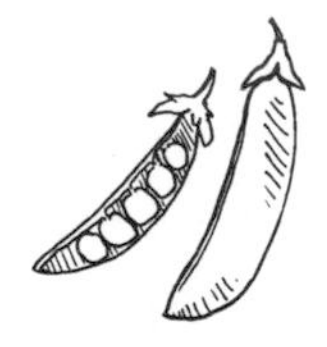

Sweet Pea

Peas are a wonderful source of nutrition. They have fiber, protein and several vitamins and minerals, including many of the B vitamins, iron and vitamin C. These nutrients work together to provide energy, making a handful of peas a great pick-me-up snack!

Pea & Celery Salad

1 (10 oz.) pkg. frozen garden peas, thawed
1/4 cup minced red onion
4 ribs celery, diced (2 cups)
1/2 tsp. Dijon-style mustard
1/2 cup Arugula Pesto Salad Dressing (p. 44)

Toss together peas, onion and celery. **Stir** mustard into arugula dressing; **add** to vegetables and stir.

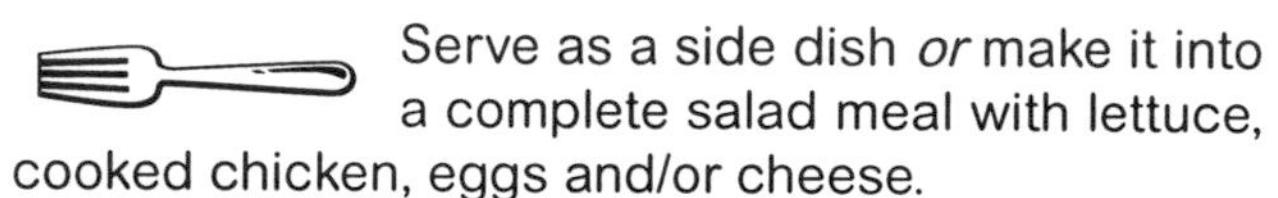

Serve as a side dish *or* make it into a complete salad meal with lettuce, cooked chicken, eggs and/or cheese.

Yield: 4 side salads   4 cups

Analysis/Serving:
Calories: 129 (Fat Cal 61)   Fat: 6.8g (1g Sat)   Cholesterol: 0mg
Sodium: 140   Carbs: 12g (4g Fiber 6g Sugar)   Protein: 3.8g

Peppers — Hot (Chili)

Instead of just being a lot of hot spice, hot peppers can add flavor and definition to meals. There are many varieties, including red chilies, chipotles, jalapeños, carrot chilies, Anaheim, ancho and cayenne peppers. They are a rich source of vitamins and minerals, but it is their amount of capsicum that determines both the intensity of their heat and the strength of their health benefits.

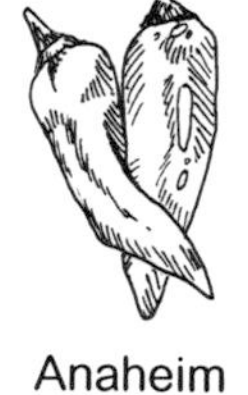

Anaheim
(hot pepper)

Benefits: Capsicum is good for heart health, easing congestion, reducing inflammation, reducing pain and – contrary to popular belief – preventing ulcers. Most of the capsicum is in the seeds and membranes of peppers, but even peppers from the same plant can vary in their level of heat.

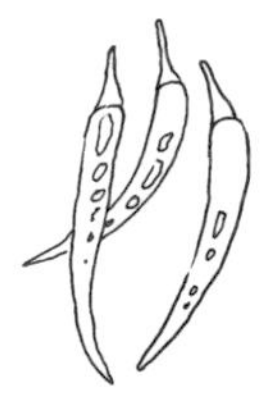

Cayenne
(hot pepper)

Using: For a milder taste, remove seeds. However, this reduces the health benefits. The flavor of peppers often reduces the need for sodium and sugar. Many enjoy using sour cream to "cool down" the heat of a peppery dish. A glass of milk can do the same. It is the casein protein (from milk) that counteracts the heat of the capsicum.

Handling Hot Peppers: The capsicum can cause a burning sensation on skin and in eyes. Wash hands, cutting board and knife after handling, and avoid touching your eyes. Many wear plastic gloves during preparation.

Peppers — Sweet

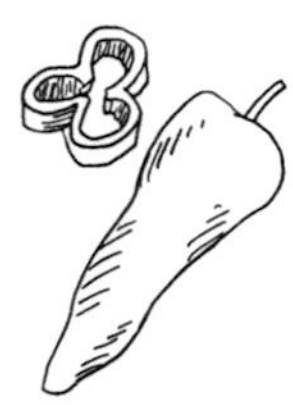
Cubanelle Sweet Pepper

Abundantly rich in nutrients, sweet peppers are an extremely healthy food and come in a variety of colors. Generally the lighter the color, the milder the taste. This is true of the mild Cubanelle/Italianelle, our favorite pepper for stuffing. The red bell is the most flavorful and the most nutritious.

Stuffed Peppers

Peppers can be stuffed with almost anything and served as the main course or as a side dish. Below are two easy stuffing ideas.

- Mix together leftover Quinoa Pilaf (p. 179) with shredded cheese.
- Sauté some chopped onions and celery in a small amount of oil until tender. Add some minced fresh thyme, rosemary and garlic toward the end of sautéing time. Combine with cooked brown rice, leftover chunks of Scarborough Fair Turkey Breast (p. 162) and shredded cheese.

Preheat oven—375°. Baking sheet with sides.

Cut Cubanelle/green bell peppers in half lengthwise, remove seeds and **steam** for 5–7 minutes, or until almost tender. Cool in bowl of room temperature water long enough to handle. Drain. **Fill** with a stuffing mixture. Place stuffed-edge up on a baking sheet. **Bake** 10–15 minutes, or until 160° internal temperature.

Peppers Sweet & Hot

Shopping Tips:

Choose peppers with glossy, tight skins, deep, vibrant color and no wrinkles or black spots.

Storage Tips:

Peppers are best stored in a crisper drawer, wrapped in a paper bag or towel. (Plastic may cause moisture, speeding spoilage.)

Hot whole peppers can be frozen. Remove just before using; they are easier to mince when slightly frozen.

Sliced bell peppers can be frozen without blanching.

Vitamin C

One cup of red bell pepper slices contains 175 mg. of vitamin C. That's two and a half times the amount found in a whole orange!

Simmer Them Whole

Hot peppers can be simmered whole in dishes. Their rich flavor comes through without the heat (e.g., 100).

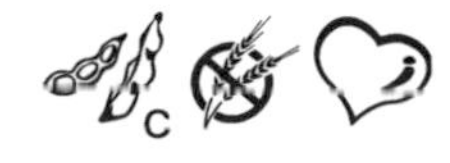

Potato

Shopping Tips:

Potatoes should be firm, free of decay, without sprouts and without greenish tint (may indicate the presence of toxins).[14]

Storage Tips:

Store potatoes in a cool, dark place (e.g., sack), away from onions. Storing potatoes below 33°F (e.g., in the fridge) causes their starches to turn to sugar. Some say that returning them to reasonable temperatures will allow their sugars to revert back to starch. Exposure to sunlight causes toxins to form.

Recipes Using:

- Topped Baked Potato
- Kale/Chard Potato Bake
- Cabbage Patch Soup

Keep the Peel!

Potato with the peel has twice as much fiber as potato without the peel. (**Safety Note**: Nonorganic potatoes may have chemical residues, so do not eat their peels. Organic vegetables should be scrubbed thoroughly to remove any possible bacteria.)

Potato

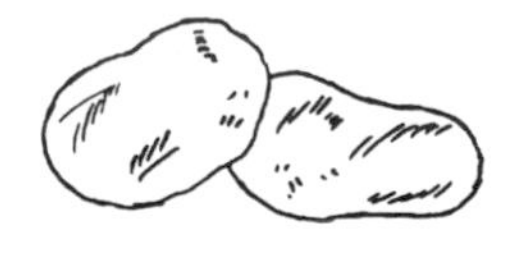

Potatoes have a reputation for being starchy and high in carbs. However, scientists are uncovering new information about their nutritional value. The number of phytonutrients and antioxidants known to exist in potatoes is growing daily, including some nutrients that are rarely found in other plants.

So do away with trans fats found in many fried varieties (chips, fries) and limit fatty additions to baked potatoes and casseroles (sour cream, cheese, bacon). Use sodium in moderation, and count your carbs as needed. But don't be afraid to try a variety of flavorful ways to serve this easy complement to many meals. Potatoes can be a healthy part of your diet!

Oven Fries

Prep: ~5 minutes Bake: 20–25 minutes.

Enjoy creating your own personal flavor. Some ideas include chili powder and crushed red pepper, Italian seasonings with a garnish of Parmesan cheese (add after baking) and our favorite: garlic powder and fresh or dried thyme.

1 1/2 lb. russet or fingerling potatoes
(cut into 1/2-inch fry wedges)
4 tsp. High-Heat oil
Salt, pepper and other seasonings (see above)

Preheat oven: 425°/450° (convection/conventional).
Baking pan (stainless steel or preheated cast iron).

1. Spread potatoes in a single layer on baking pan. **Drizzle** evenly with oil. Sprinkle with seasonings. Using your hands, **toss** to coat.
2. **Bake** for 20–25 minutes, or until as crispy as you desire, stir about 15 minutes into baking.

Yield: 4 servings

Estimated Analysis/Serving:
Calories: 165 (Fat Cal 41) Fat: 4.6g (0.4g Sat) Cholesterol: 0mg
Sodium: 143mg Carbs: 30g (2.3g Fiber 1.1g Sugar) Protein: 3.4g

Encouraging Children

By the time many children reach toddlerhood, they've developed preferences and opinions about food. New textures, tastes and smells are often not attractive to them. Introducing new flavors takes time, patience and creativity. Here are some ideas.

Try, Try Again: It often takes several tries before we decide if we like something. If your child doesn't care for a food, try it again another time. Or try cooking it in a different way or pairing it with another food. (Dorie doesn't usually care for sweet potatoes, but she enjoys them with pork or sausage.)

Take Advantage of the Moment: Often kids express an interest in something they see. "What's that, Mommy?" Seize the moment and say, "Let's get some and try it out." A young child might show interest in what the "big people" are eating. If it's safe and appropriate, serve some to the child.

Model Enthusiasm: When you're excited about something, your kids notice. Even if they don't agree that the food tastes good, they know that someone likes it and maybe one day they will too.

Take Things in Stride: When food becomes an emotional ordeal, everyone suffers. Most children have phases when they are picky – some more so than others. Help them make good choices within their parameters and encourage them to keep trying new things.

Talk About How to Make Good Choices: Discuss with your children how you make some of your choices – it will help them to accept the choices more readily, and it models the process for them. Dorie's seven-year-old son surprised her one day after a birthday party by saying, "Mommy, can I please have some cheese? I had a lot of sugar and now I really need some protein!"

Keep Kids Involved: Ask kids to help with menu planning, grocery shopping, gardening, preparing and serving food. Dorie's kids enjoy having their own small shopping list at the store – especially if they helped to create it!

Little Chefs

Origin of Foods Game

Hang a world map near your dinner table. On occasion, choose a fruit, vegetable, herb or spice and find out its country of origin. Children can then write it on the map.

Here is one to start: Basil is native to India.

A Meal Planning Game

List favorite family foods according to food groups. Then make a game out of creating healthy meals by selecting foods from each group. Choose some created meals to actually prepare. (See our websites, p. 242, for links to guides on meal planning.)

Garden Fun

An herb garden is a great way for the whole family to be involved in food preparation. Basil is an easy one to start with — it grows quickly, is easy to pick, will last all summer and even keeps away mosquitoes!

Radishes

Shopping Tips:

Bulbs should be firm with bright color and few blemishes. Leaves are not long but should be bright and fresh.

Storage Tips:

Store leaves separately from the root. Both parts may be stored in plastic bags in the refrigerator. Leaves will last for a day or two; the roots will last longer.

Serving Suggestions:

- Include on a relish tray.
- Slice, dice or shred and use to spice up salads.
- Chop and stir in to dips (e.g., Confetti Dip, p. 42).
- Add to stir-fries and soups. Also, for added nutrition, include the green leaves when fresh and available.

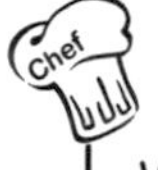

Make Them Crisp

Want to crisp up your radishes? Soak in ice water for about an hour before serving.

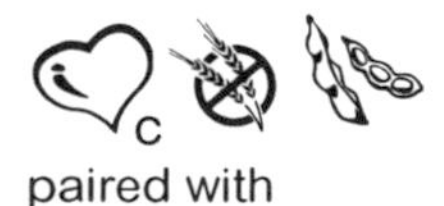

paired with

Radishes

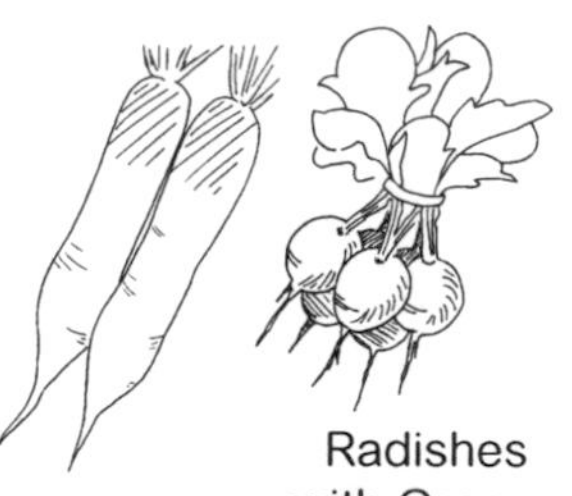

Daikons without tops

Radishes with Greens

The radish has a distinctive peppery flavor that sweetens when cooked. It provides an easy way to liven up the color and flavor of salads and veggie trays. There are many varieties. Daikon radishes are a pearly white root that can be as long as your arm.

Veggie Burgers

Mix: 15 minutes

2 eggs, slightly beaten
1/4 tsp. salt
1/3 cup walnuts (chop while shredding veggies)
1/4 cup flaxseed meal
1 cup cooked brown rice
1/2 small red onion, shredded
4 cups shredded vegetables Sondra uses:
2 ribs celery, 3 med. carrots, 1 med, green bell pepper and 1 small daikon radish (or a few red)
6 Tbsp. soy protein isolate (p. 89)

Preheat griddle to slightly cooler than when water dances when sprinkled on surface.

1. In bowl, **combine** all ingredients except soy protein together. **Sprinkle** soy protein evenly over mixture and **stir** to combine.
2. Lightly **oil** preheated griddle. **Dip** mixture onto griddle. Flatten and shape into 4-inch patties. **Cook** 3–4 minutes on each side, or until golden brown and vegetables are tender.

Serve as sandwich on whole grain bun. Complement meal with fruit.

Freeze extra. Great quick meals for singles.

Yield: 8 (4-inch) burgers 4 servings

Analysis/Serving:
Calories: 273 (Fat Cal 114) Fat: 12.7g (1.4g Sat) Cholesterol: 106mg
Sodium: 399mg Carbs: 21.5g (5.6g Fiber 3.9g Sugar) Protein: 20.6g

Spinach

A Bunch of Spinach

A tasty addition to salads, sandwiches, soups and casseroles, spinach can be enjoyed raw or cooked. Because it easily absorbs flavors and spices, it enhances many dishes with more than its own flavor. It is rich in many phytonutrients, including thirteen flavonoids. It also contains some iron. Winter spinach has a stronger taste than spinach grown in the summer months.

Spinach Dip

S→T: 5 minutes (after thawing) + chilling time

1/2 (10 oz.) pkg. frozen chopped spinach
2 green onions (scallions)**, sliced**
1 lg. or 2 small cloves garlic, crushed
1/8 tsp. salt
8 oz. Neufchâtel cheese (sidebar on p. 42)
OR 1 cup low-fat sour cream

Thaw and drain spinach. **Press** water out in colander (or squeeze out in towel). In small food processor, finely **chop** onion and garlic. **Blend** in salt, Neufchâtel cheese (or sour cream) and spinach.

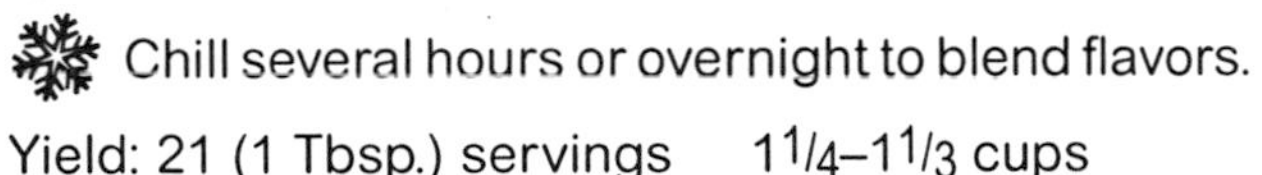
Chill several hours or overnight to blend flavors.

Yield: 21 (1 Tbsp.) servings 1 1/4–1 1/3 cups

Dividing Frozen Spinach

- **For Box:** Cut in half on cutting board with a sharp knife.
- **For Bag:** Squeeze bag in center to break apart the portion you need.
- Wrap unused portion and store in freezer.

Spinach

Shopping Tips:

Choose spinach with crisp, green leaves. It has the best flavor in the spring and fall. Spinach that is slimy or bruised has begun to decay.

Storage Tips:

Wrap loosely and store in a plastic bag in refrigerator. Do not wash before storing because it will spoil quickly.

Serving Suggestions:

- Use as salad greens.
- Ribbon-cut or use frozen chopped for a beautiful addition to soups, stews and casseroles.

Easy to Hide

Spinach virtually disappears in casseroles, thus increasing nutrition without turning away those who don't like vegetables.

Recipes Using:

- Hamburger Soup
- Wilted Spinach Salad
- Fancy Scrambled Eggs
- Southwestern Casserole
- Shepherd's Pie Makeover

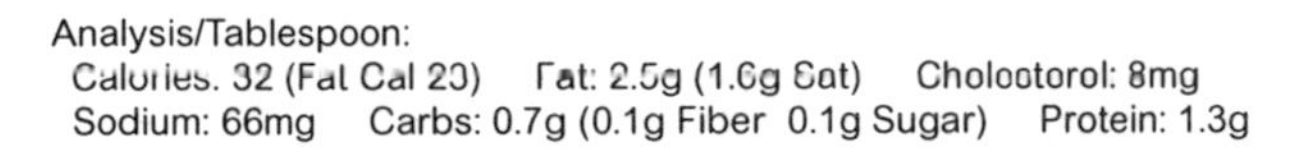
Analysis/Tablespoon:
Calories: 32 (Fat Cal 23) Fat: 2.5g (1.6g Sat) Cholesterol: 8mg
Sodium: 66mg Carbs: 0.7g (0.1g Fiber 0.1g Sugar) Protein: 1.3g

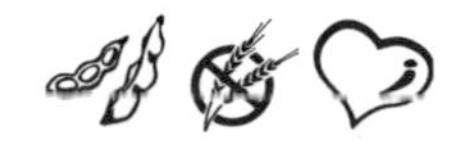

Squash Summer Varieties

Shopping Tips:

The most flavorful summer squash is small to medium in size. It should be glossy and heavy for its size.

Storage Tips:

Protect summer squash since it is easily bruised and punctured. It will keep for about a week if refrigerated in a plastic bag. May be blanched and frozen.

Recipes Using:

- Beef Barley Soup
- Chunky Garden Spaghetti Sauce
- 20-Minute Stir-Fry Dinner

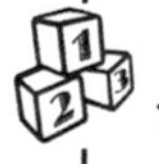

Seasoning Blends for Squash Side Dish

Parsley Blend
1/2 tsp. dried parsley
1/4 tsp. garlic powder
1/4 tsp. paprika

Italian Blend
1 tsp. dried oregano
1/2 tsp. dried basil
1/4 tsp. garlic powder
1 pinch crushed red pepper

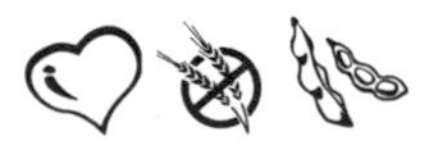

Squash—Summer Varieties

A wonderful addition to summer's bounty, there are many varieties of summer squash. Zucchini, crookneck and straightneck are three of the most popular; pattypan is our personal favorite. All summer squash has mild flesh that can be eaten along with the peel and seeds. The skin is fragile, so, unlike winter squash, summer squash cannot be stored for a long time.

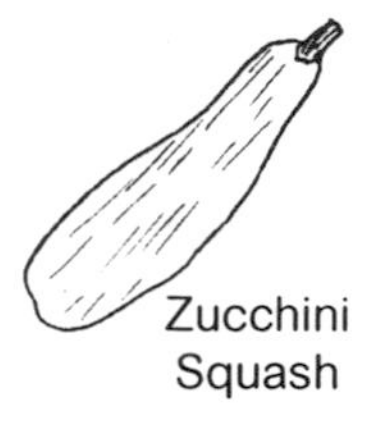

Zucchini Squash

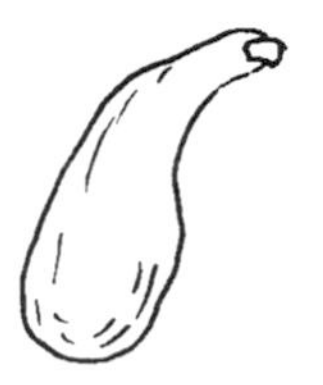

Crookneck Squash

With a strong showing of phytonutrients, summer squash is a healthy addition to any meal or snack. It is much more flavorful when just picked.

Seasoned Squash Side

S→T: 12 minutes

Seasoning (see sidebar for 2 suggested blends)
Salt and pepper as desired
1 tsp. High-Heat oil
2 cups sliced summer squash
(pattypan, yellow or zucchini)
2 Tbsp. minced red onion
1 Tbsp. raw sunflower seeds

1. In bowl, **combine** your choice of seasoning blend (see sidebar), salt, pepper and oil. **Add** squash and onions. **Toss** to coat. (If desired, prepare earlier in the day, cover and refrigerate so the flavors marry.)
2. In preheated skillet, **sauté** for 5 minutes to sear the squash on almost all sides, stirring regularly. Add sunflower seeds during last few minutes.

Yield: 2 servings (4 vegetable servings)

Analysis/Serving:
Calories: 70 (Fat Cal 44) Fat: 4.9g (0.6g Sat) Cholesterol: 0mg
Sodium: 78mg Carbs: 5.8g (2g Fiber 2.6g Sugar) Protein: 2.6g

Preparing Patty Pan Squash:
Cut squash into fourths, remove core and slice or dice.

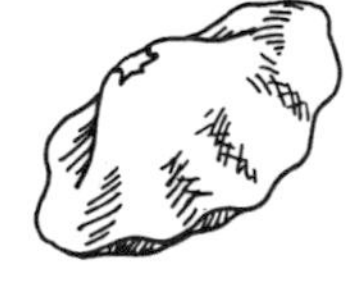
Pattypan Squash

Seasoned Squash Dinner

S→T: 30-minute meal

1 Tbsp. Medium-Heat oil
1/8 tsp. salt
Seasonings (see sidebar)
6 cups sliced squash
 (pattypan or yellow)
1 lg. onion, sliced (2 cups)
2 med. green peppers, sliced (2 cups)
2 (or more) **cloves garlic, minced**
2 cups Bean-Corn Salsa (p. 91)
 OR Marinara Sauce (p. 90)
4–6 oz. shredded cheese (see sidebar)

1. In large bowl, **combine** oil, salt and dried seasonings (see sidebar), holding fresh basil, cilantro or parsley. **Add** squash, onions and peppers. **Stir** to coat vegetables with spices. (May marinate a couple hours or overnight.)
2. In large skillet, **sauté** vegetables 5–10 minutes, stirring often. **Stir** in garlic and half of the fresh basil, cilantro or parsley (if using) during the last few minutes.
3. **Add** salsa or marinara sauce, cover and simmer 5–10 minutes. Remove from heat and **top** with cheese and remaining fresh herbs. Cover and allow to **set** for 5 minutes.

If desired, serve dinner with Grilled Chicken Rub (p. 145) or Seared Tofu (p. 158) using less cheese.

Yield: 4 meal servings or many side servings

Squash Summer Varieties
(continued)

Serving suggestions:

- Slice/dice for salads.
- Cut into sticks for fun finger food.
- Use for stuffings and bread.
- Add to stir-fry, pasta or spaghetti sauce.
- Excellent when sautéed.
- Large squash will gain flavor as it is cooked.

Squash Dinner Seasonings and Cheese Ideas

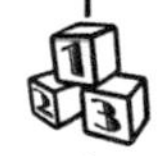

With Bean-Corn Salsa:

1 1/2 tsp. chili powder
1 tsp. ground cumin
1 handful fresh cilantro (or parsley), minced
Monterey Jack cheese

With Marinara Sauce:

2 tsp. dried oregano
1 tsp. dried basil (or use fresh ribbon cut)
1/4 tsp. crushed red pepper
Mozzarella cheese
Serve over al dente whole-grain pasta.

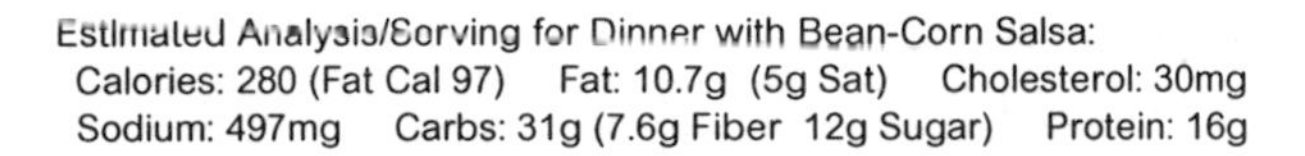
Estimated Analysis/Serving for Dinner with Bean-Corn Salsa:
Calories: 280 (Fat Cal 97) Fat: 10.7g (5g Sat) Cholesterol: 30mg
Sodium: 497mg Carbs: 31g (7.6g Fiber 12g Sugar) Protein: 16g

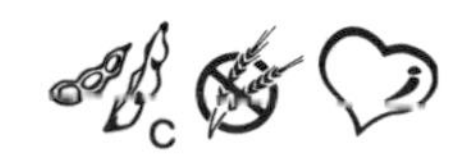

Squash—Winter Varieties

Winter squashes come in many shapes and sizes. Harvested at the end of the growing season, their tough skin will protect them for long periods of storage – some will keep for up to six months! They contain several phytonutrients, have high amounts of vitamin A and are a good source of omega-3 fatty acids as well as other vitamins and minerals.

Acorn, butternut, pumpkin and spaghetti squash are featured on the next five pages..

Acorn Squash

With green and orange skin, acorn squash makes a beautiful centerpiece before it is cooked. The yellow flesh has a slightly sweet and somewhat nutty flavor.

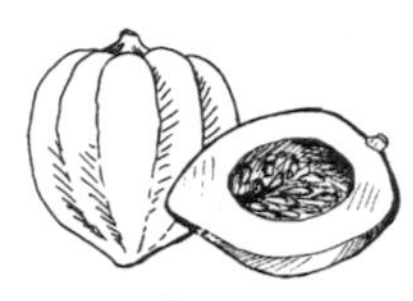

Acorn Whole/Half

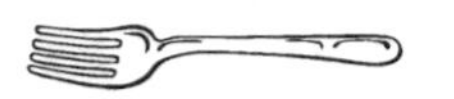

Complement the meal with green beans; the flavors go together really well.

Fancy Twists

A Natural "Bowl": When scooping out the squash, leave some squash inside the shell (~¼ inch) so the shell remains intact. Then fill shells with sausage and squash mixture. Bake for 10–15 minutes. Place filled shells directly on serving plates.

Fancy Flowers: Undercook squash slightly, slice horizontally into flower-shaped rings and fill the center of rings with sausage mixture. Bake 15–20 minutes, or until squash is tender.

Acorn Squash & Sausage Bake

S→T: 1 hour

2 (1 lb.) acorn squash
12 oz. ground chicken/turkey sausage, hot or sweet (p. 232)
1½ cups chopped onion

Preheat oven—400°, then 325°. 8x8 baking dish.

1. Place whole squashes in baking pan. **Roast** for about 30 minutes, or until squash gives a bit when gently pushed with the thumb.
2. *Meanwhile,* in skillet, **sauté** onions with sausage, stirring regularly.
3. When squash is done, remove from oven, cool slightly and lower oven temperature. Cut squash in half (vertically), remove seeds and **scoop** flesh into skillet. (If squash is stringy or dry, first blend with an immersion blender until creamy and smooth.) **Stir** to combine with sausage and onion mixture.
4. **Transfer** to baking dish. **Bake** 10–15 minutes.

Yield: 4 servings

Analysis/Serving:
Calories: 197 (Fat Cal 62) Fat: 6.9g (1.7g Sat) Cholesterol: 65mg
Sodium: 506mg Carbs: 18.8g (5g Fiber 4.8g Sugar) Protein: 15.4g

Butternut Squash

A bell-shaped squash with deep-orange flesh, butternut squash is a milder winter squash and stores well. Because the skin is thin and light, we leave it on when dicing; it almost disappears when cooked. This method saves time and adds nutrition to the meal.

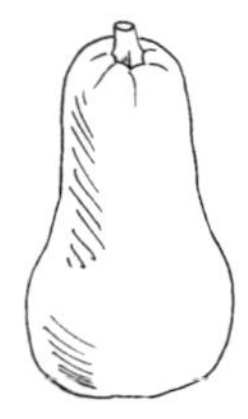

Butternut Squash

Roasted Butternut Squash

S→O: 10 minutes Roast: 25 minutes

2 cups diced butternut squash (~½-inch)
1/4–1/2 cup diced onions
2 tsp. High-Heat oil
1/8 tsp. salt
1/2 tsp. dried parsley
1/2 tsp. ground cinnamon
1/4 tsp. ground cumin
1/4 tsp. allspice
Freshly grated nutmeg (~1/8 tsp.)

Preheat oven—400°.
Baking pan (stainless steel or preheated cast iron).

1. Spread squash and onions in a single layer on baking pan. **Drizzle** evenly with oil. Mix seasonings in small bowl; sprinkle on squash. Stir to **coat**.
2. **Roast** for 25 minutes, or until vegetables are tender; stir about 15 minutes into baking.
3. **Optional Apple Version:** Sprinkle diced apple with allspice and ground cinnamon. Stir into squash during the last 10 minutes.

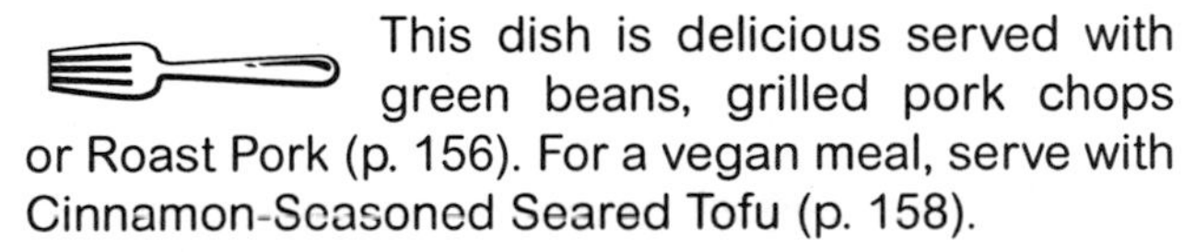

This dish is delicious served with green beans, grilled pork chops or Roast Pork (p. 156). For a vegan meal, serve with Cinnamon-Seasoned Seared Tofu (p. 158).

Yield: 2 servings 1 3/4 cups

Squash Winter Varieties

Shopping Tips:

Good winter squash will have a hard, dull skin. They should be firm and heavy for their size.

Storage Tips:

Store away from direct light, out of extreme heat and extreme cold. (Ideal storage temperature is 50° to 60°.)

Once squash is cut, wrap it in plastic and refrigerate. It can be frozen, uncooked. Cooked, mashed squash also freezes well.

Serving Suggestions:

Winter squash can be roasted whole and served as a side dish or used in casseroles and baking (pp. 39, 82 and 160).

continue p. 86 (sidebar)...

Recipes Using Butternut Squash:

- Fall Harvest Stews
- Apple Squash Bake

3 lb. butternut squash yields ~8 1/2 cups diced/sliced squash with peel

Analysis/Serving:
Calories: 110 (Fat Cal 39) Fat: 2.1g (0.4g Sat) Cholesterol: 0mg
Sodium: 140mg Carbs: 19g (3.6g Fiber 4g Sugar) Protein: 1.8g

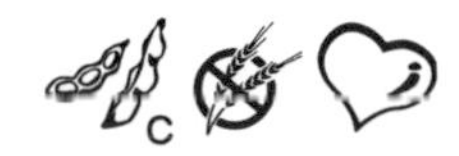

Pumpkin

Shopping Tips:

If you are choosing to puree your own pumpkin, look for small, "sugar" varieties that are free of soft spots.

If you are purchasing canned pumpkin, avoid brands with added ingredients (e.g., syrup).

Storage Tips:

Leftover pureed pumpkin (fresh or from a can) can be stored, covered, in the refrigerator for several days. It can also be frozen for several weeks.

Pumpkin Seeds:

Commercially available pumpkin seeds are harvested from a special kind of pumpkin grown in South America. Good for colon health, the seeds are also a good source of protein, omega-3 fatty acids, iron, zinc, phosphorus and vitamin D. They also contain calcium and vitamin B. Easier to digest if they are lightly roasted, they add a nice crunch to stir-fries and salads.

Pumpkin

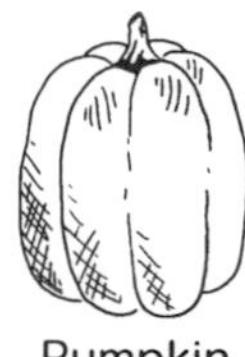
Pumpkin

As a low-fat, low-sodium, no-cholesterol food, pumpkin has a lot of flavor and is packed with nutrients, rich in vitamin A and potassium. Pureed pumpkin is one of the few canned foods in which little nutritional value is lost during the canning process. Pumpkin is good for regulating blood sugar and easing asthma. Enjoy adding the fullness of its flavor and the richness of nutrients to a variety of foods.

15-Minute Pumpkin Soup

S→T: 15 minutes

1 Tbsp. Medium-Heat oil
1/2 med. onion, chopped (~1/2 cup)
1 Tbsp. brown rice flour
1/16 tsp. salt
1 tsp. ground cinnamon
Freshly grated nutmeg
1 cup broth—vegetable or chicken
1 (15 oz.) can pumpkin
8 oz. (1 cup) half and half cream
OR heavy whipping cream

1. In saucepan, **sauté** onion in oil until tender.
2. **Add** flour to skillet; whisk while cooking for a minute. (Add a bit of broth if needed.) Whisk in seasonings. Gradually add broth, whisking to blend. **Whisk** in pumpkin, stirring often while heating through. Gradually **add** or half and half (or cream) while whisking. **Heat** slowly to serving temperature, whisking often.
3. Taste. If more seasoning is needed, start with freshly grated nutmeg; then try a little salt.

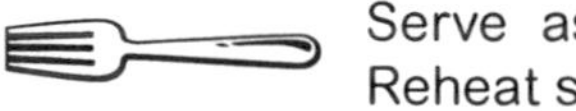
Serve as appetizer or side dish. Reheat slowly.

Yield: 6 servings ~3–3 1/4 cups

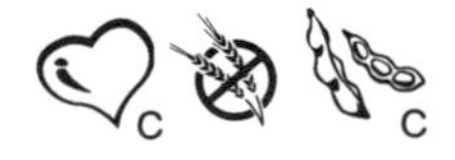

Analysis/Serving: (using half and half/heavy cream)
Calories: 134/218 (Fat Cal 77/169) Fat: 8.6/18.8g (4/11g Sat) Cholesterol: 18/59mg
Sodium: 128/130 Carbs: 10/11g (3.1g Fiber 4/3g Sugar) Protein: 1.5/1.7g

Getting Great Taste and Nutrition

Because pureed pumpkin is smooth and complements a variety of breads and baked goods, it is a great way to boost the vegetable consumption of picky eaters. A perfect example: many people who do not like vegetables love these Pumpkin Cookies with chocolate chips.

Pumpkin Cookies

S→O: 20 minutes   Bake: 12 minutes

Flour Choices: (choose one)
- 2 1/4 cups "white" whole-wheat flour
- OR 2 1/2 cups whole-grain spelt flour
- OR 2 1/4 cups Gluten-Free Flour Mix (p. 27)

1/2 cup soy protein isolate (p. 89)
4 tsp. baking powder
1/2 tsp. baking soda
1/2 tsp. salt
2 tsp. ground cinnamon (omit with choc chips)
1/3 cup Medium-Heat oil
2/3 cup honey
1/2 cup unsweetened applesauce
1 tsp. vanilla
1 (15 oz.) can pumpkin
1 cup semi-sweet chocolate chips (*or* raisins)
1 cup walnuts, chopped (optional)

Preheat oven—350°. Lightly **oil** baking sheets.

1. In bowl, **whisk** dry ingredients together.
2. In separate bowl, **whisk** together oil, honey, applesauce, vanilla and pumpkin. Add to dry ingredients. **Mix** to moisten. **Stir** in chocolate chips, raisins and/or walnuts.
3. **Drop** with rounded teaspoons on prepared baking sheets, then lightly flatten with fork or back of spoon. **Bake** 12 minutes. Immediately remove to cooling rack.

Yield: ~5 dozen

Analysis/Cookie: (Chocolate Chip/Raisin)
Calories: 64/59 (Fat Cal 20/12)   Fat: 2.2/1.3g (0.7/0.2g Sat)   Cholesterol: 0mg
Sodium: 71/72mg   Carbs: 9.3/9.5g (1/1g Fiber 5/5.4g Sugar)   Protein: 1.8/1.8g

flour mix, vanilla, chocolate chips, raisins

Pumpkin
(continued)

Recipes Using:
- Pumpkin Pancakes
- Pumpkin Pie Smoothie
- Pumpkin Pie
- Pumpkin Cupcakes
- Pumpkin Cheesecake
- 15-Minute Pumpkin Soup

Freezing Cookie Dough

These cookies are best eaten freshly baked. Unbaked dough can be stored in the refrigerator for a day or frozen. If desired, shape dough into four logs, wrap and freeze. Then slice when slightly thawed. Before baking, allow dough to come to room temperature while preheating oven.

Squash
Winter Varieties
(continued)

Healthy Bites

Vitamin A: One cup of winter squash typically contains over 7,000 IU of vitamin A.

Lung Cancer Risk: Beta-cryptoxanthin is a carotenoid found in winter squashes (especially pumpkin) and has been linked with lowering the risk of lung cancer. Vitamin A also reduces the risk of lung cancer, so the two coupled together (as they are in winter squashes) make a great team.

Save Flavor and Nutrients: Often winter squash is cut in half before roasting, or it is vented by cutting slits. This, however, allows the moisture in the squash to escape, taking nutrients and flavor with it. Roasting the squash whole brings out a heightened flavor and retains the nutrients.

$1\frac{3}{4}$ lb. (~7" long) spaghetti squash = ~3 cups cooked

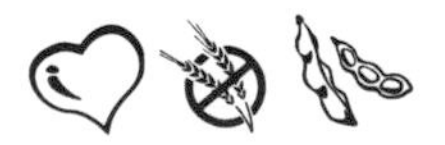

Spaghetti Squash

Spaghetti squash has a sweet flavor. It is delicious served with butter and your favorite seasoning or topped with pesto or tomato sauce.

Seasoned Spaghetti Squash

Oven temperature—375°; then 350°.

1. Place whole spaghetti squash (~2 lbs.) in baking pan. Add small amount of water. **Roast** 60–75 minutes, or until the shell yields to gentle pressure (this will be a little underdone). (You may cut it in half before cooking, but it is hard to cut raw, and nutrients and flavor are easily lost.) Remove from oven, reduce temperature to 350°. Allow to cool 10 minutes for easier handling.
2. **Remove squash from shell**: Cut squash in half lengthwise. With scissors (or grapefruit knife), cut strands that attach to the seeds; then scoop seeds out. With two table forks, pick at the squash as it separates from shell into strands that resemble spaghetti. Spread evenly in baking dish.

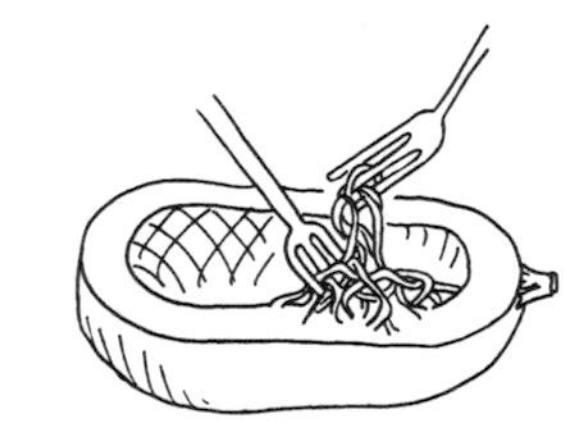
Pulling out Strands of Spaghetti Squash

3. **Season** squash with salt, freshly ground black pepper, 1 tablespoon unsalted butter and desired seasoning (or pesto just before serving). Below are our favorites (used individually):
   - 1/2 cup freshly minced parsley
   - 2 tsp. dried dill
   - 2 tsp. dried thyme
4. Return to oven. **Bake** uncovered for 20 minutes, or until hot and tender (but not mushy).

❄ Freeze extra before Steps 3 and 4.

Yield: 4 servings ~3 cups

Spaghetti Squash Casserole

S→T: 45 minutes + extra time for squash to bake

3 cups cooked spaghetti squash
1 tsp. garlic powder
2 tsp. dried oregano
1 tsp. dried basil
1 lb. lean ground beef
1 1/2 cups chopped onion
2 ribs celery, diced (1 cup)
1 med. green bell pepper, diced (1 cup)
1/4–3/8 tsp. salt (use lower amount with cheese)
1/4 tsp. dried crushed red pepper flakes
2 tsp. dried oregano
1 tsp. dried basil
4 cloves garlic, minced
1 handful flat-leaf parsley, minced (~1/4 cup)
1 (15 oz.) can diced tomatoes (with salt)
1 (15 oz.) can diced tomatoes (no salt added)
Parmesan cheese (optional)

Preheat oven—375°. 9x13-inch baking dish.

1. **Roast** squash according to method on previous page. **Spread** squash strands evenly in baking dish. **Season** squash with garlic powder, first listing of oregano and basil and a light sprinkle of salt and black pepper.
2. *Meanwhile,* in large skillet, **"Chop & Drop"** ground beef, onions, celery, bell peppers, seasonings, fresh garlic and parsley.
3. **Add** tomatoes (hand crush when adding) and **simmer** covered for at least 15 minutes, stirring occasionally.
4. **Pour** sauce evenly over squash. **Bake** to serving temperature. Sprinkle with Parmesan cheese if desired.

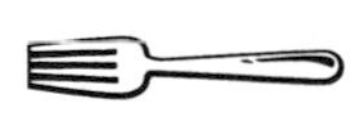

Serve with garlic toast and mixed greens salad. Warms up nicely.

Yield: 6 servings

Squash Winter Varieties
(continued)

More Facts:

Squashes originated in Central America and were first taken back to Europe by Christopher Columbus.

Winter squash does not typically contain pesticide residues.

Freezing Tips for Spaghetti Squash and Casserole

Completed casserole can be prepared and frozen unbaked for a month.

Sondra often prepares the recipe in two (8-inch) square baking dishes, freezing one dish unbaked for an easy dinner later.

Cooked squash and meat-tomato mixture can also be frozen separately.

Recipe can be made with previously baked, frozen and thawed spaghetti squash.

Analysis/Serving:
Calories: 234 (Fat Cal 92) Fat: 10.2g (3.6g Sat) Cholesterol: 46mg
Sodium: 381 Carbs: 18.3g (3.4g Fiber 8.6g Sugar) Protein: 17.6g

Sweet Potato

Shopping Tips:

Choose firm sweet potatoes without cracks or bruises. Nonorganic sweet potatoes often have been treated with wax or dye, so if you use them, peel them first.

Storage Tips:

Sweet potatoes should be kept in a cool, dark place, not in plastic, and out of the refrigerator.

Serving Suggestions:

Sweet potatoes can be enjoyed baked, mashed, roasted or steamed. They are great paired with pork.

Recipes Using:

- Southern-Style Shepherd's Pie
- Fruit Glazed Sweet Potatoes

Point of Confusion:

Many think of the moist, orange variety of sweet potatoes as yams, and they are often labeled that way in the store. However, true yams are native to Africa and are of a different family.

Sweet Potato

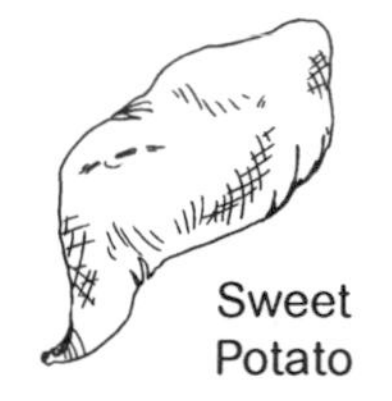

Sweet potatoes are rich in several vitamins and minerals. They also have a unique protein that has great antioxidant properties. Because of their ability to stabilize and control blood sugar, sweet potatoes are classified as an antidiabetic food. The more than four hundred varieties vary in size, shape, color and texture.

Baked Sweet Potato

Preheat oven—400°.

Scrub and dry. Rub High-Heat oil on the skin. Pierce several times with a fork. Bake 30–45 minutes until tender. Serve with salt, pepper and Omega Butter (p. 192). Some use sour cream.

Candy Fries

Prep: ~6 minutes Bake: 35–45 minutes.

12 oz. sweet potato, 1/2-inch fry wedges
(peeling optional but crispier with peel)
2–3 tsp. High-Heat oil
1/2 tsp. onion powder
Salt and pepper

Preheat oven: 425°/450° (convection/conventional).
Baking pan (stainless steel or preheated cast iron).

1. Spread potatoes in a single layer on baking pan. **Drizzle** evenly with oil. Sprinkle with seasonings. Using your hands, **toss** to coat.
2. **Bake** 30–45 minutes, or until as crispy as you desire without burning them. Stir after baking for 15 minutes; then stir occasionally.

Note: Sweet potatoes vary in their moisture content. This recipe works best with drier varieties.

Yield: 2 servings

Analysis/Serving of Candy Fries:
Calories: 171 (Fat Cal 41) Fat: 4.6g (0.4g Sat) Cholesterol: 0mg
Sodium: 83mg + varies Carbs: 30.5g (4.5g Fiber 6.5g Sugar) Protein: 2.4g

Soy Protein Isolate

There is much ongoing research about the benefits of soy. While some people may need to use soy sparingly (allergies, difficulty with oxalates or difficulty with goitrogens – see p. 218), there is evidence supporting the idea that soy can be beneficial to our health. Soybeans can be enjoyed whole, or the protein from the soybean can be purchased and used in a powdered form. Soy protein isolate is a higher quality form of protein than soy protein concentrate.

Sweet Potato Cakes

Mix: 15 minutes

2 eggs
1/2 tsp. salt
~1 lb. sweet potato, shredded
(~3 cups semipacked)
Wedge of onion (~1/4 cup)
(shred with sweet potato)
6 Tbsp. soy protein isolate (see sidebar)
OR brown rice flour

Preheat griddle to be slightly cooler than when water dances when sprinkled on surface.

1. In bowl, lightly **beat** eggs with salt. **Stir** in potatoes and onions. **Sprinkle** soy protein (or flour) evenly over mixture. **Stir**.
2. **Oil** preheated griddle. **Dip** mixture onto griddle. Flatten and shape into 3-inch patties. **Cook** 3–4 minutes on each side, or until golden brown and vegetables tender.

Serve with grilled pork chop (or grilled nitrate-free ham steak) and green beans.
Serve at breakfast with lean sausage patty.
Serve for brunch with Roasted Asparagus.

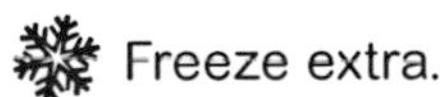

Freeze extra.

Yield: 5 servings [2 (3-inch) cakes/serving]

Analysis/Serving:
Calories: 149 (Fat Cal 24) Fat: 2.7g (0.6g Sat) Cholesterol: 85mg
Sodium: 345mg Carbs: 17g (2.5g Fiber 3.8g Sugar) Protein: 13.4g

Soy Protein Isolate

How do brands vary?

Numerous soy protein products are available, and they vary in quality and nutrition. A quality soy protein isolate will be manufactured:

- using certified non-GMO soy protein
- without the use of alcohol or heat
- to retain nutrient benefits during cooking/baking
- without the addition of excessive sodium or sugar

The soy protein isolate that we are most comfortable with is unsweetened and produced by the Shaklee Corporation. See our websites (p. 242) for more information.

Soy protein has been shown to:[15]

- lower blood pressure
- lower cholesterol
- provide energy
- protect against heart disease
- increase bone health
- stabilize blood sugar
- promote intestinal health
- protect against diabetic-related diseases

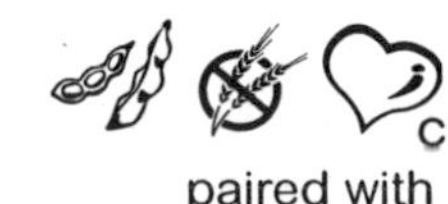

paired with

Tomato

Shopping Tips:

Choose tomatoes that are smooth, with no bruises or cracks. Ripe tomatoes will give slightly when you press gently with your thumb. Generally the deeper the color, the richer the nutrients.

The high acid content of tomatoes can lead to the corrosion of metal. In canned tomatoes, this can cause whatever the can is made of to leak into the fruit. Not all countries have standards prohibiting the use of lead in their cans, so we advocate purchasing canned tomatoes that were produced in the United States.

Storage Tips:

Tomatoes keep for several days at room temperature. If overripe, they can be kept in the refrigerator for 1–2 days. To speed up the ripening process, place the tomato in a paper bag. Adding a banana or apple will make the process even faster (the ethylene gas emitted by these aids in the ripening process).

Tomato

Though technically a fruit, tomatoes are typically enjoyed in the fashion of vegetables. The many variations of tomatoes offer subtle differences in taste. Tomatoes have high amounts of lycopene, a carotenoid that fights cancer and heart disease. It is the blend of lycopene with other phytonutrients that make the tomato so beneficial to our health.

Marinara Sauce

S→T: 30 minutes (20 minutes is semi-inactive)

1 tsp. Medium-Heat oil
1 med. onion (finely chop in food processor)
1/4 cup diced carrots
2 cloves garlic, crushed
5/8 tsp. salt
2 tsp. dried oregano
4 tsp. dried basil
1 tsp. dried parsley
1/4 tsp. sage
Scant 1/4 tsp. black pepper
1 (28 oz.) can Tuscan-style, low-salt tomatoes
(see sidebar on p. 137)
2 tsp. olive oil
1 tsp. sweetener—honey, agave nectar

1. In large saucepan, lightly **sauté** onions in Medium-Heat oil. *Meanwhile,* finely **chop** carrots and garlic in mini food processor; add to onions; **sauté** with salt and seasonings.
2. Remove from heat; add tomatoes; with immersion blender, **puree** sauce. Return to heat, cover and **simmer** 10 minutes. **Add** olive oil and sweetener, cover and simmer 5 minutes.

For a vegetarian dinner, heat tofu in Marinara Sauce. Serve over pasta.

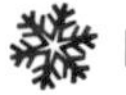
Freeze extra

Yield: 14 (1/4 cup) servings   3 1/2 cups

Analysis/Serving:
Calories: 32 (Fat Cal 9) Fat: 1g (0.2g Sat) Cholesterol: 0mg
Sodium: 107mg Carbs: 5g (1g Fiber 1.2g Sugar) Protein: 0.7g

Salsa

Mix: < 10 minutes

1 (15 oz.) can fire-roasted diced tomatoes with green chilies
1/2 cup finely chopped red onion
2 cloves garlic, minced
2 tsp. freshly squeezed lime juice
2 Tbsp. minced fresh parsley
OR minced fresh cilantro
OR 2 tsp. dried parsley

Mix all ingredients. Chill.

Yield: 2 cups

Analysis/4 Tablespoons:
Calories: 17 (Fat Cal 0) Fat: 0g (0g Sat) Cholesterol: 0mg
Sodium: 185mg Carbs: 3.6g (0.6g Fiber 1.8g Sugar) Protein: 0.5g

Bean Salsa

Follow Salsa recipe with following changes:

- **Double the amount of onions**
- **Add 1 (15 oz.) can black beans** (with added salt) (may desire to drain off some liquid)

Yield: 3 cups

Analysis/4 Tablespoons:
Calories: 44 (Fat Cal 0) Fat: 0g (0g Sat) Cholesterol: 0mg
Sodium: 144mg Carbs: 8.5g (1.7g Fiber 1.7g Sugar) Protein: 2.4g

Bean-Corn Salsa/Vegetarian Tacos

Sauté 1 cup frozen corn for about 5 minutes. **Add** to Bean Salsa.

For Tacos: Simmer to desired consistency. Serve in soft tortillas with toppings such as shredded lettuce, low-fat shredded cheese, low-fat sour cream or low-fat unsweetened plain yogurt and/or Guacamole (p. 47).

Yield: 4 cups

Analysis/4 Tablespoons:
Calories: 43 (Fat Cal 0) Fat: 0 (0g Sat) Cholesterol: 0mg
Sodium: 108mg Carbs: 8.4g (1.4g Fiber 2g Sugar) Protein: 2.7g

Tomato
(continued)

Some Recipes Using:

- Pepper-Corn Chili
- Green Bean Basil Salad
- Fancy Hamburgers

Healthy Bites

Hidden Ingredients: Tomatoes are enjoyed raw or cooked, diced, pureed and juiced. All forms of tomatoes are healthful additions to our diets. If they come packaged as sauces, juices or condiments, check for added sugars and sodium.

Lycopene: There is typically three times as much lycopene in organic ketchup as there is in nonorganic brands.

Fiber: Tomatoes are a good source of fiber. One cup of fresh tomatoes provides almost two grams of fiber. The fiber is reduced by half if the skin is removed.

Salsa Storage Hint

Each salsa keeps for several days. Extras may be frozen.

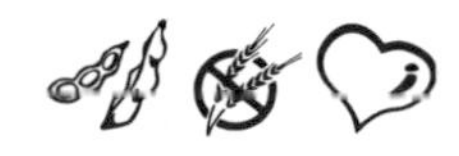

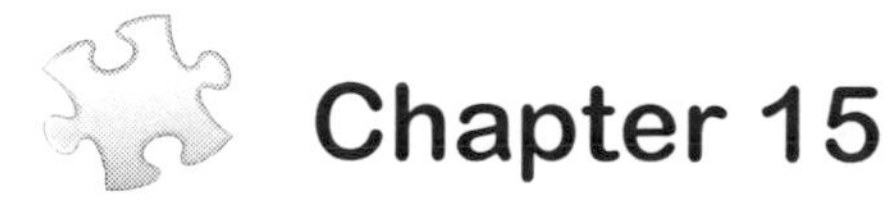

Chapter 15

Condiments

Condiments, such as salad dressings and spreads, add flavor and variety to our food. Many brands and flavors are commercially available. However, since many purchased products contain added salt, sweeteners (especially corn syrup), partially hydrogenated oils and a variety of preservatives and artificial flavorings, they are often not healthy choices. Typically they are high in sodium and, usually, high in fat and/or sugar. Often they are high in calories. A healthy sandwich or salad can quickly become a health hazard. Making your own condiments is often a quick and tasty solution. They can be cheaper and healthier, without sacrificing flavor.

Less Healthy Options Add Up

Sandwich Condiments: 1 tablespoon of the typical mayo adds 90 calories, 10 g. of fat and 90 mg. of sodium to your meal. Most restaurants put at least 2 tablespoons on a typical sandwich. Add to that 2 teaspoons of mustard and you add another 130 mg. of sodium.

Instead, try 1 tablespoon of Basil Pesto. You get great flavor, the nutrition of the greens and you add only 52 calories, 4.7 g. of fat and 48 mg. of sodium.

Salad Dressings: Adding 1 tablespoon of a typical salad dressing to a side salad adds over 200 mg. of sodium. Use one of our 5-minute recipes and you add only 10 to 60 mg. of sodium.

Condiment recipes are found on the following pages:

- Bean Salsa + Bean-Corn Salsa (p. 91)
- Dips
  - Bean Dip (p. 149)
  - Confetti Dip (p. 42)
  - Hummus (p. 49)
  - Spinach Dip (p. 81)
- Fruit Pancake Syrup (p. 188)
- Guacamole (p. 47)
- Lemon-Butter Sauce (p. 43)
- Marinara Sauce (p. 90)
- Omega Butter (p. 192)
- Pesto (p. 93)
- Salad Dressings
  - Arugula Pesto (p. 44)
  - Balsamic Vinaigrette (p. 70)
  - Citrus Vinaigrette (p. 97)
  - Dijon (p. 99)
  - Guacamole (p. 47)
- Salsa (p. 91)

Pesto

Mix: 10 minutes or less + toasting nuts

1/4 cup nuts— pine, English walnuts, almonds
Vegetable/herb leaves
Choose one or a mixture, using mostly leaves. Measure packed except watercress.
- 2 cups fresh basil (p. 220)
- 2 cups fresh arugula (p. 44)
- 2 cups fresh cilantro (p. 220)
- 2 cups flat-leaf parsley (p. 221)
- 2 cups fresh spinach (p. 79)
- 1 bunch watercress (p. 69)

2 cloves garlic, cracked
1/8–1/4 tsp. salt
Freshly grated nutmeg
1 1/2 tsp. freshly squeezed lemon juice
2–4 Tbsp. olive oil
2–4 Tbsp. water (optional)
Parmesan cheese (optional)
(use lower amount of salt)

1. **Toast** nuts in a 200° oven for 5–8 minutes, or until fragrant, stirring a couple of times.
2. **Rinse** and **spin-dry** vegetable/herb(s).
3. Add nuts and garlic to food processor (or blender). **Process** until finely chopped. Add vegetable/herb, salt, nutmeg and lemon juice. **Process** until finely choppped. While processing, **stream** in oil, then water to desired consistency (see sidebar, Healthy Bites).
3. When serving, stir in Parmesan cheese as desired.

❄ Freeze extras (without cheese) in ice cube tray. After frozen, transfer cubes to food storage bag. Thaw before using.

Yield: ~11 (1 Tbsp.) servings 2/3 cup

Serving Suggestions:

Serve the thinner consistency pesto over:

- whole-grain pasta cooked al dente
- cooked vegetables, such as summer or spaghetti squash

Use the thicker consistency pesto as a:

- dip for raw vegetables
- sauce for pizza
- spread for sandwiches

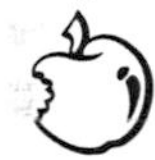

Healthy Bites

Less Oil: For a healthier version, use half water and half oil.

Without Cheese: The amount of water and oil used depends upon your taste and consistency desired. Adding Parmesan cheese thickens the pesto. Use lesser amounts of oil and/or water for a thicker pesto without cheese.

Less Green Taste

To cut the "green" taste, especially in frozen pesto, stir in a little Dijon-style mustard.

Analysis/Tablespoon for Basil Pesto (without Parmesan cheese):
Calories: 52 (Fat Cal 41) Fat: 4.6g (.52g Sat) Cholesterol: 0mg
Sodium: 48mg Carbs: 1g (0.4g Fiber 0.2g Sugar) Protein: 0.7g

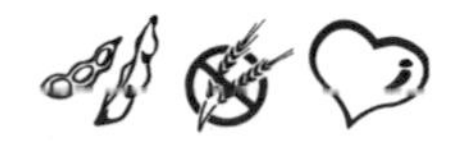

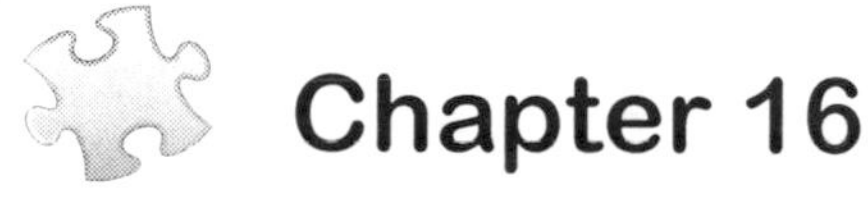

Chapter 16

Making a Meal with Salads

While salads are often enjoyed on the side, they can also be a wonderful, quick, nutritious and versatile meal. Because almost anything can go into them, they do not need a lot of advanced planning and are a great way to use up what's in your refrigerator. They are easy to alter for family members with different tastes, and the combinations are endless, making for a delightful variety of entrée-type meals.

The recipe below offers ideas to create a total meal-in-a-salad. You are limited only by your imagination. The seven pages following offer additional salads with complementary salad dressings that make complete quick, easy and nutritious meals.

Helpful Hints

Involve the whole family: Everyone can help choose and prepare items to go in the salad. Or place a variety of items in the center of the table and let everyone create their own.

Potluck Treat: Ask everyone to bring a favorite salad ingredient and then throw it all together for a tasty community-built meal.

Meal-in-a Salad

Starch Choices: (~½ cup/serving if desired)
- Whole-grain pasta, cooked al dente
- Cooked brown rice

Nonvegetable Protein Choices: (when choosing portion size, consider sodium and saturated fat)
- Baked/poached salmon, flaked
- Cooked poultry chunks
- Hard cooked eggs, sliced or crumbled
- Low-fat cheese (shredded or cubed)
- Shredded pork or beef
- Nitrate-free ham, sliced or diced

Vegetable Protein Choices:
- Canned beans (e.g., black, garbanzo), drained
- Edamame beans (p. 101)
- Nuts (e.g., walnuts, pecans, almonds)
- Peas, fresh or frozen (thawed)
- Seeds (e.g., pepito/pumpkin, sesame, sunflower)
- Seared Tofu (p. 158)

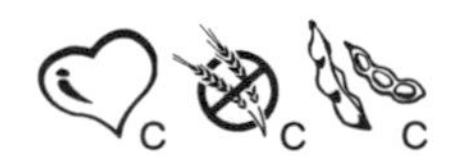

salad choices continue ...

Vegetable Choices: (~2 cups/serving)
(shredded, sliced or diced)

- Artichoke hearts, drained
- Asparagus (blanched or lightly roasted)
- Avocado
- Beet (raw/roasted)
- Broccoli (blanched)
- Cabbage (red/green)
- Carrots
- Cauliflower (blanched)
- Celery
- Corn, frozen whole kernel (thawed)
- Cucumber
- Kohlrabi
- Leeks
- Onion (any color)
- Peppers (any color)
- Radishes
- Potatoes (roasted)
- Shallots
- Summer squash
- Tomatoes

Fruit Choices:

- Apple, diced or sliced
- Berries, fresh or frozen (thawed) (blueberries, raspberries, blackberries, huckleberries, sliced strawberries)
- Citrus fruit, sectioned and diced
- Grapes
- Mangos or peaches, fresh or frozen (thawed)
- Pomegranate
- Raisins or other dried fruit (such as cranberries, blueberries, currents)

Greens: (choose a variety to add color, texture and nutrition to your meal)

- Arugula
- Chard and kale (tiny leaves)
- Mixed greens (pp. 68–69 for ideas)
- Spinach and/or baby spinach

Fresh Herb Choices:

- Basil (green or purple)
- Cilantro
- Dill
- Parsley

Prepare and gently **toss** your choice of ingredients. Stir in the greens or serve on a bed of greens. Garnish with fresh herbs. **Drizzle** with salad dressing (pp. 44, 47, 70, 97 and 99) or purchased healthier-choice salad dressing. **Toss** to coat ingredients. Serve immediately.

Helpful Hints

Prepare for Leftovers: Add salad dressing only to the portion you plan to eat so remaining salad can serve as a ready-to-go lunch the next day. Salad dressing can be carried to work or school in a small container (e.g., an empty spice jar).

Quick-Fix Ideas: Wash and chop veggies (e.g., carrots and peppers) or hard-cook eggs the night before.

"Cool" Packed Lunch Idea: Dice ham or other leftover cooked meats and freeze in snack-sized baggies. Pack frozen for travel lunch salad (thaws by lunchtime and doubles as an icer).

Sondra's Favorites

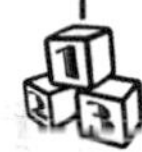

Romaine lettuce, celery, chicken, Roasted Beets (p. 50), blueberries and walnuts with Citrus Vinaigrette Salad Dressing (p. 97).

or

Top mixed salad greens with Pea & Celery Salad, sliced hard-cooked egg and a little extra Arugula Pesto Salad Dressing (p. 44).

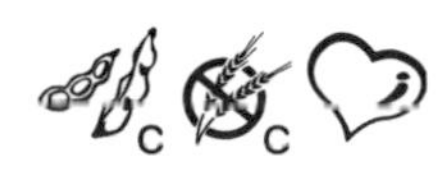

Fresh Ginger

Purchase Tips:

Ginger can be purchased in many forms. The healthiest and most flavorful is the ginger root, found in the produce section of the grocery store. Most ginger sold in the United States is mature, with a tough skin that needs to be peeled.

Storage Tips:

Keep unpeeled fresh ginger in the refrigerator for about a week. It can be frozen for several months.

Preparing Fresh Ginger:

Peel and mince like you would garlic (p. 60).

Healthy Bites

Natural Solution: Ginger relieves motion sickness. In one study, it proved superior to Dramamine.[1]

Health Benefits: Ginger helps reduce inflammation, contains several antioxidants and is wonderful for relieving stomach upset.

Ginger

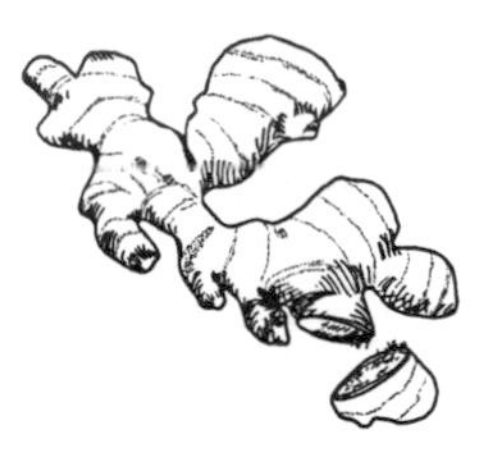
Fresh Ginger

Ginger adds a distinctive spicy flavor to Asian dishes, baked goods, beverages and smoothies as well as vegetable and fruit dishes. There are several varieties; the flesh may be colored red, yellow, white or brown.

Asian Salmon Salad

Prep: 5 minutes Marinate: 1 hour or longer
Bake: 20–25 minutes

This quick and easy recipe was developed by the inspiration and help of many people —from a cooking class at a local health food store to the clerks at that store helping Sondra to find a sauce free of corn syrup and finally us trying several versions. In the end the recipe turned out easier, quicker and healthier (especially lower in added sugars and sodium) than the original. Our hats off to many! Enjoy!

1 lb. wild Alaska salmon fillets
1–3 tsp. minced fresh ginger
6 Tbsp. Polynesian sauce (next page sidebar)
Romaine lettuce (3 cups per salad)
Frozen blueberries, thawed (1/4 cup/salad)
Citrus Vinaigrette Salad Dressing
(1 tablespoon per salad)

Oven temperature—350°

1. **Do-Ahead Marinate:** Cut fillets into serving-sized pieces. Score each pieces 3–4 times on nonskin side. Place skin side down in casserole dish. Sprinkle with ginger and evenly drizzle Polynesian sauce over fillets. Using the back of spoon, spread sauce and ginger evenly over fillets. Cover and marinate overnight or at least 1–2 hours in refrigerator.

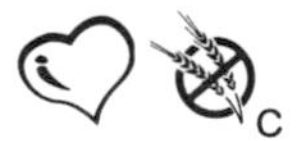

Analysis/Serving
Calories: 306 (Fat Cal 114) Fat: 12.7g (2.3g Sat) Cholesterol: 51mg
Sodium: 342mg Carbs: 18g (5g Fiber 11.1g Sugar) Protein: 26.7g

2. **Bake** uncovered at 350° until fish flakes easily (about 20–25 minutes). (If desired, broil or grill the marinated salmon instead of baking.) Peel skin off. **Flake**.
3. **Assemble** salad by layering lettuce, salmon, blueberries and dressing.

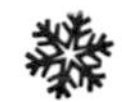 Freeze extra cooked fish.

Yield: 4 meal servings

Citrus Vinaigrette Salad Dressing

Excellent when tossed with a salad consisting of lettuce, fruit and nuts. (Our favorite is blueberries and walnuts. We thaw frozen wild Maine blueberries.)

1 Tbsp. raw apple cider vinegar
1 Tbsp. honey
1/4 cup 100% orange juice
1 tsp. garlic powder
3–4 pinches xanthan gum (p. 70; sidebar)
1/4 cup olive oil

In bowl, **whisk** together all ingredients except oil. **Whisk** while streaming in oil; continuing to whisk until opaque. Lightly **season** with salt and pepper as desired.

 Drizzle over Asian Salmon Salad or any mixed greens salad just before serving.

Store in refrigerator for 2–3 weeks. Empty glass jars/bottles (e.g., purchased salad dressing bottles, spice jars) make excellent containers. Allow leftover to come to room temperature before serving.

Yield: 15 (2 tsp.) servings ~2/3 cup

Healthy Bites

Choosing a Sauce: A good Polynesian or hoisin sauce adds sweetness and flavor without large amounts of sugar or sodium. For a serving (2 tablespoons), the options range from 350 to 800 mg. of sodium, from 30 to 80 calories, and from 2 to 14 g. of sugar (that's seven times as much!). Sweetener choices also vary from corn syrup to cane sugar to honey with added fruit juice (of course, using honey and fruit juice is best). See page 231.

Choosing Fish: Fish provides an excellent source of protein, is low in saturated fats and is high in omega-3 fatty acids. Unfortunately, there are reasons to be cautious. Fish found in wild waters can contain high levels of mercury, while fish raised on farms often have high levels of antibiotics. (High-mercury-containing fish to avoid include shark, swordfish, king mackerel, tilefish and some kinds of tuna.) We encourage you to keep abreast of current research while enjoying small amounts of fish regularly.

Lettuce Fun Fact:

In China, where it symbolizes good luck, lettuce is served for celebrations such as New Year's and birthdays.

Analysis/Serving (2 tsp.):
Calories: 39 (Fat Cal 32) Fat: 3.6g (0.5g Sat) Cholesterol: 0mg
Sodium: 9mg Carbs: 1.7g (0g Fiber 1.6g Sugar) Protein: 0g

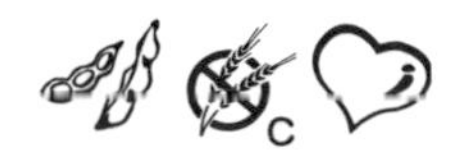

Helpful Hints

Dry Bread Crumbs: These are easy to make using Ezekiel or whole-grain bread (see p. 191 for purchasing tips or p. 190 for Hearty Homemade Bread recipe). Tear slices into pieces. Leave out overnight or place in 200° oven for 20 to 30 minutes. Finely grind dry pieces in mini food processor, alternating between chop and grind buttons.

Do-Ahead Tips. Prepare any of the following in advance:

- Bread crumbs
- Breading mixture (this is Step 2)
- Steps 1, 2, 3 and 4. Refrigerate until ready to cook (do this no more than 24 hours in advance).
- Chicken can be breaded and frozen. Bake straight from freezer in preheated oven, allowing approximately 5 minutes extra baking time or thaw and bake.

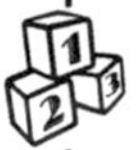

Gluten-Free

Replace bread crumbs with 2/3 cup puffed brown rice cereal (finely chopped in food processor).

Pecan Crusted Chicken Salad with Dijon Salad Dressing

S→O: 20 minutes   Bake: 20–25 minutes

1 lb. boneless, skinless chicken breasts/tenders

Breading Mixture:

- **1/2 cup pecans, finely chopped**
- **1/2 cup dry bread crumbs** (see sidebar)
- **1/2 tsp. dried oregano** (crushed)
- **1/2 tsp. dried thyme** (crushed)
- **1/4 tsp. salt**
- **1/4 tsp. garlic powder**
- **1/4 tsp. onion powder**
- **1/4 tsp. dry mustard**
- **1/4 tsp. paprika**
- **1 shake cayenne pepper**
- **Freshly ground black pepper**

Dipping Mixture: (choose one)

- 1 egg, lightly beaten
- OR 1 Tbsp. Medium-Heat oil (see Step 3)

Romaine lettuce (3 cups per salad)

Dijon Salad Dressing (1 tablespoon per salad)

Preheat oven—375° (convection or conventional).
Baking pan

1. **Cut** breasts into strips and then crosswise or cut tenders in half crosswise, making finger-length pieces. Rinse. Dry with paper towels.
2. In bowl, **stir** together breading ingredients, crushing oregano and thyme with fingers. Lay a piece of waxed paper on kitchen counter; pour some breading on it.
3. **Dipping mixture**:
   In separate shallow dish, whisk egg. Dip dry chicken strips, turning to coat all sides.
   Or dip dry chicken strips into a small amount of oil, turning to coat all sides.

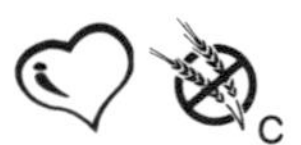

Analysis/Serving: (Using Ezekiel Bread and Egg)
Calories: 341 (Fat Cal 164)   Fat: 18.2g (2.6g Sat)   Cholesterol: 89mg
Sodium: 303mg   Carbs: 17g (6.2g Fiber 4.3g Sugar)   Protein: 29g

4. **Breading**: Transfer each "dipped" chicken strip to breading mixture. Roll and press the breading onto chicken to coat all sides. Place single layer on baking pan (tucking under any small pieces).
5. **Bake** for 20–25 minutes in preheated oven, or until 180° internal temperature.

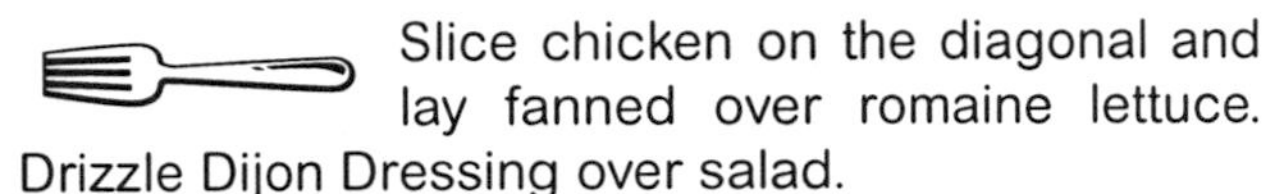

Slice chicken on the diagonal and lay fanned over romaine lettuce. Drizzle Dijon Dressing over salad.

See sidebar for more serving ideas.

Yield: 4 meal servings

Dijon Salad Dressing

3 Tbsp. Dijon-style mustard
2 Tbsp. freshly squeezed lemon juice
1 Tbsp. raw apple cider vinegar
1 Tbsp. sweetener—agave nectar or honey
1/4 tsp. onion powder
1/4 cup olive oil

In bowl, **combine** all ingredients except oil. **Whisk** while streaming in oil; continuing to whisk until opaque. Lightly **season** with salt and pepper if needed.

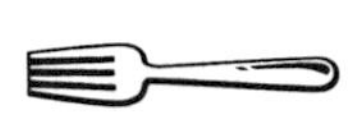

Drizzle over Pecan Crusted Chicken Salad or any mixed greens salad.

Also, use as a dipping sauce for Oven-Fried Chicken Chunks (p. 144).

❄ Store in refrigerator for 2–3 weeks. Empty glass jars/bottles (e.g., purchased salad dressing bottles, spice jars) make excellent containers. Allow leftover to come to room temperature before serving.

Yield: 30 (2 tsp.) servings ~2/3 cup

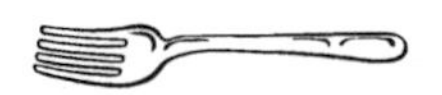

May serve Pecan Crusted Chicken as main entrée, drizzling sauce over strips or using dressing as a dipping sauce.

If desired, bread bone-in chicken pieces, allowing extra time to bake.

Complement the meal with steamed broccoli and/or Glazed Carrots.

Helpful Hints

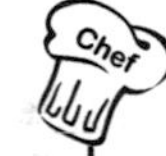

Food Safety: Throw away extra breading that comes in contact with raw chicken. Any other unused breading mixture may be frozen.

For Small Families and Singles: Use oil option for dipping so small amounts can be prepared without wasting egg.

Little Chefs

Children can help to dip and bread the chicken.

Meat Thermometer

A kitchen thermometer is a perfect tool to confirm that meat is cooked to the safe internal temperature.

Analysis/Serving (2 tsp.):
Calories: 35 (Fat Cal 31) Fat: 3.4g (0.5g Sat) Cholesterol: 0mg
Sodium: 38mg Carbs: 1.2g (0g Fiber 1.1g Sugar) Protein: 0g

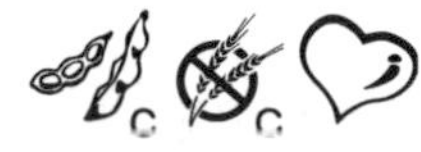

GF - vinegar, mustard

Healthy Bites

Adjusting Salt for Beans: If you use canned black beans without salt, increase salt to 1/2 teaspoon, taste and add more if needed.

Adjusting Salt for Spices: Increasing spices allows you to reduce the salt without compromising flavor.

Lowering Carbs: If you desire a lower carb meal, enjoy one taco with tortilla and one as a taco salad.

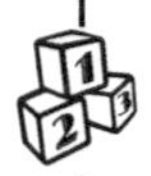

Spice It Up Spice It Down

For a spicier version, dice the red chili peppers.

For a milder version, omit crushed red pepper.

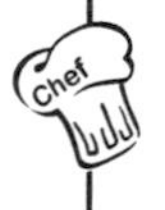

Variety Is the Spice of Life

For a family with varied tastes, prepare as suggested, omitting crushed red pepper. After it simmers, set some meat aside for those with a milder preference.

Remove whole chilis and mince. Add minced chilis and crushed red pepper to meat mixture remaining in skillet. Stir well.

Tacos and Taco Salad

S→T: 30 minutes or less

1 lb. lean ground meat (beef or turkey)
1 lg. onion, chopped (2 cups)
1/4 tsp. salt
1 tsp. each: dried leaf oregano, chili powder
1/2 tsp. each: crushed red pepper, cumin
4 cloves garlic, minced
1 (8 oz.) can tomato sauce (optional)
1 (15 oz.) can black beans (with added salt)
(drain beans, reserve liquid, add liquid as needed)
2–4 whole (uncut) **red chili peppers** (optional)
Soft whole-grain tortillas

Topping & Garnish Ideas:
Shredded cheddar and/or Monterey Jack cheese
Diced fresh tomatoes (or drained canned)
Thinly sliced romaine lettuce
Diced onions
Sliced black olives
Easy Guacamole (p. 47)
Salsa (pp. 91 or 153)
Low-fat sour cream (or plain unsweetened yogurt)

1. In skillet, "**Chop & Drop**" meat, onion, seasonings and garlic. **Stir** in tomato sauce, beans (with liquid as needed) and optional whole chili peppers. (If omitting tomato sauce, use more bean liquid.) **Simmer** uncovered for 12–15 minutes until liquid is absorbed, stirring often. **Remove** whole peppers.
2. Meanwhile, prepare toppings.

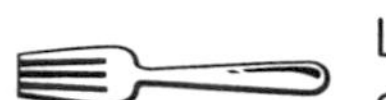

Layer taco mixture and toppings on one side of tortilla. Fold and enjoy. Makes a great sauce for Taco Pizza (p. 170) or to top a Baked Potato (p. 21).

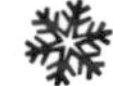 Freeze extra.

Yield: 15 (1/3 cup) tacos   5 cups

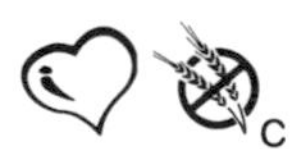

Analysis/Taco (meat mixture only):
Calories: 94 (Fat Cal 28) Fat: 3.1g (1.2g Sat) Cholesterol: 20mg
Sodium: 76mg Carbs: 8g (1.6g Fiber 1.4g Sugar) Protein: 8.3g

Creating a Taco Salad ...

To create a taco salad, simply serve taco mixture on a bed of greens with your favorite toppings lightly sprinkled on the top (see p. 68 for green ideas). If desired, serve with tortilla chips (p. 143).

Leftovers make for a great lunch that can be carried to work or school the next day.

Remaining taco mixture can also make for a healthy snack. Stir in a bit of salsa and/or low-fat sour cream to make it of dipping consistency and enjoy with tortilla chips (p. 143).

Wilted Spinach Salad

Photo on Front Cover

S→T: 30 minutes or less

1 (10 oz.) pkg. frozen shelled edamame
1/2–1 pint grape tomatoes (halve all or some)
1 bunch spinach (wash, spin-dry, ribbon-cut)
1/2 med. red onion, minced
1 clove garlic, minced
Peel and juice from 1 lemon
1 Tbsp. flaxseed oil
Salt and freshly ground black pepper

1. In saucepan, **simmer** beans in small amount of water until tender. Season.
2. *Meanwhile,* prepare and **layer** tomatoes, spinach, onions, garlic and lemon peel in large bowl. **Add** hot cooked beans. **Cover** bowl and set aside, allowing steam to wilt the spinach and release flavor from the lemon peel. **Drizzle** lemon juice and oil over salad, lightly season. **Toss**. Serve within 24 hours.

Complement meal with whole-grain crackers and/or fresh fruit.

Yield: 2 complete meals

Estimated Analysis/Serving:
Calories: 330 (Fat Cal 136) Fat: 15.1g (1.4g Sat) Cholesterol: 0mg
Sodium: 291mg Carbs: 31g (10.6g Fiber 9.7g Sugar) Protein: 21.6g

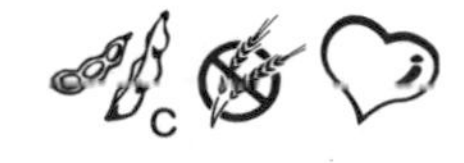

Edamame Beans
(green soybeans)

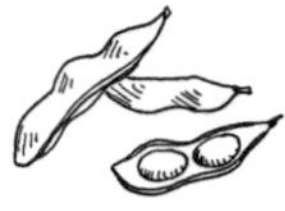

Edamame in Shells

Shopping Tips:

Edamame, or fresh soybeans, can be purchased fresh or frozen. Frozen varieties come both shelled and unshelled. Edamame that is not frozen should be in its shell when purchased. Shells should be a bright green, without blemish.

Canned soybeans come in several varieties, with or without additional salt. Canned soybeans have the same nutritional value as dry soybeans.

Storage Tips:

Fresh edamame should be refrigerated and is best used within 2–3 days. Frozen edamame keeps for several months.

The Difference in Syrup

Not all products labeled "maple syrup" are the same. One popular brand contains no maple syrup at all but is comprised of corn syrup, high-fructose corn syrup, salt, artificial flavors and preservatives.

Though admittedly higher in sugar, pure maple syrup has 24 times less sodium, is easier to digest and has several naturally occurring minerals.

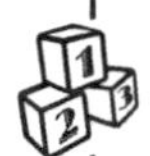

Different Tastes

Use more or less oil, vinegar, juice and/or maple syrup to suit your taste.

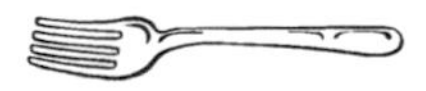

- Use cooked chicken chunks or goat (or other) cheese in place of the eggs.
- Garnish with cilantro/ parsley before serving.
- Makes a delicious side dish with grilled chicken (like serving cranberry relish with turkey).
- Finely chop salad in food processor to serve as salsa or relish.

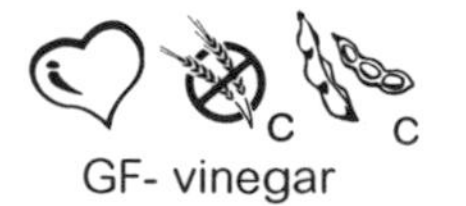

GF- vinegar

Beet Salad

S→T: 45 minutes (25 minutes total active time) + chilling

Recipe adapted from Bob's favorite beet recipe at Friendly Farm, Iowa City, Iowa.

1 1/2 cups diced unpeeled beets (~10 oz.)
High-Heat oil
Salt and pepper
3/4 cup chopped onion
1 clove garlic, minced
1 Tbsp. each: lime juice, red wine vinegar and 100% pure maple syrup
Fruit Choices:
1 mango, peeled and diced
1 nectarine, diced
1 cup frozen mangos
1 cup diced frozen peaches

Hard-cooked eggs, diced (1–2 per salad)
Romaine lettuce (3 cups per salad)

Preheat oven—375°.
Baking pan (stainless steel or preheated cast iron)

1. **Roasting**:
   - Place beets in cast-iron skillet, drizzle with approximately 1 tablespoon of oil. Season with salt and pepper and toss to coat beets. Roast for 10 minutes.
   - Stir in onions and a little more oil, if needed. Continue to roast for 10 minutes.
   - Stir in garlic and roast for 5 more minutes until beets and onions are al dente.
2. **Cool** slightly.
3. In bowl, **whisk** together lime juice, vinegar and maple syrup. **Stir** in cooled beets and fruit. **Chill**.

Assemble Salad: lettuce, beet/fruit mixture and diced egg.

Yield: 4 servings ~2 cups

Analysis/Serving:
Calories: 207 (Fat Cal 82) Fat: 9.1g (1.9g Sat) Cholesterol: 212mg
Sodium: 191mg Carbs: 24.5g (6.1g Fiber 16g Sugar) Protein: 9.8g

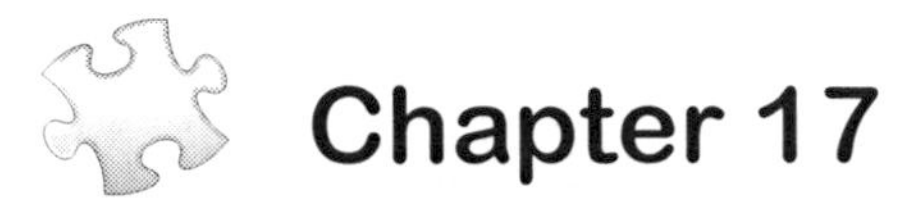

Chapter 17

Breakfast and Brunch Ideas

"Eat breakfast like a king, lunch like a queen and dinner like a pauper." The old saying has a lot of truth to it. Breakfast should be a prime source of energy and nutrients as we head into the day. However, it's often hard to take time to eat — or to eat well. Breakfasts that are high in sugar and low in protein lead to headaches and the inability to concentrate later in the morning. Breakfasts that are devoid of fat leave us hungry well before lunch. Here are some ideas for how we can we eat a nutritious breakfast, even if it's in a hurry. For our recommendations on healthier-choice ingredients, see the Healthier Choices Shopping Guide.

Eight Ways to Have a Healthy Breakfast:

1. **Capitalize on fiber.**
   - Stir Granola (p. 208) into thawed frozen or fresh fruit or yogurt.
   - Eat a whole-grain muffin or bread (pp. 186–187 and 190–191).
   - Put oatmeal ingredients in the slow cooker the night before – you wake up to breakfast and everyone can eat whenever they are ready!
   - Add oat bran or wheat bran to cooked cereals such as oatmeal.
   - Stir flaxseed meal and/or wheat germ into cold cereals or use as a garnish on hot cereals.
   - Add flaxseed meal and/or wheat germ to smoothies or a dish of yogurt.
   - Enjoy a Granola or Protein Bar.
   - Add whole fruits and vegetables.

continue ...

Syrup Facts

- Two tablespoons of a typical blueberry syrup add 22 g. of sugar and 200 calories to your breakfast, without adding any fiber.
- Make your own syrup in less than 15 minutes (see p. 188) and add only three to four grams of sugar (an 85% decrease) and 19 to 24 calories (a 90% decrease).

Plus you get 0.6 g. of fiber and all the nutritional value of real blueberries while avoiding the corn syrup and preservatives.

2. **Avoid highly sugared cereals and pastries.**
   - To wean off high-sugar cereals, buy two kinds (one high sugar and one low or no sugar) and mix them for an overall lower-sugar breakfast. Mix three-fourths high and one-fourth low, then go to two-thirds high and one-third low; then half-and-half . . . . Or purchase very-low or no-sugar cereal and add your own sugar, gradually cutting back until little is needed.
   - Add fruit to cereal for sweetness (wash and cut the night before).
   - Choose plain hot-cooked cereals. Add your own sugar, gradually using less.
   - Consider adding honey, brown rice syrup, 100% maple syrup and/or dried fruit to cereal in place of cane sugar (see Sweetener Glossary).
   - Enyoy Granola (p. 208) with some fruit and/or milk.
   - Enjoy Blueberry Coffee Cake; assemble the night before and bake in the morning as you get ready for the day (pp. 184–185).
3. **Choose proteins that are low in saturated fat.**
   - Enjoy an egg dish with vegetables.
   - Occasionally choose a small amount of chicken (not pork) sausage.
   - Try low-fat yogurt with Granola (p. 208) or yogurt smoothies.
   - Have a soy protein smoothie.
   - Add low-fat milk to cereal.
   - Have a Granola or Protein Bar (pp. 112–115).
   - Enjoy some Spinach Dip (p. 79) with a whole-grain bagel.
4. **Include some healthy fat.**

   Why:
   - Since fat slows digestion, small amounts at breakfast keep us feeling "full" longer.
   - Eating fats packaged with proteins (nuts, eggs, low-fat cheese, small portions of meat) leaves us satisfied without feeling "stuffed" like when we eat fats packaged with lots of carbohydrates.
   - It's best to consume most of your fats early in the day, when you have time to burn them for energy, instead of allowing them to convert to body fat.

   How:
   - Try Omega butter on toast.
   - Enjoy some yogurt or a slice of cheese.
   - Cook some eggs, or have hard-boiled ones ready in the fridge.
5. **Eat – even if it's in the car (though it's ideal to sit down at home).**
   - Keep Protein or Granola Bars in freezer (pp. 112–115).
   - Keep baggies filled with low-sugar Granola (p. 208) or finger-food cereals (e.g., O's or squares) packed and ready to grab.
   - Take a piece of toast or English muffin with Hummus (p. 49), heathlier-choice nut butter or all-fruit jelly or jam.
   - Enjoy a muffin (pp. 186–187).
   - Make a breakfast egg sandwich (pp. 108–109).

6. **Try some vegetables and fruits.**
   - Bake extra sweet potatoes for dinner. After they cool, peel and puree them with an immersion blender. Add ground ginger and 100% orange or apple juice to taste. Heat for breakfast.
   - Enjoy Sweet Potato Cakes (p. 89).
   - Try a Pumpkin Pie Smoothie (p. 106).
   - Add vegetables (e.g., peppers, spinach. leeks) to Fancy Scrambled Eggs (p. 109).
   - Add vegetables (e.g., tomatoes, bok choy, onions) to Breakfast Squares (p. 108).
   - Make extra roasted potatoes for dinner and save some to reheat and serve as "hash browns" with eggs.
   - When preparing dinner the night before, chop some vegetables for the next morning (e.g., leeks, onions, tomatoes, spinach, other greens). Use them for an omelet or a sautéed side to accompany any entrée.
   - Who says breakfast has to be traditional? Do not hesitate to use a favorite vegetable dish to jump-start your day!
7. **Offer choices.**
   We all like to choose, so have two or three options available. It could be as simple as having two different fruit choices for adding to cereal.
8. **Decide the night before.**
   When we plan ahead, we are more likely to go through with healthier eating. So decide what you'll eat and get it ready ... then enjoy it the next morning!

Rice 'n' Fruit

Combine and heat cooked brown rice, milk (any variety), dried fruit and a little honey for an easy, delicious and healthy breakfast.

All about Juice

Choose a whole fruit rather than juice when possible. A half cup of orange juice contains the juice of three oranges but only one-tenth the fiber of a single orange.

When you do enjoy juice with your breakfast:

- Limit it to about six ounces – the size of a typical juice glass. That's just enough to get a good taste of the juice and enough nutrients to be beneficial without overdoing the sugar.
- Eat before you drink. That way you don't fill up on juice before consuming other food.
- Choose 100% juice; avoid added sugars and flavorings.
- Look for variety and capitalize on the fruits with high antioxidant levels – try pomegranate or a cranberry or blueberry blend.

Yogurt, Fruit & Nuts

Mix plain or vanilla yogurt with fresh or thawed frozen fruit, chopped nuts, flaxseed meal and/or wheat germ for breakfast, snack or dessert.

If you are using sweetened yogurt, combine it with unsweetened. Begin with three-fourths sweetened and one-fourth plain, gradually using more plain.

Smoothies

Smoothies can be a great way to personalize your breakfast and create a meal that can travel with you. Some blenders are now sold with single-serving jars that detach and double as a mug, often fitting right into the cup holder of a car.

To create a smoothie, chose a fruit, a thickener (low-fat milk, low-fat yogurt, soy protein, nut milk) and a sweetener (juice, honey, agave nectar – but remember that there may be sweeteners in the yogurt or milk). If desired, add fiber (wheat germ, flaxseed meal, fiber blend) or soy protein isolate. You may also want to add seasonings (e.g., extracts, ground spices) and/or flavorings (e.g., cocoa). Ice cubes can be added as you blend it to make it cold, or simply use frozen fruit. The combinations are endless.

As you enjoy smoothies, there are numerous ways to transition away from higher sugars with empty calories and toward lower sugars with more nutrients.

- Include more fruit.
- Move away from sweetened yogurts and milks (you might mix half and half).
- Use different types of sweeteners and in smaller amounts. (If some family members desire more sweetener than others, allow them to stir small amounts into their individual serving rather than making the whole recipe with more sugar.)

Pumpkin Pie Smoothie

Mix: 10 minutes

This smoothie was inspired by Sondra's local health food store. They used banana; she chose applesauce. They used vanilla sweetener; she chose honey with vanilla extract. Use these ideas to create your own favorite.

1/2 cup frozen peaches or mangos (if measuring thawed, use half the amount)
1/2 cup unsweetened applesauce OR applesauce-apricot blend
1/2 (15 oz.) can pumpkin (best if chilled)
2 Tbsp. flaxseed meal
3/4 tsp. ground cinnamon
1/8 tsp. allspice
2 pinches salt
Freshly grated nutmeg
1 tsp. vanilla extract
1 Tbsp. sweetener—honey, agave nectar, pure maple syrup, sugar
2 cups milk (unsweetened soy, low-fat cow)

Add all ingredients in order listed to blender. **Blend** for 30 seconds or until smooth.

Yield: 4 (1 cup) servings   4 cups

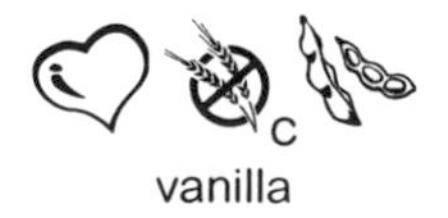

Analysis/Serving:
Calories: 117 (Fat Cal 28) Fat: 3.1g (0.3g Sat) Cholesterol: 0mg
Sodium: 64mg Carbs: 16g (4.2g Fiber 10g Sugar) Protein: 4.8g

Egg Cookery

The inexpensive egg is generally quick and easy to prepare and offers high-quality protein with a wide variety of nutrients, including high amounts of vitamins A and E as well as riboflavin and folate.

Proper handling of eggs is critical to reduce the risk of salmonella poisoning: (1) Keep eggs refrigerated at all times. (2) Discard cracked or broken eggs. (3) Cook completely, scrambling until no liquid remains and baking until internal temperature is 160° and a knife inserted comes out clean.

The Perfect Hard-Cooked Egg

1. Gently place cold eggs in saucepan. Add room temperature water to cover. Add a sprinkle of salt to help prevent shells from cracking.
2. Bring to gentle boil, remove from heat source and cover for 15 minutes, allowing the hot water to carryover-cook.
3. Refrigerate in uncracked shell for up to a week.

Top Ten Ways to Enjoy Eggs in Moderation

1. Try Fancy Scrambled Eggs.
2. Enjoy Breakfast Squares.
3. Eat Breakfast Pizza.
4. Top salads with hard-cooked eggs. Great on Beet Salad!
5. Add hard-cooked eggs to pasta or potato salads with pesto for dressing.
6. Use in a sandwich or tortilla wrap.
7. Fix them with roasted potatoes, peppers and onions.
8. Have them scrambled, for dinner, with asparagus and fresh fruit.
9. Enjoy your favorite way with pancakes. Complement with a vegetable and/or fruit side dish.
10. Eat them fried, with a slice of whole-wheat toast and a glass of pomegranate juice.

Healthy Egg for Heart Debate

Over the years, there has been much debate about the nutrition of eggs, especially when it comes to heart health.

Some of the benefits of eggs include:

- high-quality protein
- natural vitamin D
- quality antioxidants (especially lutein and zeaxanthin)
- choline (for brain function)
- unsaturated fats

It is true that eggs are high in cholesterol (over 200 mg. per egg). However, scientists are discovering that the way the body handles the cholesterol of an egg is not likely to affect the heart.[1] Moreover, numerous nutrients in eggs are likely to help the heart.[2] More research needs to be done, and those with diabetes are still being cautioned to limit consumption of eggs. Until we have more information, we recommend the moderate consumption of eggs; certainly don't ignore them!

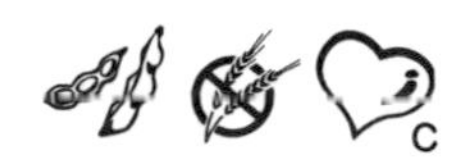

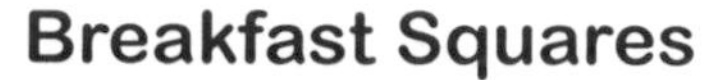

Breakfast Squares

S→O: 10 or more minutes   Bake: 30–40 minutes

This recipe provides the how part of the preparation. You determine what goes inside. Have fun and enjoy! The recipe can be divided by four and baked in single-serving bowls.

4 eggs, slightly beaten
1/2 cup milk (low-fat cow, unsweetened soy)
Seasoned garlic salt (p. 222) or other seasonings/fresh herbs (e.g., chives)
Any combination of 3–4 vegetables and/or meats (see below for some ideas)

Preheat oven—350°. **Oil** an 8x8-inch dish.

1. In bowl, **combine** eggs, milk, seasoning and desired vegetables (except tomatoes) and meats together. **Pour** into prepared dish.
2. **Bake** 30–40 minutes, or until puffy and golden brown and 160° internal temperature.
3. Allow to **set** 5 minutes. Cut into 4 squares.

To create your own "breakfast muffin to go," place square on toasted whole-grain English muffin. Or serve with Salsa (p. 91 or 153).

Yield: 4 servings

Vegetable and Meat Ideas

- 1 cup spinach (fresh baby or frozen)
- 1 cup diced tomatoes (canned or fresh) (sprinkle on top instead of stirring in)
- 1/2 cup diced sweet peppers
- 1/2 cup sliced mushrooms
- 1/2 cup other vegetables (e.g. onion, bok choy)
- 1/4 lb. ground sausage, cooked and drained (p. 232)
- 1/2 cup diced nitrate-free ham
- ~1 cup Sausage-Pepper-Onion Mix (p. 110)

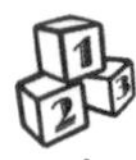

"Cheese, Please"

- Stir in two ounces of shredded low-fat cheese before baking.
- Or, sprinkle shredded low-fat cheese over top of eggs near the end of baking.

Do Ahead

- Do Step 1 the night before. Cover and store in refrigerator.
- In morning, gently stir with fork before baking.
- Bake while you prepare for the day.

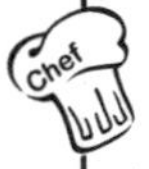

Different Tastes

If you are serving people with different tastes, add vegetables or meats to individual portions after pouring the egg mixture into the baking dish. For example, sprinkle sausage on half and tomatoes on half.

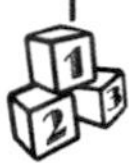

Our Favorite

- Fresh spinach
- Tomatoes
- Red onion
- Seasoned garlic salt (p. 222)

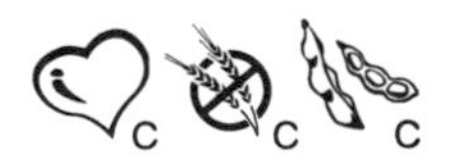

Analysis/Serving: (Our Favorite)
Calories: 112 (Fat Cal 47) Fat: 5.2g (1.8g Sat) Cholesterol: 214mg
Sodium: 256 Carbs: 8.5g (0.9g Fiber 8.2g Sugar) Protein: 8.4g

Fancy Scrambled Eggs

Many ingredients can be added to scrambled eggs to make this traditional breakfast favorite a fast, delicious and healthy meal for any time of the day. Here are some suggestions:

Vegetables

Bell peppers, diced
Cabbage, chopped or shredded
Garlic, minced
Green onions, sliced
Hot peppers, minced
Leeks, sliced
Mushrooms, sliced
Onion, chopped
Tomatoes, diced
Shallots, chopped
Zucchini, diced

Seasonings

Chili powder
Fresh herbs (e.g., parsley, cilantro, chives)
Freshly ground black pepper
Garlic powder
Red pepper flakes
Salt
Seasoned salt

Greens

Arugula, torn or chopped
Baby bok choy, chopped
Chard, torn or ribbon-cut
Spinach, torn or ribbon-cut

Meats & Cheeses

Low-fat cheese, shredded
Nitrate-free ham, diced
Cooked sausage, ground or sliced (p. 232)

Toppings

Low-fat cheese, shredded
Salsa
Tomatoes, diced, crushed or sautéed

1. In skillet, **sauté** vegetables and meats in small amount of oil until tender.
2. In bowl, **whisk** together eggs and seasonings. Add to skillet, stirring while **cooking** as with scrambled eggs.

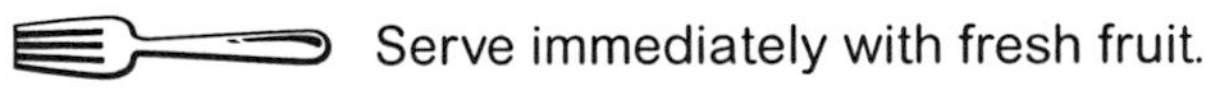
Serve immediately with fresh fruit.

For a fun twist, serve as a tortilla wrap. Use whole-grain or veggie tortilla (e.g., tomato, spinach).

Favorite Combos

Garden:
- Peppers
- Tomatoes
- Onions (any variety)
- Parsley

Deluxe:
- Tomatoes
- Bell peppers
- Sausage
- Onions
- Mushrooms

Farmers:
- Ham
- Cheese
- Spinach
- Onions

Dorie's Favorite:
- Leeks
- Baby bok choy
- Seasoned garlic salt (p. 222)

Sondra's Favorite:
- Leeks (or shallots)
- Spinach
- Cooked brown rice
- Seasoned garlic salt (p. 222)

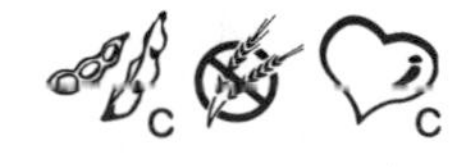

Breakfast Pizza

S→O: 5 minutes after crust and filling are ready
Bake: 25–30 minutes

1/2 pizza dough recipe (p. 168)
Filling of your choice (see below & next page)
4 oz. Monterey Jack cheese, shredded
4 eggs, slightly beaten
1/2 cup milk (low-fat cow, unsweetened soy)

Preheat oven—325°. **Oil** 9x13-inch dish.

1. In prepared dish, **push** (or roll, see equipment tip) dough out on bottom and ¼-inch up on sides. In a warm place, **proof** dough for 20–30 minutes.
2. *Meanwhile,* prepare filling.
3. With fork, **poke** holes in bottom of proofed crust.
3. **Layer** filling mixture and then cheese evenly over crust.
4. **Combine** eggs and milk (plus seasonings if using). **Pour** over cheese.
5. **Bake** in preheated oven 25–30 minutes, or until knife inserted in center comes out clean of egg (melted cheese may be on knife). Allow to **set** 5 minutes before slicing and serving.

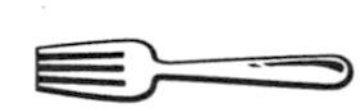

If desired, garnish with hot sauce or salsa.

Yield: 6 servings

Sausage-Pepper Breakfast Pizza

Use half batch of Sausage-Pepper-Onion Mix (see sidebar) and follow directions in above recipe using sausage mix as filling.

One-Handed Rolling Pin

A roller with a vertical handle works well for rolling out pizza dough.

Sausage-Pepper-Onion Mix

12 oz. ground chicken sausage, hot or sweet (p. 232)
1 lg. onion, chopped (2 cups)
1 (10 oz.) pkg. tri-color frozen peppers, diced OR 1 1/2 cups diced bell peppers

In skillet, **"Chop & Drop"** sausage, onions and peppers, sautéing until sausage is fully cooked. (Note: no oil is necessary since the fat from the sausage cooks the vegetables. If the skillet gets too dry, add some water.)

Freeze extra.

Yield: ~2 cups.

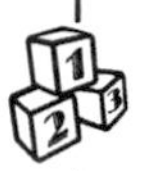

Other Filling and Seasoning Ideas

- Sliced mushrooms
- Baby spinach leaves
- Sautéed bok choy
- Seasoned garlic salt and/or fresh herbs.

Analysis/Serving:
Calories: 301 (Fat Cal 127) Fat: 14.1g (5.5g Sat) Cholesterol: 184mg
Sodium: 425mg Carbs: 32.4g (3g Fiber 10.7g Sugar) Protein: 18g

C C C

GF - see our websites (p. 242) for tips on using gluten-free pizza mixes with these recipes.

Southwestern Chicken Breakfast Pizza

Prepare Filling: ~12 minutes

8 oz. raw chicken chunks (small pieces)
1 med. onion, chopped (1 cup)
Salt, pepper, garlic powder
1 cup frozen corn
1/4 cup sliced olives (optional)
1 (15 oz.) can diced tomatoes w/ green chilies
OR 1 1/2 cups salsa (p. 91 or 153)

1. **Sauté** seasoned chicken and onion in water (see p. 61), stirring often until completely cooked. **Add** the corn when chicken is about half cooked.
2. **Stir** in olives and tomatoes (or salsa).
3. Follow directions on previous page to complete the Breakfast Pizza.

Ham-Leek-Asparagus Breakfast Pizza

Prepare Filling: ~12 minutes

1 cup sliced leeks
1 (10 oz.) pkg. frozen asparagus (cut 1/2-inch)
1/2 tsp. garlic powder
1 cup diced nitrate-free ham (5 oz.)

1. **Sauté** leeks, asparagus and garlic powder in water (see p. 61), stirring often until tender.
2. Follow directions on previous page to complete the Breakfast Pizza, sprinkling vegetable mixture, then ham for the filling.

Spicy Southwestern Bean Breakfast Pizza

Stir 1/4 cup sliced olives into 1 1/2 cups of Bean-Corn Salsa (p. 91). Follow directions on previous page for assembling.

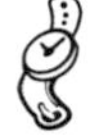

Advanced Prep

The pizza crust dough can be prepared in advance.

Simply shape it in the baking dish, allowing it to proof for 20 minutes. Cover and refrigerate. Allow it to come to room temperature before continuing with recipe.

or

Prepare Crust in Advance: Instead of using oil, line the baking dish with parchment paper (have the paper come up on two sides). Then do Steps 1 and 3 as described in recipe on previous page. Bake in preheated oven for 5 minutes. Immediately transfer crust to cooling rack. After cool, wrap and freeze. Thaw; continue with recipe as written.

Analysis/Serving for Southwestern Chicken
Calories: 350 (Fat Cal 129) Fat: 14.3g (4.8g Sat) Cholesterol: 183mg
Sodium: 595mg Carbs: 38.7g (3.2g Fiber 13.8g Sugar) Protein: 22g

Analysis/Serving for Ham-Leek-Asparagus
Calories: 300 (Fat Cal 120) Fat: 13.3g (5g Sat) Cholesterol: 176mg
Sodium: 365mg Carbs: 32.6g (3.3g Fiber 11.9g Sugar) Protein: 19g

Analysis/Serving for Spicy Southwestern Bean
Calories: 301 (Fat Cal 120) Fat: 13.3g (4.5g Sat) Cholesterol: 182mg
Sodium: 440mg Carbs: 36g (3.4g Fiber 11g Sugar) Protein: 16g

C C C

GF - see page 110.

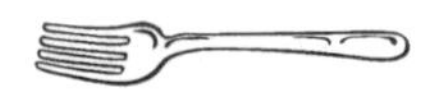

The Granola Bars on these two pages and the Protein Bars on the following two pages make great:

- after-school snacks
- breakfast on the go
- school lunches
- gifts (see below)

Gift Giving

Granola or Protein Bars make great gifts. Consider them for:

- mission trips
- college or high school student care packages
- exam week care packages
- holiday gifts bags

Little Chefs

Great recipe for children to be involved:

- measuring
- packing bags (lunches, snacks, gifts/care packages)
- decorating bags or cards to go inside
- helping with mixing
- helping with pressing batter into pans

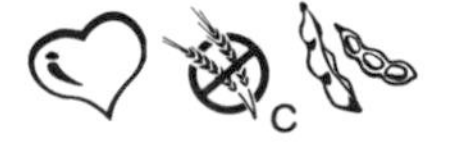

Chocolate Chip Crispy Granola Bars

S→O: 15 minutes   Bake: 15 minutes (10 minutes for GF)

1/2 cup raisins (or dried apricots; ~3 oz.)
1/2 cup semi-sweet chocolate chips
1/2 cup quick oats
3/4 cup brown rice crispy cereal
OR cocoa brown rice crispy cereal
1/8 tsp. salt (optional)
2 Tbsp. flaxseed meal
1/4 cup raw sunflower seeds
1/4 cup raw pumpkin seeds
1/3 cup sweetener—brown rice syrup, honey or agave nectar
1/2 cup healthier-choice "nut" butter
(peanut, almond or cashew)
1–3 Tbsp. water (depends upon thickness of "nut" butter)

Fruity Crispy Granola Bars

- Omit chocolate chips.
- Use a total of 1 cup (~ 6 oz.) raisins or dried fruit.
- Decrease sweetener to 1/4 cup.

Granola Bars

- Omit brown rice crispy cereal.
- Use 1 1/4 cups quick oats.
  (Can make either "Chocolate Chip" or "Fruity")

Gluten-Free Granola Bars

- Omit oats.
- Use 1 1/4 cups gluten-free (cocoa) brown rice crispy cereal.

(Can be made either "Fruity" or "Chocolate Chip")

Kid-Friendly Granola Bars

Some people, especially children, do not like large pieces of nuts or seeds. If this is your situation, grind the seeds with the dried fruit and chocolate chips. Or omit the seeds and use a total of 1/3 cup additional quick oats and/or crispy rice cereal.

Directions for all granola bars.

Preheat oven—325°.
At Step 3, **oil** an 8x8x2-inch glass baking dish.

1. Place dried fruit and chocolate chips (if using) in bowl of mini food processor/chopper. Cover and **process** until semi-finely chopped. (Raisins and apricots get gummy if processed alone. If not using chocolate chips, add the flaxseed meal and/or the sunflower and pumpkin seeds with the raisins before processing.)
2. In large bowl, place fruit mixture, oats and/or crispy rice cereal, salt, flaxseed meal and seeds (if not ground with fruit). **Stir** to combine. **Drizzle** sweetener evenly over the mixture. **Spoon** nut butter as evenly as possible over mixture. **Mix** with rubber spatula.
3. Oil hands while preparing baking dish. With oil-coated hands, continue to **mix** until well combined, gradually adding water as needed to get batter to hold together.
4. Transfer batter into prepared baking dish. Spread batter evenly and **press** firmly with hands. **Bake** in preheated oven 15 minutes (only 10 minutes for gluten-free versions).

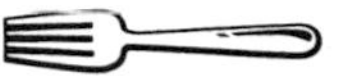 Allow to cool in baking dish. Cut 4x2.

 Package individually in snack-sized plastic bags. Store in refrigerator. If keeping over a week, store in freezer.

Yield: 8 servings/bars.

Great Math!

There are many things to measure in this recipe. And do kids ever love to measure and pour! Talk with your child about the measurements: how many ¼ cups would make a ½ cup? 1¼ cups? Your child will be learning fractions without even knowing! If you have a small kitchen scale, allow your child to weigh out ½ cup of raisins. Is it close to 3 ounces? Even if your little one is just watching from a backpack on your back, have her count with you as you pour things in.

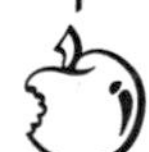

Healthy Bites

These granola bars are higher in fiber and protein than the typical packaged granola bar (often by a third) and much lower in sodium (often by three-quarters).

A Little Fat Is Good

The modest amount of fat in these granola bars is important if they will be used as a breakfast food.

Analysis for one Chocolate Chip Crispy Granola Bar/Fruity Crispy Granola Bar:
Calories: 320/284 (Fat Cal 147/119) Fat: 16/13g (3/2g Sat) Cholesterol: 0mg
Sodium: 81/74 Carbs: 37/34g (4/4g Fiber 21/18g Sugar) Protein: 8/8g

Analysis for one Granola Bar (Chocolate Chip/Fruity):
Calories: 339/304 (Fat Cal 152/123) Fat: 17/14g (3/2g Sat) Cholesterol: 0mg
Sodium: 66/59 Carbs: 40/37g (5/5g Fiber 21/18g Sugar) Protein: 9/9g

Analysis for one Gluten-Free Granola Bar (Chocolate Chip/Fruity):
Calories: 307/271 (Fat Cal 145/116) Fat: 16/13g (3/2g Sat) Cholesterol: 0mg
Sodium: 91/84 Carbs: 37/33g (4/4g Fiber 21/18g Sugar) Protein: 8/7g

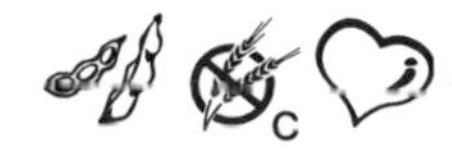

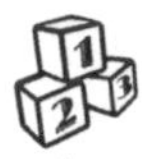

Other Flour Choices

1/4 cup whole-wheat pastry flour

- - - - -

1/4 cup + 2 Tbsp. whole-grain spelt flour

Doubling the Recipe

This recipe successfully doubles, using three whole eggs. The easiest method with double the ingredients is as follows:

- Perform Step 1 as described.
- In bowl, whisk together flour, soy protein, flaxseed meal, baking powder and salt. Set aside.
- Use stand mixer with flat beater.
- In mixer bowl, whisk together oil, sweetener and eggs.
- Add flour mixture; mix on low to just combine.
- Add fruit mixture; mix on low to just combine.
- Proceed with Step 3 using a 9x13x2-inch baking dish. Bake 22 minutes. Cut bars 8x2 for 16 servings.

Protein Bars

S→O: 15 minutes Bake: 18 minutes

1/2 cup raisins (~3 oz.)
1/2 cup dried apricots (~3 oz.)
1/2 cup walnuts
1 cup regular *or* quick oats
1/4 cup "white" whole-wheat flour
(see sidebar for other flour options)
1/2 cup soy protein isolate (p. 89)
2 Tbsp. flaxseed meal
1 tsp. baking powder
1/8 tsp. salt
1 Tbsp. Medium-Heat oil
1/4 cup sweetener—honey *or* agave nectar
1 whole egg
1 egg white *or* yolk

Preheat oven—325°.
At Step 3, **oil** an 8x8x2-inch glass baking dish.

1. Using chopper blade, **process** dried fruit and nuts in food processor until finely chopped. Add oats and process to coarsely **chop**. (If using quick oats, process only to mix).
2. **Sprinkle** dry ingredients (flour, soy protein, flaxseed meal, baking powder and salt) evenly on top of fruit mixture. Process to **combine**. **Drizzle** oil, sweetener and egg evenly over batter. **Process** to gently combine.
3. Oil hands while preparing baking dish. With oil-coated hands, continue to mix until well combined; transfer to baking dish. **Spread** evenly; **press** firmly. **Bake** in preheated oven 18 minutes, or until toothpick comes out clean and bars are just golden brown around edges.

 Allow to cool in baking dish. Cut 4x2.

 See next page sidebar for storage hints.

Yield: 8 servings/bars

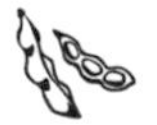

Analysis/Bar:
Calories: 268 (Fat Cal 83) Fat: 9.6g (1.1g Sat) Cholesterol: 40mg
Sodium: 199mg Carbs: 33.7g (3.5g Fiber 20.4g Sugar) Protein: 13.3g

Gluten-Free Protein Bars

S→O: 15 minutes   Bake: 18 minutes

1/2 cup raisins (~3 oz.)
1/2 cup dried apricots (~3 oz.)
1/2 cup walnuts
1/4 cup Bob's Red Mill Gluten-Free Baking MIx
1/2 cup soy protein isolate (p. 89)
2 Tbsp. flaxseed meal
1 tsp. baking powder
1/8 tsp. salt
1/4 tsp. xanthan gum
1 Tbsp. Medium-Heat oil
1/4 cup sweetener—honey or agave nectar
1 large egg
1 cup gluten-free brown rice crispy cereal

Preheat oven—325°.
At Step 4, **oil** an 8x8x2-inch glass baking dish.

1. Using chopper blade, **process** dried fruit and nuts in food processor until finely chopped
2. **Sprinkle** dry ingredients (flour, soy protein, flaxseed meal, baking powder, salt and xanthan gum) evenly on top of fruit mixture. Process to **combine**. **Drizzle** oil, sweetener and egg evenly over batter. **Process** to gently combine.
3. Transfer batter to bowl. **Mix** in cereal.
4. Do Step 3 as described in Protein Bars (p. 114).

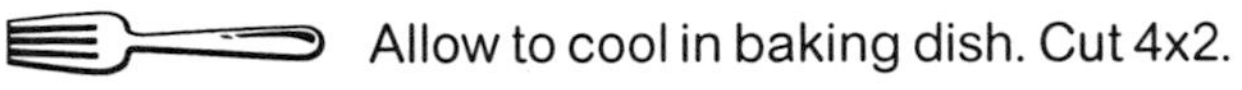

Allow to cool in baking dish. Cut 4x2.

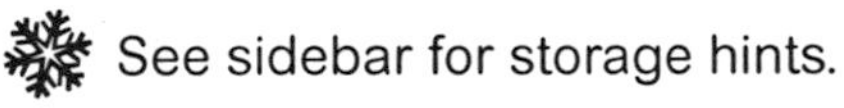

See sidebar for storage hints.

Yield: 8 servings/bars

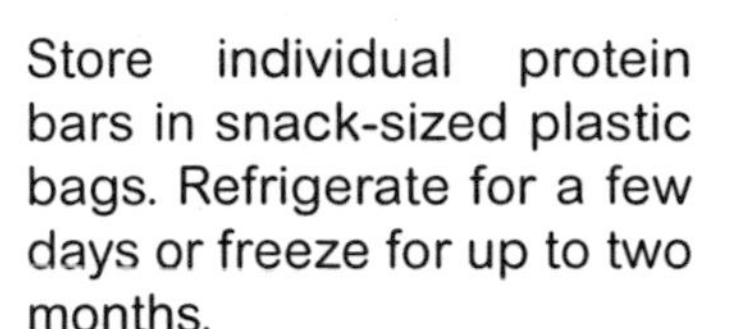

Storage Hint

Store individual protein bars in snack-sized plastic bags. Refrigerate for a few days or freeze for up to two months.

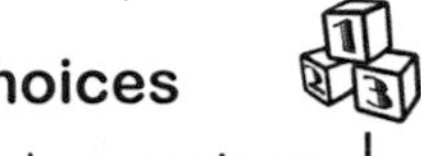

Fruit Choices

These protein bar recipes have been tested with all raisins and with prunes in place of either raisins or apricots.

Healthy Bites

Check the Ingredients: Many companies are using artificial sweeteners in place of sugar in their protein bars so that they can claim fewer calories. We strongly discourage the consumption of artificial sweeteners (p. 17).

Gluten free, not flavor free! In an attempt to make up for lost flavor when removing gluten-containing grains, many companies increase the levels of fat and sugar. Our protein bars are typically lower in fats and sugars and higher in protein ... and the taste is still great!

Analysis/Bar:
Calories: 242 (Fat Cal 78)   Fat: 9g (1g Sat)   Cholesterol: 40mg
Sodium: 219mg   Carbs: 29.9g (2.4g Fiber 20.3g Sugar)   Protein: 11.6g

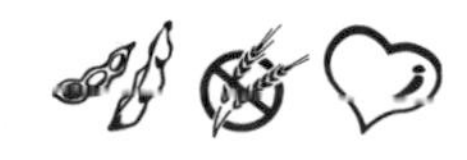

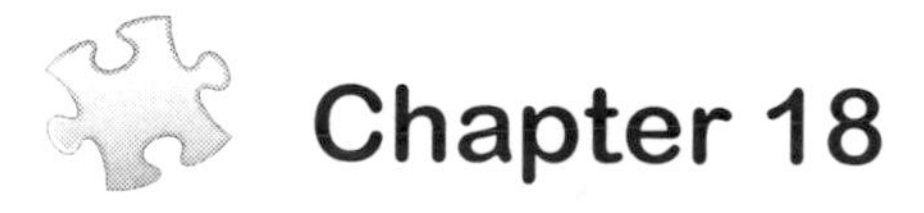

Chapter 18

Travel Lunches

Eating away from home can be a challenge, especially if it's something we have to do every day at work or school. Eating out can be expensive, is not always practical and is rarely as healthy as eating at home. But packing a lunch when we're rushing to leave for the day isn't always easy. There are many prepackaged foods, from entrées to snacks and desserts. But these are often high in sodium, sugar and saturated fat.

The trick to making travel lunches (or other meals) quickly and in a healthy manner comes with developing a list of things you and your family like and finding ways to have those things easily accessible for you to grab and go.

Here are some ways to use your dinner preparation the night before to prepare the travel meal for the next day.

Cook extra so you can take the leftovers. Before you do the dinner dishes, package lunch-sized portions of the meal in containers that can travel. Put them in the fridge for the next morning or the freezer for whenever they are needed. Some of our recipes that make great lunches the next day include the following:

- Any salad – pages 74 and 96–102 (carry dressing in small container)
- Any soup (some are good cold; others can travel in insulated container) – pages 118–132
- Any oven-fried chicken – pages 98 and 144
- Any roast (beef, pork, poultry) – pages 156–157
    - o Slice for a sandwich (can freeze in baggies for sandwiches whenever)
    - o Ground in mini food processor for base for sandwich wraps – page 160
    - o Dice or shred for a salad
    - o Warm up and eat as you did the night before
- Many casseroles (if you have a way to warm them) – pages 133, 134, 138 and 150.

Cook extra so you can prepare something new for the next day:

- Make extra Oven Fries (p. 76) so you have enough to make Roasted Potato Salad (see easy method on p. 45).
- When slicing vegetables or fruit for soups, casseroles and salads, slice extra and put them in baggies for the next few days.

- When washing salad greens, wash a few extra and put them in a small carry dish. It will be all set for creating a salad with leftovers or things in the fridge. (Assemble salad while your dinner cooks or just before doing the dinner dishes.)

Use your meal prep time to cook something additional:

- While dinner is cooking or baking, hard-cook some eggs for a salad.
- While cooking, eating and doing dishes, poach or bake a chicken breast for salads or sandwiches.

"Extras" to keep on hand that can round out any travel lunch (also, see chapter twenty-three):

- Breads, including tortillas for cool sandwich wraps (see p. 191 for breads and p. 153 and 160 for sandwich wrap ideas)
- Nitrate-free ham slices and luncheon meats (for healthier-choice brands, see p. 231)
- Yogurt (see Yogurt, Fruit & Nuts on p. 105)
- Granola
- Sliced raw vegetables
- Fresh fruits
- Unsweetened applesauce
- Pretzels (see p. 166)
- Whole-grain crackers
- Sliced or cubed low-fat cheese
- Baggies of nuts or seeds. If purchasing roasted, compare labels to get lowest added sodium and sugars. We recommend purchasing raw and toasting them yourself (see sidebar). To save money, purchase nuts and seeds in larger quantities and individually bag in snack-sized baggies.
- Bags of trail mix. It's cheaper to create your own (see sidebar) and then you control the quality of ingredients. Bag in snack-sized baggies.

Seasoned Nuts-Seeds

Toasting: See Step 1 on Pesto recipe (p. 93) on how to toast nuts. Harder or denser nuts (such as almond and Brazil nuts) or mixed nuts will take a little longer toasting time.

Flavoring: Mix up a few spices and/or crushed dried herbs (crush between your fingers) with water and syrup-type sweetener (e.g., honey, brown rice syrup, agave nectar). The water is to dilute the sweetener so you can coat the nuts and seeds without raising the empty calorie nutrition of them. Use caution if adding salt. We use very little and let the spices and herbs offer the flavor.

Coating: Place nuts and seeds in a single layer on baking sheet with sides. Drizzle sweetener mixture evenly over them while stirring to coat. Stir about every ten minutes during both toasting and cooling time so they do not stick together.

Trail Mix

Combine Granola (p. 208; adding nuts/seeds and little more water before baking), unsweetened, unsulfured dried fruit and/or semi-sweet chocolate chips.

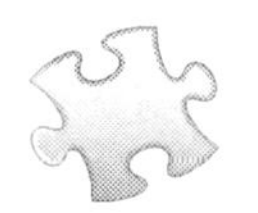

Chapter 19

Soups, Stews and Casserole Meals

Soups and stews are wonderful, warm comfort foods in the winter, and some soups offer a light meal in the dog days of summer. Soups, stews and casseroles can offer a great way to use "the extras," provide a hearty, nutrient-dense meal in and of themselves (or with a side dish, such as salad or fruit) and can be prepared in large quantities to freeze and enjoy on those "no time" days. Enjoy creating and eating.

Choosing a Soup Base

There are many packaged broths and creamy soups available. One of the most important things to consider when purchasing a soup base is the type of ingredients included. Many contain numerous preservatives, additives and flavorings, including MSG and corn syrup. By contrast, there are also many soups and broths, several of them organic, that use only vegetables, poultry/meat (if appropriate), seasonings/spices and oil. You can taste the difference in quality and feel better about the food you are consuming.

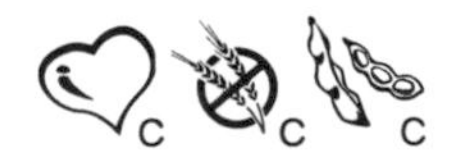

Quick Basic Soup

Base Choices:

Lower sodium broth—chicken, beef, vegetable
Canned tomatoes
Prepared cream soups (see sidebar)

Protein Choices:

Chicken or turkey chunks (raw or cooked)
Roast beef or pork (shredded, cooked)
Edamame beans (p. 101)
Peas, fresh or frozen
Tofu

Vegetable Choices: (dice/slice/shred)

Asparagus, frozen
Broccoli
Cabbage (green/napa)
Carrots
Celery
Frozen mix (p. 232)
Green beans
Leeks (p. 67)
Onion (any color)
Radishes (offers a slight sweet flavor; red/purple radishes color broth slightly)
Summer squash

Starch Choices:

Corn, frozen whole kernel
Potatoes (diced)
Whole-grain or gluten-free pasta (any shape)

Last-Minute Choices:
Freshly minced garlic (may divide)
Tomatoes (cherry/grape; whole/sliced)
Spinach (baby leaves or ribbon-cut)

Sauté onions with raw meat and seasonings in oil or some of the broth. **"Chop & Drop"** other vegetables. Add liquid (combo of broth and water). If using, add cooked meats. **Simmer**, so flavors "marry" and vegetables cook until tender. (Potatoes may need to be pushed down into the liquid to speed their cooking process.) Add dry pasta during last 6–12 minutes (or whenever your brand will be cooked al dente). **Add** last-minute choices, cooked pasta and fresh herbs during last 2–3 minutes. If desired, garnish freshly snipped chives.

Slow Cooker Chowder

Prep for slow cooker: 10 minutes

1 lb. raw chicken breast chunks
1 small onion, chopped (1/2 cup)
1 cup sliced or diced carrots
Salt, pepper, dried parsley
1 (10 oz.) pkg. frozen broccoli cuts
1/2 (10 oz.) pkg. frozen corn
1 (32 oz.) pkg. creamy potato leek soup (p. 230)

Standard-size slow cooker

In skillet, **sauté** chicken, onions, carrots and seasonings in oil until browned. **Add** to slow cooker along with other vegetables and soup. **Cook** on LOW for 3–4 hours.

Serve with shredded cheese stirred in or sprinkled on top.

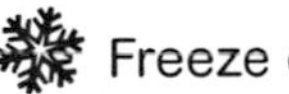

Freeze extra.

Yield: 6 servings

Analisis/Serving:
Calories: 206 (Fat Cal 36) Fat: 4g (.5g Sat) Cholesterol: 42mg
Sodium: 429mg Carbs: 23g (4.4g Fiber 6.2g Sugar) Protein: 19g

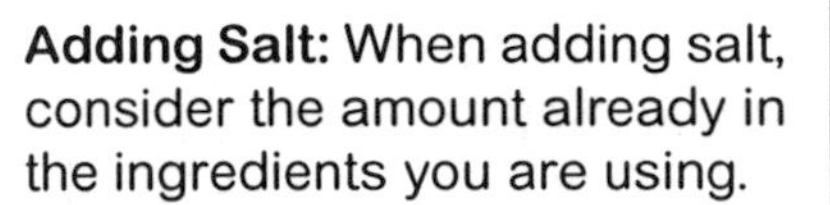

Sodium

Adding Salt: When adding salt, consider the amount already in the ingredients you are using.

Soups/Broths: Many packaged soups and broths have close to 1000 mg. of sodium per cup. We have found that some brands are now offering options with between 100 and 200 mg. per cup, providing enough salt for flavor but not so much that it is unhealthy.

Tomatoes: At the time this book is going to print, most canned tomatoes contain ridiculously high levels of sodium (often 800–1000 mg. per cup), yet the "no salt added" versions lack flavor. Until the industry finds a good compromise, we suggest using a mixture (when possible) of salted and "no salt added" tomatoes. It is also easier to get by with the unsalted tomatoes in recipes that are spicier and/or that simmer longer. If you are using both broth and tomatoes in the same recipe, try the lower sodium broth with the salted tomatoes. Sondra has found a brand of Tuscan-style tomatoes that were low in sodium but high in flavor. They make great Italian dishes (see p. 137).

Beans: See page 123 for information on choosing beans.

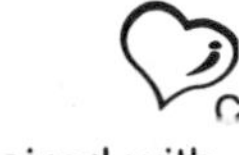

paired with

Appeal to Kids

- Reduce kale to 3 cups.
- Double the amount of carrots and chicken.
- Use chicken thighs for richer flavor.
- Omit dill if children do not like green flecks on their food (add dill for adults later).
- Scoop out pieces of carrot, chicken and/or kale for your children to eat with whole-grain pasta or brown rice.

Healthy Bites

Good for the Eyes: Kale contains both lutein and zeaxanthin, key nutrients for eye health and the prevention of macular degeneration.

Autumn Treat: Kale is sweetest after a good frost.

Heart Health: Carrots are a rich source of beta-carotene, an antioxidant proven to reduce blood cholesterol levels and reduce the risk of heart disease.

Grilled Chicken Kale-Carrot Soup

S→T: 45 minutes

This recipe includes a range on the quantity of salt; use less if including rice or pasta or adding crackers (see next page for making healthier choices). Also, sometimes a little more salt is needed if carrots or kale are not at their prime flavor.

2 cups low-sodium chicken broth
3 cups water
1 small onion, finely chopped (1/2 cup)
4 med-sized kale leaves, ribbon-cut (4 cups loosely packed)
1/4–3/8 tsp. salt
1 tsp. dried dill
Freshly ground pepper, as desired
2 med. carrots, sliced/diced (1 cup)
8 oz. raw chicken thighs or breasts/tenders (cut into small chunks)
1 cup water

1. In large pan, bring broth, 3 cups of water, onion, kale and seasonings to boil. Reduce heat, cover and **simmer** for 15 minutes. Add carrots and **simmer** an additional 15–20 minutes.
2. *Meanwhile,* in skillet **sauté** chicken (seasoned lightly with salt and dill) in a teaspoon of oil, stirring occasionally to brown evenly. **Add** to soup. **Deglaze** skillet with the final cup of water. Add to soup.

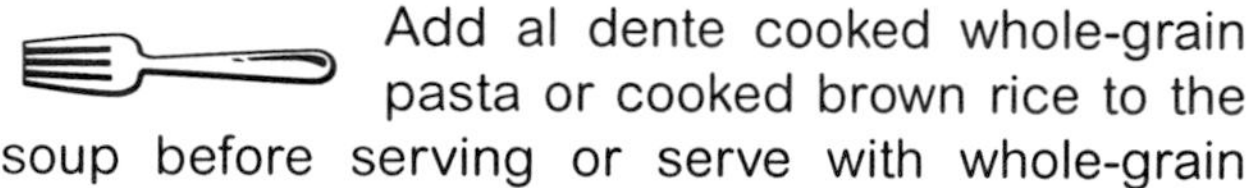

Add al dente cooked whole-grain pasta or cooked brown rice to the soup before serving or serve with whole-grain bread, whole-grain crackers and/or cheese.

Complement the meal with fresh or frozen fruit with a drizzle of plain yogurt.

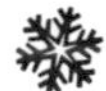 Freeze extra.

Yield: 3 servings 6 cups

Analysis/Serving:
Calories: 190 (Fat Cal 54) Fat: 6g (1g Sat) Cholesterol: 66mg
Sodium: 430–518 Carbs: 16.4g (3.3g Fiber 3.1g Sugar) Protein: 19.1g

Beef Barley Soup

Prep for slow cooker: 25 minutes Cook: 6–10 hours

Beef barley soup is a popular comfort food; however, a typical purchased version can contain 1,300 mg. of sodium per a one and half cup serving. This recipe, packed with nutrition and flavor, has 69% less sodium.

1 Tbsp. High-Heat oil
3/4 lb. round beef steak (bite-sized pieces)
1 lg. onion, chopped (2 cups)
1/2 cup dry hulled barley (rinse and drain)
1/2 tsp. salt
2 tsp. dried thyme
1 Tbsp. Worcestershire sauce
2 cloves garlic, minced
4 cups water (divided)
2 cups beef broth
2 ribs celery, sliced (1 cup)
2 cups sliced carrots
3 cups thick half-sliced zucchini squash
1 (10 oz.) pkg. frozen green beans
1 med. leaf kale, ribbon-cut (1 cup packed)
1 handful fresh parsley, minced (~1/4 cup)

Standard-sized Slow Cooker

1. In skillet, "**Chop & Drop**" beef through garlic in oil to brown meat and toast barley. Transfer to slow cooker. Add 1 cup of the water to skillet. Heat while whisking to **deglaze** the pan. Add to slow cooker.
2. *Meanwhile,* prepare and add remaining ingredients with 3 cups of the water to slow cooker. **Cook** on LOW for 6–8 hours; if desired, keep on warm for up to for 2 hours.

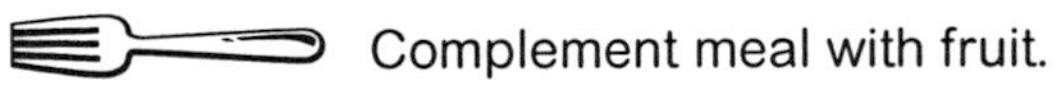
Complement meal with fruit.

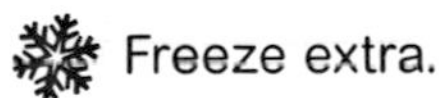
Freeze extra.

Yield: 8 (1 1/2-cup) servings 12 cups

Adding Crackers to Soup

Many people enjoy having crackers with their soup. Crackers can be a healthy addition to a meal, providing we make some simple choices:

- **Which cracker?** Typical oyster crackers and saltines list twelve to fifteen ingredients (many of them preservatives) and 170 mg. of sodium per handful. Some healthier brands have only four to six ingredients and 60 mg. of sodium.
- **Waiter, there's salt in my soup!** If you plan to enjoy soup with crackers, remember that they usually contain high amounts of sodium. When tasting for seasoning, go for a little less than you think is needed, knowing more will come from the crackers.

Seasoned Croutons (p. 190) can be used in soup in place of crackers.

Helpful Hint!

Soup can be prepped and refrigerated in the removable crock of a slow cooker the night before. Allow 8 to 10 hours for cooking the next day.

Analysis/Serving
Calories: 198 (Fat Cal 53) Fat: 5.9g (1.5g Sat) Cholesterol: 45mg
Sodium: 399 Carbs: 21.9g (5.3g Fiber 5.2g Sugar) Protein: 15.9g

Timing

Step 1: 5 minutes. Do the night before serving.

Step 2: 10 minutes (use food processor to prep onions and garlic). Do this in the a.m.

-- OR --

To save time in the morning, prep onions and garlic and measure out seasonings the night before when washing beans.

Immersion Blender

An immersion blender offers a safe, easy way to blend foods directly in the cooking pan.

For easy clean-up, choose a unit that separates, allowing the portion that touches the food to be washed in the dishwasher.

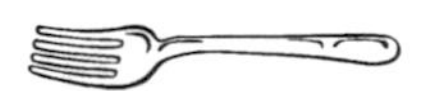

Garnish Ideas

- Diced onion
- Frozen peas, thawed
- Salsa (p. 91 or 153)
- Low-fat sour cream or low-fat plain unsweetened yogurt
- Shredded low-fat cheese

Slow Cooker Black Bean Soup

Prep for slow cooker: 15 minutes (see sidebar)

2 cups dry black beans
1 lg. onion, finely chopped (2 cups)
1 Tbsp. Medium-Heat oil
2 cloves garlic, minced
4 tsp. chili powder (divided)
2 tsp. ground cumin (divided)
5 cups water
1 Tbsp. cornstarch
1 tsp. salt

Standard-sized slow cooker

1. **Prepare Beans:** Rinse and drain beans a couple of times. Place in a 2-quart bowl. Fill with water (enough to allow beans to double). Cover and allow to soak for 8–10 hours, at room temperature or in the refrigerator.
2. Before cooking, drain off water. **Rinse** to remove the starchy substance. **Add** beans, onion, oil, garlic, half the amount of seasonings and water to slow cooker. **Stir** to combine.
3. **Slow-cook** for 8–10 hours on LOW, or until beans are tender.
4. Remove small amount of broth to a bowl. Whisk in remaining seasonings, cornstarch and salt until smooth. **Stir** into soup. Partially **puree** beans with immersion blender (see sidebar). Slow-cook 20 minutes to blend flavors. *Meanwhile,* preparing garnishes and salad.

Garnish individual servings (see sidebar). Serve with large mixed greens salad with Balsamic Vinaigrette Salad Dressing (p. 70) and fresh/frozen fruit.

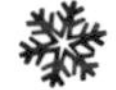

Freeze extra. Flavors are enhanced when reheated.

Yield: 6 servings   6 3/4 cups

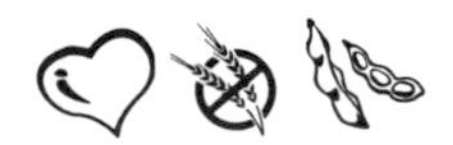

Analysis/Serving:
Calories: 273 (Fat Cal 27) Fat: 3g (0.3g Sat) Cholesterol: 0mg
Sodium: 365mg Carbs: 48.6g (16g Fiber 2.3g Sugar) Protein: 14g

Black Bean Soup

S→T: 45 minutes

1 lg. onion, finely chopped (2 cups)
Sprinkle of salt
1 Tbsp. Medium-Heat oil
4 (15 oz.) cans black beans, undrained
(with added salt; see below)
Water, if needed
2 cloves garlic, minced
4 tsp. chili powder
2 tsp. ground cumin

1. In saucepan, **sauté** onions with salt in oil until tender, stirring often.
2. **Add** beans and their liquid, partially **mashing** with fork. Add water, garlic and seasonings. Bring to boil, reduce heat, cover and **simmer** for 30 minutes to blend flavors, stirring occasionally. *Meanwhile,* prepare soup garnishes (see sidebar on previous page) and salads.

   Or add sautéed onions along with remaining ingredients to standard-sized slow cooker. Slow-cook for 3–4 hours on LOW.

Garnish individual servings and serve the same as Slow Cooker Black Bean Soup.

Yield: 6 servings 6 1/2 cups

Beans and Sodium

Canned beans come with and without salt. Those cooked and packed in salt have more flavor, but they often have high amounts of sodium. Pouring off the liquid reduces the sodium content in the recipe but also removes some of the nutrients. When unsalted cooked beans are simmered with other foods, they slowly begin to absorb those flavors and seasonings. Mashing the beans with a fork speeds up this process. (Likewise, using an immersion blender to partially puree the beans in Slow Cooker Black Bean Soup helps these beans to absorb more of the flavor of the spices.)

If you prefer the texture of whole beans, mash only the beans that have not been salted. Or pour some of the beans into the pot and mash the remaining beans in the can before adding.

Beans and Sodium continued: At the time this book went to print, some companies were beginning to use smaller amounts of salt in their salted beans. This recipe was created with the aim of having a total of from 400 to 500 mg. of sodium coming from the beans themselves. This can be achieved by using two cans of beans with added salt that contain 140 mg. of sodium per half cup serving and two cans of "no salt added" beans *or* by using four cans of lower sodium beans that contain around 80 mg. of sodium per half cup serving.

Analysis/Serving:
Calories: 300 (Fat Cal 22) Fat: 2.4g (0.2g Sat) Cholesterol: 0mg
Sodium: 197mg Carbs: 50g (11g Fiber 4.7g Sugar) Protein: 16.8g

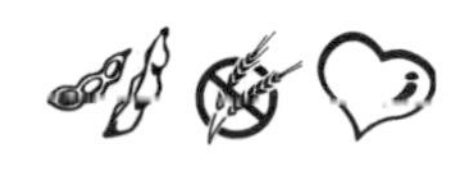

Caramelized Soups

The following is a collection of soup recipes so versatile (the method and ingredients can be changed to meet a variety of needs) and so flavorful that they are sure to satisfy a variety of taste buds. They are complete meals in and of themselves.

The secret of these soups is that each one is built on caramelizing onions and then browning the meat/poultry to absorb that flavor. Even people who do not like onions often enjoy these soups since the caramelization renders the texture and appearance of the onions virtually unnoticeable. It also brings out the natural sugars in the onions, making their flavor sweeter and more appealing to those who resist an onion taste. This rich flavor is the signature mark of these soups.

The other secret to these soups is that the meat/poultry (except for the sausage) is "marinated" in Worcestershire sauce as it is browning. It can be omitted for a gluten-free meal by adding slightly more salt (e.g., ⅛ teaspoon).

Once the flavors are established in the meat/poultry, the vegetables and liquids are added and arranged according to preference.

The cooking method can also be arranged to meet your needs:

- **Heading out for the afternoon and want to return to a home-cooked meal?** Caramelize the onions, brown the meat/poultry and combine everything in the slow cooker to simmer on **LOW for 3 to 4 hours**.
- **Putting this together during a child's afternoon nap?** Caramelize the onions, brown the meat/poultry and heat the remaining ingredients in saucepan before adding to slow cooker. Allow the flavors to "marry" for **1 to 2 hours on HIGH**.
- **Needing a meal in less than 45 minutes?** Caramelize the onions, brown the meat/poultry and then add the crunchy vegetables to sauté in the skillet. If the skillet is large enough, add the liquids and simmer until cooked through and vegetables are tender, and then add the quick-cooking ingredients (e.g., spinach, pasta). (If skillet is too small, transfer sautéed ingredients to a stockpot before proceeding.)

Food Processor

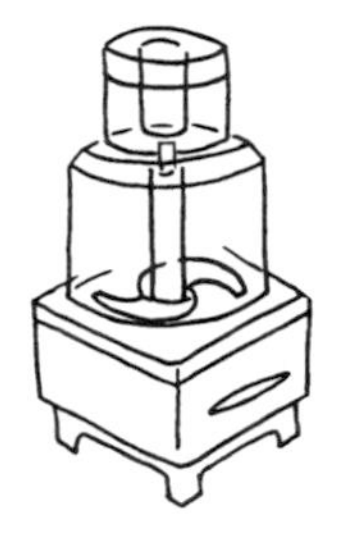

A food processor is great time saver for slicing onions, especially when doing a large quantity. It is also great to chop, slice and shred cabbage, carrots, nuts, etc. *And* it doubles as dough mixer.

Hamburger Soup

Prep for slow cooker: 30 minutes

1 Tbsp. High-Heat oil
1 1/2 lg. onions, sliced (3 cups)
1 lb. lean ground beef
3/4 tsp. salt (divided)
1/2 tsp. garlic powder
2 tsp. dried thyme
1 tsp. dried oregano
1 Tbsp. Worcestershire sauce

1 cup sliced celery
1 cup sliced carrots
1/2 (6 oz.) can tomato paste
1 cup beef broth
3 1/2–4 cups water (divided)

6 oz. dry whole-wheat pasta
1/4 (10 oz.) pkg. frozen cut spinach

Standard-sized slow cooker

1. In skillet, **sauté** onions in oil with ¼ teaspoon of the salt until semi-caramelized (approximately 15–20 minutes). **Add** meat, rest of the salt, seasonings and Worcestershire sauce, stirring often until meat is **browned**.
2. *Meanwhile*, **prepare** celery and carrots, adding to slow cooker with tomato paste and broth.
3. Transfer meat mixture to slow cooker. Add 1 cup of water to skillet. Heat while whisking to **deglaze** the pan. Add to slow cooker with remaining water. **Stir**.
4. **Cook** as desired (see p. 124 for options).
5. **Cook** pasta without salt slightly under al dente (p. 137), drain, return to pan and toss with an extra ⅛ teaspoon of salt.
6. **Add** spinach and cooked pasta during last 15–30 minutes of slow cooking.

Yield: 6 servings   7 1/2 cups without pasta

Family Appeal

This soup is designed to appeal to children while training their taste buds to enjoy vegetables. To spruce up the meal for adults, serve with a salad topped with blueberries, walnuts and Citrus Vinaigrette Salad Dressing (p. 97).

Cheeseburger Soup

Garnish each serving with shredded low-fat cheese or grated Parmesan cheese.

Tex-Mex Soup

During Step 2, toss in a little frozen corn, a can of beans (red, kidney, black) and chili powder. Omit pasta. Consider using less salt, especially if using beans with added salt.

Idea for Small Families

Prepare soup through Step 4. Divide into family-sized portions and freeze. Add spinach and cooked pasta when reheating.

Helpful Hint

Use the remaining half can of tomato paste in Meat Loaf Patties (p.155).

Analysis/Serving:
Calories: 301 (Fat Cal 99) Fat: 11g (3.3g Sat) Cholesterol: 50mg
Sodium: 574mg Carbs: 29g (5.4g Fiber 6.3g Sugar) Protein: 20.6g

Worcestershire sauce & pasta

More Caramelized Soups ...

See page 124 for understanding the secret to the rich favor to these soups.

45-Minute Meal

This is a great recipe to make on the stovetop rather than in the slow cooker.

1. Begin caramelizing onions with sausage.
2. "Chop & Drop" carrots, leeks, cabbage and potatoes into skillet with onions.
3. Add broth and simmer until carrots and potatoes are fork-tender.

Voilà! You have a complete, nutritious and tasty meal in 45 minutes.

Analysis/Serving:
Calories: 265 (Fat Cal 49)
Fat: 4.9g (1.2g Sat) Cholesterol: 49mg
Sodium: 557–627mg
Carbs: 38g (8.2g Fiber 10.7g Sugar)
Protein: 17.7g

Cabbage Patch Soup

Prep for slow cooker: 25 minutes

9 oz. hot Italian fully cooked chicken/turkey sausage links, diced (p. 232)
1 1/2 lg. onions, sliced (3 cups)
1 cup sliced leeks
4 cups chopped or shredded cabbage
1 1/2 cups sliced carrots
2 cups diced potatoes
4 cups low-sodium chicken broth (divided)
1/2 (10 oz.) pkg. frozen cut spinach

Standard-sized slow cooker

1. Place diced sausage and onion in skillet, **sautéing** onions until semi-caramelized (approximately 15–20 minutes).
2. *Meanwhile,* **prepare** leeks, cabbage, carrots and potatoes, adding to slow cooker.
3. Transfer sausage mixture to slow cooker. Add 1 cup of the broth to skillet. Heat while whisking to **deglaze** the pan. Add to slow cooker with remaining broth.
3. **Cook** as desired (see p. 124 for options). Add spinach during last 15–30 minutes.

Yield: 4 servings 8 cups

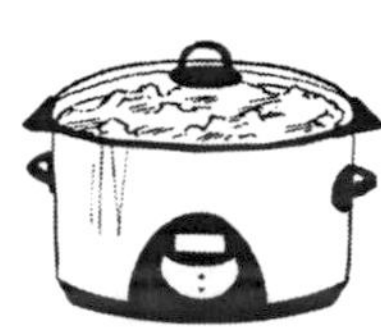

Slow cookers come in a variety of sizes and shapes, and some have programmable features. With all sizes, including the mini, a removable crock increases the convenience because food can be prepped the night before and placed in the refrigerator. A removable crock also makes clean-up easier.

Tips for Great Slow-Cooker Meals

- Oil the crock before filling for easier clean-up.
- For safety, the slow cooker should be one-half to three-fourths full.
- Generally one hour on high equals two to two and a half hours on low.
- Keep the lid on, especially during the first two hours of cooking.
- Add most seasoning during the last hour or two of cooking time.

Hearty Chicken Noodle Soup

Prep for slow cooker: 25 minutes

1 Tbsp. High-Heat oil
1 1/2 lg. onions, sliced (3 cups)
1 lb. raw skinless chicken breast chunks
1/2 tsp. salt (divided)
1 tsp. garlic powder
1 tsp. dried dill
1 Tbsp. Worcestershire sauce

1 cup sliced carrots
1 (10 oz.) pkg. frozen asparagus (cut into ~3/4 inch lengths)
2 1/2–3 cups water (divided)
2 cups chicken broth

6 oz. dry whole-grain noodle-like pasta
1/4 (10 oz.) pkg. frozen cut spinach

Standard-sized slow cooker

1. In skillet, **sauté** onions in oil with ¼ teaspoon of the salt until semi-caramelized (approximately 15–20 minutes). **Add** chicken, rest of the salt, seasonings and Worcestershire sauce, stirring often until chicken is **browned**.
2. *Meanwhile,* **prepare** carrots and asparagus, adding to slow cooker.
3. Transfer chicken mixture to slow cooker. Add 1 cup of water to skillet. Heat while whisking to **deglaze** the pan. Add to slow cooker with remaining water and broth. **Stir**.
4. **Cook** as desired (see p. 124 for options).
5. **Cook** pasta without salt slightly under al dente (p. 137), drain, return to pan and toss with an extra ⅛ teaspoon of salt.
6. **Add** spinach and cooked pasta during the last 15–30 minutes of slow cooking.

Yield: 6 servings   8 cups without pasta

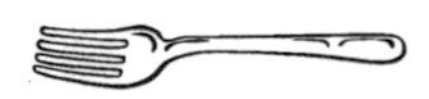

Serve soup with Side Salad (p. 69) and low-sodium dressing such as Balsamic Vinaigrette Salad Dressing (p. 70).

Hearty Chicken Rice Soup

Substitute cooked brown rice for pasta. Cook 3/4 cup of dry brown rice in 2 cups of water with little or no salt until al dente.

❄ Idea for Small Families

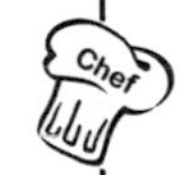

Prepare soup through Step 4, divide into family-sized portions and freeze. Add spinach and cooked pasta when reheating.

Analysis/Serving:
Calories: 249 (Fat Cal 44) Fat: 4.9g (0.7g Sat) Cholesterol: 42mg
Sodium: 530mg Carbs: 26.6g (5.8g Fiber 4.8g Sugar) Protein: 22g

Worcestershire sauce & pasta

Fall Harvest Stew

S→T: 60 minutes

The time-consuming part of these stews is preparing the ingredients. Most butchers will cube the pork for you. Veggies can be cut earlier and stored in a sealed container (not peeling squash saves time and nutrients).

1 Tbsp. High-Heat oil
1 lb. boneless pork loin roast, cubed
OR skinless chicken breast, cubed
1 1/2 cups coarsely chopped onion
1 cup sliced carrots
1 (10 oz.) pkg. frozen green beans (~2 1/4 cups)
2 cloves garlic, minced
Seasonings (see sidebar)
1 cup broth—vegetable or chicken
1 (15 oz.) can diced tomatoes (*or* see sidebar)
2 cups diced butternut squash (~½ inch)
1/8 tsp. freshly grated nutmeg
~3/4 cup mixed pepper slices (optional)
1 cup frozen chopped spinach

1. In large saucepan or skillet, begin **browning** meat in oil. "**Chop & Drop**" onions, carrots, green beans, garlic and seasonings (on sidebar), stirring occasionally.
2. **Add** broth and tomatoes (hand crush while adding). Bring to boil, reduce heat, cover and **simmer** 15 minutes.
3. *Meanwhile,* prepare remaining ingredients, clean up kitchen and **cook rice**, if serving, at appropriate time.
4. **Stir** in squash and nutmeg. Cover and **simmer** 20 minutes, or until vegetables are tender and liquid is thickened. **Stir** in peppers and spinach and **simmer** 5 more minutes.

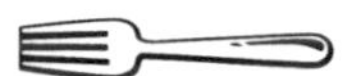

May be served over brown rice.

Yield: 6 servings 7 cups

Seasonings

1/2 tsp. salt (3/4 tsp. if not using fresh nutmeg)
1 tsp. dried thyme
1/2 tsp. ground cumin
Freshly ground black pepper, as desired

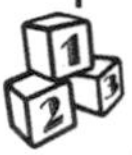

Slow-Cooker Method

1. Brown pork, onion and garlic in oil with half of the seasonings and half of the nutmeg.
2. Meanwhile, place prepared vegetables in the slow cooker.
3. Stir in the pork mixture, broth and optional tomatoes. Cook on low for 6–8 hours.
4. Stir in spinach and remaining seasonings and nutmeg 30 minutes before serving.

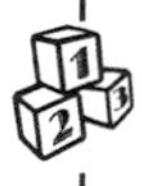

Substitutions for Diced Tomatoes

Option 1—use:
1 (8 oz.) can tomato sauce
1 cup additional broth

Option 2—omit tomatoes and increase veggies:
Carrots to 1 1/2 cups
Onions to 1 3/4 cups
Squash to 2 1/2 cups
Increase salt slightly

Analysis/Serving:
Calories: 226 (Fat Cal 67) Fat: 7.4g (2.1g Sat) Cholesterol: 42mg
Sodium: 507 Carbs: 19.7g (4.5g Fiber 7.1g Sugar) Protein: 19.4g

Fall Harvest Vegan Stew

S→T: 45 minutes (25 minutes semi-inactive time)

1 Tbsp. Medium-Heat oil
1 1/2 cups coarsely chopped onions
1 cup sliced carrots
1 (10 oz.) pkg. frozen green beans (~2 1/4 cups)
1 med. kale leaf, ribbon-cut (~1 cup)
OR spinach (see sidebar)
2 cloves garlic, minced
1/4 tsp. salt
1/2 tsp. ground cumin
1 tsp. curry powder
1 tsp. ground cinnamon
1/4 tsp. cloves
Freshly ground black pepper
1 cup vegetable broth
1 cup water
2 tsp. liquid aminos
2 cups diced butternut squash (~½ inch)
1/8 tsp. freshly grated nutmeg
2 (15 oz.) cans beans with liquid (see sidebar)

1. In skillet or large saucepan, **"Chop & Drop"** onions, carrots, green beans, kale, garlic and seasonings (salt through black pepper) in oil.
2. **Add** broth, water and liquid aminos. Cover and **simmer** 10 minutes.
3. *Meanwhile,* dice squash and **cook** rice at the appropriate time.
4. Add squash, nutmeg and beans. Cover and **simmer** for 25 minutes, or until vegetables are tender and liquid is thickened by the cooked vegetables. **Stir** as needed to prevent sticking, especially if using white kidney-cannellina beans.

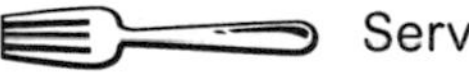 Serve over brown rice.

Yield: 6 servings ~7 cups

Healthy Bites

Making a Meal: Serving this stew over rice makes it a complete protein.

Hidden Peel: Amazingly, the peel on the squash becomes tender and blends well in these stews.

Variations

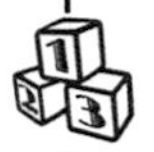

Substituting Spinach for Kale: Use one or more cups of fresh ribbon-cut or frozen chopped spinach instead of kale, adding the spinach during the last five minutes of cooking.

Beans: This recipe has been tested using unsalted garbanzo beans and unsalted white kidney-cannellina beans.

Meal Complement: For more protein, serve with low-fat cottage cheese and optional sliced tomatoes.

Analysis/Serving without rice:
Calories: 238 (Fat Cal 41) Fat: 4.6g (0.4g Sat) Cholesterol: 0mg
Sodium: 288 Carbs: 40g (10g Fiber 4.5g Sugar) Protein: 10.8g

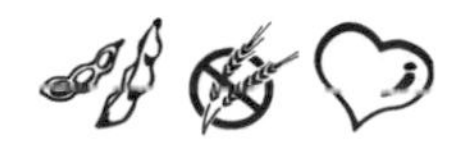

Bell Peppers

For a beautiful color and best flavor, use at least one each red, green, yellow and orange pepper.

You can also use two (ten ounce) packages of tricolored frozen peppers

Using Raw Poultry

Raw poultry chunks may be used; simply brown with onions and peppers.

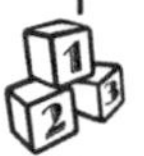

Variations

Substituting Spinach for Kale: Use 2 cups of frozen chopped spinach (or fresh ribbon-cut spinach) instead of kale. Add spinach during last 5 minutes instead of in Step 1.

Adding Beans: Some have enjoyed the addition of canned or cooked beans (e.g., black, red, black soy, pinto).

Pepper-Corn Chili Soup

Photo on Front Cover

S→T: 45 minutes (20 minutes inactive time)

A colorful and flavorful way to warm up on a cold day, this chili recipe is quite versatile. You can use Thanksgiving's extra roasted turkey, serve the chili vegan and/or introduce your family to tofu by combining both tofu and poultry.

To make the preparation of this soup go faster, use frozen vegetables (onions, peppers and spinach – see sidebar) or chop vegetables earlier in the day. (A manual or enclosed chopper makes this process much faster – and allows the kids to safely help. See sidebar, next page.)

1 Tbsp. Medium-Heat oil
1 lg. onion, chopped (~2 cups)
4–5 lg. bell peppers, diced (4–5 cups) (sidebar)
1–2 jalapeño peppers, minced (seeds optional)
2 cloves garlic, minced
5–6 small kale leaves, ribbon-cut (~2 cups)
1 tsp. chili powder
1 tsp. ground cumin
1/4 tsp. salt
1 (10 oz.) pkg. frozen whole kernel corn
1 (15 oz.) can fire-roasted crushed tomatoes
1–2 cups water
2 cups low sodium broth—chicken or vegetable
2 cups cooked turkey/chicken chunks
OR diced tofu (~12 oz.)
OR combo of poultry chunks and tofu

Jalapeño (hot pepper)

1. In large skillet, "**Chop & Drop**" onions, peppers, garlic, kale (or use optional Step 3) and seasonings in oil.

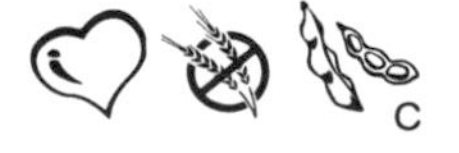

Analysis/serving:
Calories: 348 (Fat Cal 42) Fat: 4.7g (1.2g Sat) Cholesterol: 47mg
Sodium: 389 Carbs: 31g (4.6g Fiber 13g Sugar) Protein: 19g

2. **Add** remaining ingredients (corn, tomatoes, water, broth, poultry and/or tofu). Bring to boil, reduce heat, cover and **simmer** at least 20 minutes, stirring occasionally.
3. **Optional:** Thinly ribbon-cut kale and add during last 5 minutes of simmering time instead of in Step 1. Sondra prefers this method when using lacinato kale (p. 65).

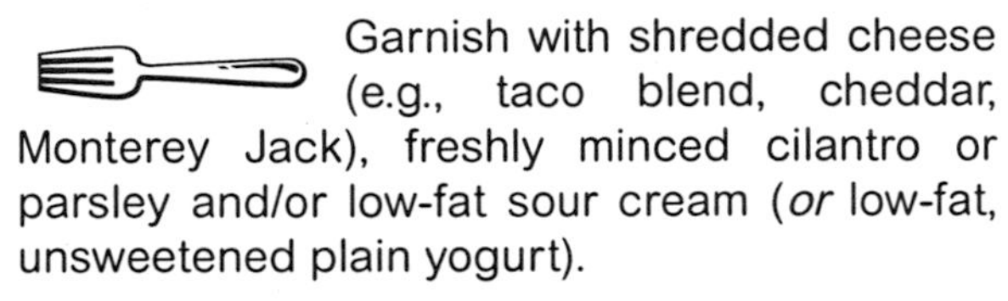

Garnish with shredded cheese (e.g., taco blend, cheddar, Monterey Jack), freshly minced cilantro or parsley and/or low-fat sour cream (*or* low-fat, unsweetened plain yogurt).

Serve with carrot sticks/chips.

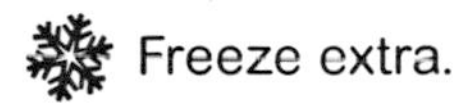 Freeze extra.

Yield: 6 servings ~10 cups

Little Chefs Enclosed Choppers

Some types of manual choppers make great cooking tools for kids. Food lies on a metal grid and is chopped/diced when you push the plastic lid down over the grid. Kids can chop without the risk of being cut by a knife!

The brand we use measures while chopping, mincing and slicing. We use it for chopping onions and peppers for this and other recipes. It's great for dicing potatoes, and the mincing blade is ideal for mincing onions for Southern-Style Shepherd's Pie.

Top Ten Reasons Why Soups, Chilies and Stews Make Great Travel Lunches

1. They are easy to make in large quantities, creating easy leftovers.
2. Most freeze well, making it easy to have several "frozen lunches" in the freezer ready to go.
3. Most freeze well in sealing bags. They do not take up much space since they lie flat in the freezer. They are quick to thaw, especially when packaged individually. If warming on location is a possibility, pack soup frozen; it will serve as an icer, helping to keep foods safely cold, yet it will thaw by lunchtime.
4. They travel well in insulated mugs; there's no need to worry about warming them away from home.
5. Your protein, vegetables and grains can all be in one entrée.
6. It's easy to pack them with nutrition providing energy for the rest of the day.
7. There are many variations, so you can have them several days in a row without feeling like you're eating the same thing.
8. They're comforting – a nice touch when away from home.
9. We can't eat them easily in the car or at the computer, so they force us to slow down for a few minutes and eat.
10. They taste great!

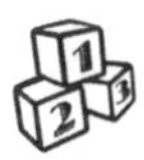

Other Meat Options

- Chicken breasts/ tenders, diced
- Lean pork loin, diced

If you use the following meat options, the simmering time in Step 2 needs to be at least 50 minutes or use slow-cooker method.

- Beef stew — cut 1-inch cubes into quarters
- Beef or venison round steak, diced

Optional seasonings tested using diced tomatoes with green chilies:

1/2 tsp. salt
2 tsp. chili powder
1 tsp. dried oregano
2 tsp. ground cumin
1/8 tsp. black pepper
1–2 jalapeño peppers, minced

Beans & Salt

Our favorite kinds of beans are listed in the recipe. Most any canned beans will work. Enjoy finding your favorite.

If using beans canned with salt, reduce salt in the recipe to 1/4 teaspoon.

The spicier the chili is, the less salt is required.

Hearty Meat & Veggie Chili

S→T: 1 hour + 10 minutes (40 or more minutes inactive)

1 Tbsp. High-Heat oil
1 lg. onion, chopped (2 cups)
3/4 lb. raw sirloin steak chunks
3/4 tsp. salt
1 Tbsp. chili powder
2 tsp. dried oregano
2 tsp. ground cumin
1/2 tsp. cayenne pepper
1/4 tsp. crushed red pepper
1/8 tsp. black pepper
4 cloves garlic, minced
1 cup broth—beef, chicken, vegetable
1 (14 oz.) can fire-roasted crushed tomatoes
2 Tbsp. tomato paste
1 cup frozen cut green beans
1 cup sliced carrots (option to finely chop)
1 (10 oz.) pkg. frozen tri-color peppers, diced (or ~2½ cups fresh)
1 (15 oz.) can black beans, undrained (no salt added)
1 (15 oz.) can red beans, undrained (no salt added)
1 Tbsp. brown rice flour
1/2 (10 oz.) pkg. frozen cut spinach (5 oz.)

1. In large saucepan or skillet, "**Chop & Drop**" onions, steak, seasoning and garlic in oil, stirring occasionally to brown meat evenly.
2. **Add** broth, tomatoes with liquid, tomato paste, green beans, carrots and peppers. Bring to boil, reduce heat and **simmer** partially covered for 20 minutes, stirring occasionally.
3. Pour ½ cup of liquid from beans into small bowl. Whisk in flour; reserve for Step 5.
4. **Add** beans with remaining liquid. **Simmer** uncovered for 25 minutes, stirring as needed.

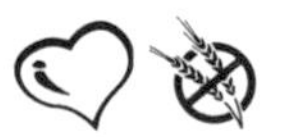

Analysis/Serving:
Calories: 267 (Fat Cal 55) Fat: 6.1g (1.4g Sat) Cholesterol: 44mg
Sodium: 481 Carbs: 32g (8g Fiber 6.6g Sugar) Protein: 20g

5. Add reserved liquid with flour and spinach, **simmer** for 5 minutes.
4. Taste and add more seasonings as desired. Simmer a few minutes to blend flavors.

Garnish with low-fat cheese and/or low-fat sour cream (*or* low-fat, unsweetened plain yogurt).

Complement meal with Side Salad and fresh or frozen fruit with an optional drizzle of low-fat yogurt.

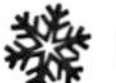 Freeze extra.

Yield: 8 servings ~9 cups

Chicken Vegetable Bake

S→O: 5 minutes Bake: 25–45 minutes

1 lb. chicken breast or tenders, chunked
OR 2 cups cooked chicken chunks
Garlic powder
Freshly ground black pepper
1 or 2 (10 oz.) pkg. stir-fry Thai blend frozen vegetables (p. 218)
1 cup chopped onion, if desired
1 (16 oz.) pkg. creamy potato-leek soup (p. 232)
1 cup Seasoned Croutons (p. 190) (optional)
OR whole-grain stuffing mix (optional)

Preheat oven—350°. **Oil** a 9x13-inch baking dish.

1. **Place** chicken in baking dish. **Season**. **Layer** vegetables over chicken. **Pour** soup evenly over layers. **Stir** gently. **Top** with croutons or stuffing mix, if desired.
2. **Bake** uncovered 25–45 minutes (depending on whether you are using raw or cooked chicken). May start even if oven is still preheating.

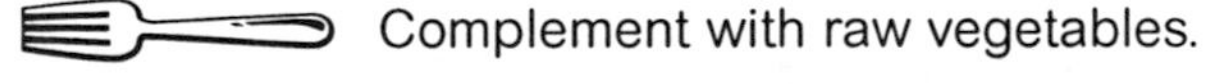

Complement with raw vegetables.

Yield: 4 servings (cut in half or double with ease)

Chili Slow-Cooker Method

Many do not have over an hour to tend to the simmering chili, and many may like to use the less expensive (less tender) cuts of meat but still make great chili. Using the slow cooker is an easy answer.

Simply do Step 1 as described. Add it with the remaining ingredients, except spinach, to the removable crock of a slow cooker. Cover and refrigerate.

In the morning, place crock in slow cooker. Slow cook on LOW for 8–10 hours.

When you get home, stir in the frozen spinach. Turn to HIGH setting. In 20 minutes or less the chili is ready.

This gives you time to make a salad with bagged lettuce, whip up one of our 5-minute salad dressings (our favorite is Citrus Vinaigrette, p. 97; top salad with blueberries and walnuts), cut fresh fruit or pull frozen fruit, set the table and gather the family for a comforting meal together.

Analysis/Serving:
Calories: 242–261 (Fat Cal 43) Fat: 4.8g (0.8g Sat) Cholesterol: 63mg
Sodium: 374–397 Carbs: 22–26g (5–6g Fiber 5–6g Sugar) Protein: 26g

Helpful Hints

Do-Ahead: Shepherd's Pie can be prepared earlier in the day or the night before. The whole pie can be prepared ahead or just the meat mixture. It can also be prepared several days to weeks ahead of time and frozen.

Time Saver: Use enclosed chopper (p. 131) to chop onions and celery for meat mixture and mince onions for topping.

Casserole Dishes: May be prepared in two (8x8x2-inch) square baking dishes or two (9-inch) pie pans. Serve one and freeze the other.

Freeze Extra:

(1) Freeze in casserole dish, topped with potatoes for two to four weeks. Thaw overnight in refrigerator and bake until heated through.

Or (2) freeze meat mixture only. Thaw. Spread cold mixture in casserole dish. Place in oven while preheating and while preparing potato topping. Remove from oven to top with mashed potatoes; continue baking until heated through.

Shepherd's Pie Makeover

There are many ways to make Shepherd's Pie. Often recipes contain few vegetables and include "extras," adding unnecessary calories and fats. We prefer to pack the sauce with the flavor and nutrition of several vegetables. We offer the option of adding spinach to the topping, which not only adds flavor and nutrition but also makes it look pretty (especially when mixed with orange sweet potatoes). These topping variations can be served on their own and are included as sides in some menus of the Quick-Fix chapter.

Use our recipe as is or as help in creating a healthier version of your own recipe.

Southern-Style Shepherd's Pie

S→T: 1 hour

This is a Southern twist on an English standard. The recipe was inspired by Rachael Ray's 30-Minute Meals.

1/2 lb. lean ground pork or lamb
1/2 lb. lean ground beef
1 1/2 cups chopped onion
1 cup thinly sliced celery *or* carrots
3/8 tsp. salt
Freshly ground black pepper
2 tsp. dried parsley
2 lg. collard leaves, ribbon-cut (1 cup packed)
1/2 (10 oz.) pkg. frozen green beans (~1¼ cups)
Freshly grated nutmeg
1 cup beef broth
1/4 cup water

2 tsp. brown rice flour
1/4 cup water
1/2 cup frozen peas

Topping Ingredients:
- **1 1/2 lbs. sweet potatoes, diced** (we use peel)
- **1 cup minced onion**
- **1/8 tsp. salt**
- **Freshly ground black pepper**
- **Freshly grated nutmeg**
- **2 Tbsp. milk** (low-fat cow, unsweetened soy)
- **1 Tbsp. unsalted butter**

Oven temperature—400°. Preheat at Step 3.
9x13x2-inch casserole dish (or see sidebar)

1. In large skillet, **"Chop & Drop"** ground meats, onions, celery (or carrots), salt, pepper and parsley, stirring often to brown meat evenly.
2. *Meanwhile,* **prepare** collards for filling and sweet potatoes and onions for topping.
3. **Preheat** oven. To skillet, **add** collards, green beans, broth and ¼ cup water. Bring to boil, reduce heat, cover and **simmer** 15 minutes, or until vegetables are tender, stirring occasionally.
3. In saucepan, **cook** sweet potatoes, minced onion, salt, pepper and nutmeg in small amount of water for approximately 15 minutes, or until tender and water is absorbed.
4. **Whisk** flour in remaining ¼ cup of water. Add to skillet with peas. Simmer for a couple of minutes while mashing potatoes. (Add butter and milk to potatoes when mashing.)
5. **Spread** meat mixture evenly on bottom of casserole dish. **Top** with mashed potatoes, spreading evenly. **Bake** in preheated oven for 10 minutes, or until heated through. (Alternately, can be broiled for 4–5 minutes.)

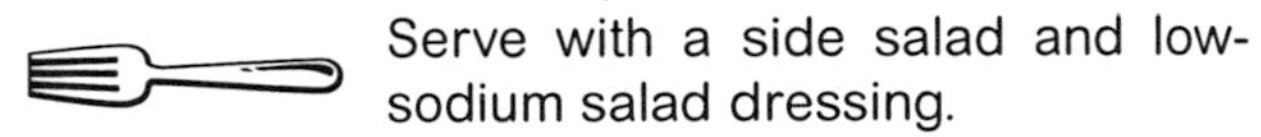
Serve with a side salad and low-sodium salad dressing.

Yield: 6 servings

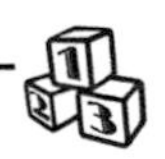

Topping Variations

When using below variations, omit collards and the ¼ cup of water in sauce.

Spinach-Red Potato

1½ lb. red potatoes, diced (we do not peel)
½ cup beef broth
1 cup frozen chopped/cut spinach

1. Steam potatoes in beef broth, seasoned with pepper until tender, adding water as needed.
2. Remove from burner, lay spinach on potatoes. Cover; allow the steam to cook the spinach.
3. Mash potatoes with a tablespoon of unsalted butter and, if needed, a splash of beef broth.

Spinach-Sweet Potato

Use sweet potato topping described in main recipe, adding spinach as described above.

Potato Masher

Potatoes with spinach (and skins) mash easier using a handheld looped-style potato masher rather than a small dice-style one.

Analysis for Southern-Style Shepherd's Pie/Serving:
Calories: 299 (Fat Cal 77) Fat: 8.6g (3.7g Sat) Cholesterol: 52mg
Sodium: 430mg Carbs: 34.9g (6.1g Fiber 9.1g Sugar) Protein: 20g

Spinach-Red Potato Estimated Analysis/Serving: (recipe serves 6)
Calories: 103 (Fat Cal 19) Fat: 2.1g (1.2g Sat) Cholesterol: 5mg
Sodium: 100mg Carbs: 18.6g (2.1g Fiber 1.4g Sugar) Protein: 2.6g

Spinach-Sweet Potato Analysis/Serving: (recipe serves 6)
Calories: 133 (Fat Cal 18) Fat: 2g (1.2g Sat) Cholesterol: 5mg
Sodium: 129mg Carbs: 26g (4g Fiber 6g Sugar) Protein: 2.5g

Spaghetti Dinner Night

Spaghetti Sauce & Pasta
(1 oz. pasta/serving)
Bread (see below)

Bread with Dinner

A slice of whole-grain bread can add 100 calories and 19 g. of carbs to your meal. So with pasta, the carbs can add up fast. Since garlic bread complements spaghetti, we recommend lower-carb meals earlier in the day so a small amount of bread is acceptable.

Garlic Bread: Warm or toast purchased whole-grain bread. Add garlic powder or salt to melted butter and brush it on the warm bread.

Breadsticks: Page 193.

Bread with Olive Oil: Dip slices of Hearty Homemade Bread in seasoned olive oil (sidebar on p. 191).

Do-Ahead

The complete spaghetti sauce (or just Steps 1 and 2, adding oil and basil when reheating) can be easily prepared the night before or on a "Do-Ahead" day and frozen until needed.

Chunky Garden Spaghetti Sauce

S→T: 45 minutes

1 lb. lean ground meat (beef or turkey)
1 1/2 cups chopped onion
1 1/2 cups diced frozen tri-color peppers
OR use fresh red, green and yellow peppers
1 cup diced summer squash
1 1/4 tsp. salt
Freshly ground black pepper
4 tsp. Italian seasoning mix
1/4 tsp. crushed red pepper flakes
4 cloves garlic, minced
1/2 cup sliced carrots
(finely chopped in food processor)
1 (28 oz.) can Tuscan-style, low-salt tomatoes
2 Tbsp. tomato paste
1 Tbsp. olive oil
3/4 oz. fresh basil, ribbon-cut (tips on p. 220)
Parmesan cheese (garnish 2 teaspoons/serving)

1. In large skillet, **"Chop & Drop"** ground meat, onions, peppers, squash, salt, black pepper, seasonings and carrots, stirring often to brown meat evenly.
2. **Add** tomatoes with liquid (hand crush while adding) and tomato paste. Bring to boil, reduce heat and **simmer** covered for 15 minutes, stirring occasionally.
3. *Meanwhile*, prepare side salad and salad dressing. Also, start water to boil for pasta.
4. Cook pasta until al dente in unsalted water (see next page). Add oil and basil to sauce; **simmer** 5 additional minutes.
5. *Meanwhile*, if serving, prepare garlic bread (see sidebar). Drain pasta; return to pan; lightly sprinkle with salt.

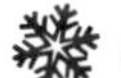 Freeze extra sauce.

Yield: 6 servings 7 cups

Analysis/Serving (sauce, Parmesan cheese, 1 ounce whole-grain pasta):
Calories: 344 (Fat Cal 117) Fat: 13g (4.7g Sat) Cholesterol: 57mg
Sodium: 592mg Carbs: 34.5g (6.3g Fiber 9.6g Sugar) Protein: 23g

Pasta Tips

Purchasing: Using whole-grain pasta is an easy way to consume whole grains. There are many brands. Our favorites are Healthy Harvest (blended) and Bionaturae (100% whole wheat). Both offer a whopping 3 g. of fiber per one-ounce serving and have a less grainy taste than some brands. Bionaturae also makes a good gluten-free blend pasta.

Serving Size: Packages usually list the serving size as two ounces. Our recipes are designed using the USDA guidelines of only one ounce per serving. We give the measurements in ounces instead of cups because various forms of pasta measure differently.

Al Dente: Cook pasta uncovered in boiling water until it is just tender yet slightly firm. We rarely cook pasta as long as the package states. Taste-test frequently during the last few minutes. Soon you will get accustomed to al dente cooked pasta.

Overcooking Pasta: The glycemic-index rating of pasta increases the longer you cook it. This means that overcooked pasta will enter your bloodstream faster (resulting in a possible sugar rush). Therefore, we do not recommend freezing foods with pasta and suggest that foods with cooked pasta be reheated at a low temperature for a short period of time.

This is also why we undercook the pasta for slow cooker soups (pp. 125 and 127), allowing the pasta to finish cooking in the slow cooker while soaking up the flavor of the soup. This method can be used in the Basic Soup on page 118 or you can add the dry pasta to the soup during the last six or so minutes of simmering time to cook pasta directly in the soup.

Cooking Without Salt: We cook pasta without adding salt to the cooking water. Instead we return the drained cooked pasta to pan and lightly season with salt and/or other seasonings; cover until ready to serve. Often this sprinkle of salt is not needed, especially with flavorful sauces such as spaghetti and marinara.

Spaghetti Sauce

Sneaky Vegetables: Some people do not like the taste, color or texture of certain vegetables. However, vegetables can be disguised by pureeing them and incorporating them into the sauce unobtrusively. In this way, their flavor can be introduced (and enjoyed) without preconceptions.

If pureeing more than one vegetable, we recommend cutting the vegetable amounts in half since pureeing them can change the texture of the sauce. If onions are a problem, try caramelizing them (p. 72).

Since carrots, red peppers and basil offer sweetness, reducing their amounts may require adding honey or agave nectar.

Reducing salt by using Tuscan-style tomatoes: Sondra's family has enjoyed using Tuscan-style canned tomatoes by Bionaturae for a real Italian flavor in spaghetti and marinara sauces. They are a low-salt product, so using other brands with salt added requires carefully watching the amount of salt you add to your sauces.

Time Saver

Use enclosed chopper (p. 131) to chop onions, peppers and squash.

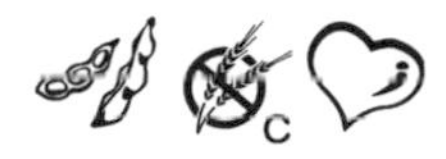

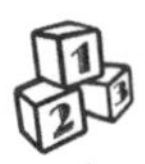

Variations

Cheese: Sprinkle 4 ounces of low-fat shredded cheddar and/or Monterey Jack cheese on the top of the meat mixture before adding cornbread batter.

Spelt Topping: Replace wheat flour in the cornbread topping with the same amount of whole-grain spelt flour, using 2 tablespoons less milk (use only 7/8 cup).

Gluten-Free Topping: Replace wheat flour with equal amount of Gluten-Free Flour Mix (p. 27) in the cornbread topping.

Helpful Hints

Smaller Families: Prepare meat mixture. Spread half in an 8x8-inch baking dish. Mix up half the topping recipe, using egg white or yolk for half an egg. Freeze rest of meat mixture.

Hot Peppers Year-Round: Freeze whole peppers in summer for fresh, hot taste year-round. See sidebar on page 75 for more information.

Southwestern Casserole

S→O: 40 minutes Bake: 15–20 minutes

This is a perfect dish to suit different tastes regarding "hot" spicy dishes. To make the least spicy dish, use mild salsa, omit crushed red peppers and simmer chili peppers whole as described but do not add them diced to meat or cornbread.

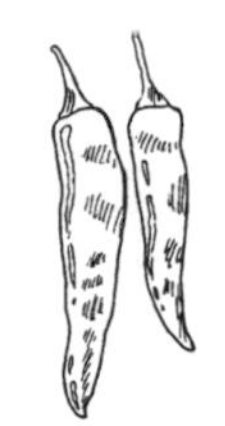

Red Chilies (hot pepper)

Meat Filling:

- **1 lb. lean ground meat** (turkey breast or beef)
- **1 lg. onion, chopped** (2 cups)
- **1/8 tsp. salt**
- **1/2 tsp. ground cumin**
- **1 tsp. dried leaf oregano**
- **1 tsp. chili powder**
- **1/4 tsp. crushed red pepper** (optional)
- **4 cloves garlic, minced**
- **1 (15 oz.) can black beans, undrained** (with added salt)
- **1–2 cups salsa** (p. 91 or 153)
- **2–4 whole** (uncut) **red chili peppers**
- **1 cup frozen corn**
- **1/2 (10 oz.) pkg. frozen cut spinach**

Cornbread Topping:

- **3/4 cup yellow cornmeal**
- **1/3 cup "white" whole-wheat flour**
- **2 tsp. baking powder**
- **1/2 tsp. salt**
- **1/4 tsp. chili powder** (optional)
- **1 egg, slightly beaten**
- **1 cup milk** (low-fat cow, unsweetened soy)
- **2 Tbsp. High-Heat oil**
- **1 Tbsp. sweetener**—honey or agave nectar
- **1/2 cup frozen corn**
- **1–2 chili peppers, diced** (from filling mixture)

Preheat oven—400°.
9x13x2-inch casserole dish

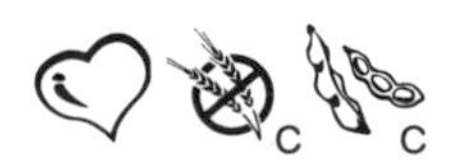

Analysis/Serving (using ground turkey breast meat; range = 1–2 cups salsa):
Calories: 313–323 (Fat Cal 71) Fat: 7.9g (0.9g Sat) Cholesterol: 58mg
Sodium: 475–565 Carbs: 41-43g (5g Fiber 9.5–10.5g Sugar) Protein: 21g

1. In skillet, **"Chop & Drop"** ground meat, onion, salt, seasonings and garlic, stirring occasionally. **Stir** in beans with liquid, salsa and whole chili peppers.
2. Bring to boil, reduce heat and **simmer** uncovered for 10 minutes. *Meanwhile,* in bowl, **whisk** cornmeal, flour, baking powder, salt and chili powder together. In separate bowl, **combine** egg, milk, oil, sweetener and corn.
3. **Remove** chili peppers from skillet and add spinach and corn. Cover and **simmer** 5 additional minutes. Dice chili peppers; add some or all to cornbread mixture and/or meat (or bean) mixture if desired.
4. **Spread** hot meat (or bean) mixture evenly in baking dish.
5. Add liquid mixture to dry ingredients for topping. **Stir** only until all dry ingredients are moistened and **pour** (and spread) evenly over filling.
6. **Bake** in preheated oven for 15–20 minutes, or until toothpick in cornbread comes out clean.

Cut 4x2. Lift each serving out with spatula.

Garnish with low-fat sour cream (*or* low-fat unsweetened, plain yogurt).

Serve with side salad or raw vegetables and/or fresh/frozen fruit. Cantaloupe, apple or applesauce is especially delicious with spicy food like this dish.

Leftovers may be frozen; thaw completely before reheating.

Yield: 8 servings

Vegetarian Version

1 Tbsp. Medium-Heat oil
1 lg. onion, chopped (2 cups)
1/8 tsp. salt
1/2 tsp. ground cumin
1 tsp. dried leaf oregano
1 tsp. chili powder
1/4 tsp. crushed red pepper
4 cloves garlic, minced
2 (15 oz.) cans black beans (with added salt) (drain one can, reserve liquid; add liquid as needed)
2–4 whole (uncut) red chili peppers
1/2 tsp. liquid aminos
1–2 cups salsa (p. 91 or 153)
1 cup frozen corn
1/2 (10 oz.) pkg. frozen cut spinach
4 oz. shredded cheese

Sauté onions and seasonings in oil for about 5 minutes, adding garlic during last minute. **Stir** in beans with liquid, whole chili peppers, liquid aminos and salsa.

Follow Steps 2 through 6 to left, sprinkling cheese on bean mixture before adding topping.

Serving option for leftovers:

Reheat casserole to serving temperature. Transfer to serving plate cornbread side down. Top with egg (fixed your favorite way). Mmm!

Analysis/Serving for Vegetarian Version (range = 1–2 cups salsa):
Calories: 343–353 (Fat Cal 86) Fat: 9.7g (2.9g Sat) Cholesterol: 36mg
Sodium: 560–650 Carbs: 50–52g (7g Fiber 10–11g Sugar) Protein: 16g

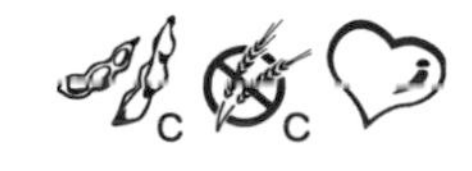

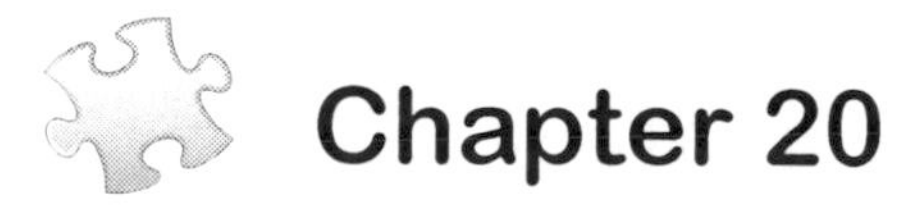

Chapter 20

Quick-Fix Meals

It's hard to find the time to cook. Whether we walk in the door tired and hungry or spend the hours before dinner attending to the demands of young children, we rarely have much time to spend in the kitchen before the evening meal. This chapter offers different options for getting dinner on the table quickly.

Start-to-Finish Quick-Fix Meals

Meals that can be on the table in 30 minutes or less from start to finish

There is no advanced preparation and often not much planning ahead, except to keep the foods needed as staples in your cabinet or refrigerator. This chapter details eight of these menus (pp. 144, 145, 147, 149, 152, 154, 155 and 158), including entrées such as oven-fried chicken, seasoned grilled chicken or pork, pizza, macaroni and cheese, salmon and meat loaf patties.

Other start-to-finish, 30-minutes-or-less meal suggestions found throughout this cookbook are as follows:

Tacos or Taco Salad (p. 100)
Wilted Spinach Salad (p. 101)
Fancy Scrambled Eggs (p. 109)
Smoothies (p. 106)
20-Minute Stir-Fry Dinner (p. 61)
Seasoned Squash Dinner (p. 81)
Sautéed Chard with Balsamic Grilled Chicken (p. 56)

Slow Cooker Quick-Fix Meals

Meals that are slow-cooked during the day

These slow-cooked meals can be prepared the night before or in the morning. Some can slow-cook all day, while others need just a few hours. Total preparation time for these meals is 30 minutes or less. This chapter details five slow-cooker meals (pp. 153, 156 and 157).

Other slow-cooker meal suggestions found throughout this cookbook are the following:

Hamburger or Cheeseburger Soup (p 125)
Cabbage Patch Soup (p 126)
Hearty Chicken Noodle Soup (p. 127)
Slow Cooker Chowder (p. 119)
Beef Barley Soup (p. 121)
Slow Cooker Black Bean Soup (p. 122)
Hearty Meat & Veggie Chili (pp. 132–133; sidebar)
Fall Harvest Stew (p. 128; sidebar)
Barley Casserole (p. 180)

Do-Ahead Quick-Fix Meals

Meals (or portions of the meal) that can be prepped at an earlier time

The menus fit into several categories:

1. Meals that can be assembled the night before or earlier in the day, allowing for baking and simmering while you relax at the end of the day or help a child with homework. An example in this chapter is Cabbage-Fish Bake (p. 150).
2. Meals in which something needs to be prepped the night before or earlier in the day. An example in this chapter is to marinate the meat for Venison Teriyaki (or Beef Teriyaki) on page 148.
3. Meals that can be ready in 20–30 minutes if one or more menu items are done in advance. Examples in this chapter are to (1) advance-prep the Fancy Hamburgers (p. 146) for a 20-minute dinner and (2) advance-prep the salad dressing and Cheese Biscuit Mix for the Easy Baked Fish dinner (p. 151).
4. Meals (or portions of meals) that can be frozen until you want to use them. Examples include making and freezing a Pizza Crust or a Shepherd's Pie.

Other do-ahead meal suggestions found throughout this cookbook are (see recipes for specific do-ahead tips):

Pizza (pp. 168–170)
Spaghetti Dinner (p. 136)
Southwestern Casseroles (pp. 138-139)
Black Bean Soup (p. 123)
Shepherd's Pie (pp. 134–135)
Pecan Crusted Chicken Salad (p. 98)
Spaghetti Squash Casserole (p. 87)
Asian Salmon Salad (p. 96)
Beet Salad (p. 102)
Breakfast Pizzas (pp. 110–111)
Breakfast Squares (p. 108)
Acorn Squash with Pork Chop (p. 180)

Making Quick-Fix Meals Work for You

The trick to making quick-fix meals truly a quick fix is to do a bit of planning. That doesn't mean you have to write out menus for the week, though that can be helpful. Planning ahead can simply mean stocking your kitchen with foods and ingredients needed for your favorite recipes. Then you can be spontaneous when deciding what to have for dinner, because the necessary ingredients are at your fingertips. Here are some ideas to get you started.

Shopping List: We often don't eat as we intended because we don't have what we need on hand. Try keeping a shopping list on your fridge door. Every time you finish something (such as a can of tomato sauce or beans), write it on the list. The next time you go to the store, buy some more so that when you next decide to make that dinner you will have everything you need. (Some people like to organize their list according to where it is located in the store. This makes shopping faster and easier.)

Do-Ahead Day: Some people like to take a block of time – a morning, an evening, a whole day – and prepare several meal items at once for their freezer. Ideas would be to make spaghetti sauce, prepare a soup, bread some chicken, make a pizza crust and assemble a casserole; five meals are ready to go for the week. (You might want to keep a list of what you put in the freezer.)

> **Idea:** Some things you make ahead might be a complete meal in and of themselves (e.g., Shepherd's Pie); others can become complete meals if you pair them with healthier-choice prepared foods. For instance, many meals would be complete with cut-up vegetables or fruit from the deli. Or grill prepared chicken or pork and serve on a sandwich-style bun with lettuce and tomato.
>
> **Idea:** Spending a morning cooking doesn't mean you can't spend it with your family. True, it's often easier to cook without the help of children. But if you can simplify what you're cooking, or limit how much needs to get done, you may feel less pressure and it will be easier to let others help. When kids help parents cook, they learn life skills, gain an understanding of the importance of contributing to household tasks and get to spend invaluable time with someone they love!
>
> **Idea:** If you need things from the store to complement what you are freezing (e.g., pasta to go with the spaghetti sauce), some family members could do the grocery shopping while others do the cooking.

Double What You Paid For: Many recipes are easy to double. For instance, if you make Pepper-Corn Chili one night for dinner, make a double batch. Enjoy one and freeze the other. You just cooked for two nights in one! Other examples would be to season extra Pork Chops (cooking some and freezing the others) or bread an extra pound of chicken chunks. Patties of all sorts are also great for this approach: make extra beef, poultry or veggie patties, wrap them individually and freeze them without cooking. They can be cooked straight from the freezer whenever desired. (Sweet Potato Cakes are handy to have on hand to pair with grilled pork chops and a vegetable – what an easy meal!)

You can also use leftover food from one night to create a new dish for the next night. For example, if you enjoy a rotisserie chicken and have some leftover, cut it up while you are doing the dinner dishes. The next night, spread it on top of some bagged lettuce, adding some chopped veggies and a bit of dressing for a "grilled" chicken salad. If desired, start whole-grain bread in the bread machine so it is ready to enjoy with the salad. This concept works well for taking lunch to work or school as well. For example, enjoy Salsa Chicken Salad one night and have the leftover chicken in a tortilla wrap for lunch the next day.

One more option is to use dinner preparation one night to prepare a key ingredient for dinner another night. For instance, if you are baking salmon for the Asian Salmon Salad, poach some extra fillets to use another night in Salmon & Pasta.

Quick-Fix Prepared Food Meals

Meals that can be on the table in a hurry, using all or mostly purchased prepared foods

The key to making these meals even healthier is choosing quality foods processed in healthy ways. In general, choose prepared food products that are free of trans fats, corn syrups, nitrates and MSG (see pp. 229–232 for more details and a more complete list). Also consider calories, fats, sodium and fiber contents listed on the label. (For more information, see p. 229 as well as chapter two). On several items below, we have highlighted some specifics in choosing a healthier-choice food.

To put a meal together, we recommend:

... choosing one main source of protein. Examples:

- Breaded fish sticks or fillets (choose whole-grain breading; avoid hydrogenated oils and additives like MSG; Natural Sea is our brand of choice)
- Chicken nuggets (choose whole-grain breading; avoid hydrogenated oils and corn syrup)
- Salmon patties (choose as little fillers as possible by comparing the ingredient list and carbohydrates per serving)
- Hot dogs (choose nitrite free and as low sodium and low fat as possible)
- Ham and other deli meats (choose nitrite free and as low sodium as possible)
- Rotisserie chicken (avoid MSG and corn syrup)
- Grain and veggie patties/nuggets (choose whole grains)
- Bean/lentil loaf (Morningstar Farms is our brand choice)

... choosing up to one source of starch:

- Frozen starchy veggies such as whole kernel corn, peas, hash browns, tater tots (choose brands with lowest added salt and sugars; avoid hydrogenated oils)
- Whole-grain pastas (p. 137)
- Blue corn chips (aim for as low sodium as possible; two of our favorite brands, Garden of Eatin and Bearitos, contain 60 mg. of sodium per 1 ounce serving)
- Whole-grain breads/rolls/buns/tortillas (p. 191)

... choosing one or more sources of other fruits and vegetables:

- Bagged lettuce, baby carrots, carrot chips, etc.
- Chopped/shredded veggies from deli
- Cut-up fresh fruit from deli
- Frozen veggies, such as broccoli, green beans, mixed bags (choose lowest sodium added as possible)
- Fresh fruit
- Unsweetened frozen fruit (choose those without corn syrup or other added sugars)
- Unsweetened applesauce (choose brands without corn syrup and no added sugars or other ingredients; our brand of choice is Santa Cruz — so sweet, no sugar is needed!)

See our websites for updates and additions to this list. We welcome your questions and comments about brands you prefer (see p. 242 for our contact information).

Oven-Fried Chicken Chunks

S→O: 12 minutes Bake: 10 (or 14) minutes

Oven-fried chicken and chunks offers a healthier way to serve fried chicken without compromising taste.

1/4 cup flour—brown rice, whole wheat pastry OR "white" whole wheat
3/8 tsp. salt
1/2 tsp. garlic powder
1/2 tsp. paprika
1/16 tsp. each: cayenne and black pepper
1 lb. boneless, skinless chicken breasts
High-Heat cooking spray (see sidebar)

Preheat oven: 425°/450° (convection/conventional). **Oil** baking sheet.

Directions for Quick-Fix Meal:

1. In bowl, **combine** flour and seasonings.
2. Rinse chicken. Cut in 1-inch long strips. Cut strips into 1- to 1½-inch pieces, forming large chunks. Place all semi-moist chunks in a plastic bag (1 gallon); spread flat in bottom.
3. Sprinkle flour mixture evenly on chicken. Hold closed (without extra air in bag). **Shake** to **coat**, ensuring all of the coating is used. Place in pan about inch apart.
4. **Spray** oil to coat. **Bake** in preheated oven until 180° internal temperature (10 min. for convection or 14 min. for conventional)
5. *Meanwhile*, prepare and start to steam broccoli and set out chips, salsa and sauce(s).

Do-Ahead: Chunks can be coated with seasoning mixture and frozen. Bake straight from frozen state in preheated oven for 5 minutes. Briefly remove from oven and spray oil to coat. Bake for 10–14 minutes longer. Do not thaw before baking.

Yield: 4 servings (Analysis allows for 1 ounce chips, ¼ cup salsa and 1 tablespoon of dipping sauce.)

Start-to-Finish Quick-Fix Menu

Do-Ahead (*)

Chicken Nuggets
BBQ sauce, ketchup or *Dijon Dressing (p. 99)
blue corn chips *Salsa
Broccoli

Cooking Spray Kitchen Spritzer

We use a refillable spray and pump bottle designed to spray oil.

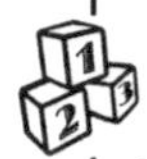

Oven-Fried Chicken

This is especially delicious served with brown rice and broccoli. Prepare/bake the same as chunks except:

- Use only brown rice flour.
- Bake at 25° lower temp.
- Use 6 to 8 bone-in, skinless chicken pieces.
- One piece at a time, add chicken to bag with a few teaspoons of seasoning on top. Shake to coat.
- Place chicken bone-side down on baking sheet.
- Bake 15 to 20 min. before spraying oil; bake about 10 min. after spraying.
- Delicious served cold.
- **Do-Ahead:** Bread, freeze, thaw and cook, loosening chicken from pan when spraying oil.

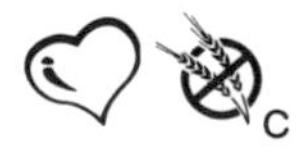

Analysis for a Serving of Chicken Nuggets/Estimate for Dinner:
Calories: 190/436 (Fat Cal 57/180) Fat: 6.3/20g (1/2g Sat) Cholesterol: 63mg
Sodium: 254/675mg Carbs: 7.9/37.5g (0.4/5g Fiber 0/5g Sugar) Protein: 24/27g

Grilled Chicken/Pork Rubs

S→T: 15– minutes

4 (4 oz.) chicken breasts (boneless, skinless)
OR lean pork chops (boneless or bone-in)
High-Heat oil
Salt, pepper, dried seasonings (see below)
1 cup low-sodium chicken broth (optional)

Preheat cast-iron skillet (or grill pan) on medium-low heat.

1. **Rinse** meat. **Dry** with paper towels. Lay on plate or piece of waxed paper. **Drizzle** oil on top side; spread with back of a spoon. **Sprinkle** with salt, pepper and seasonings; rub seasonings in with back of spoon. Using tongs or spatula, turn. Repeat oil, pepper and seasonings (not salt) to the second side.
2. **Grill** single layer in skillet (or grill pan) for approximately 4–6 minutes per side, or until no longer pink and juices run clear. If skillet becomes dry, add a splash of water or oil as needed. Thicker breasts take longer; if desired, cover pan during grilling time.
3. **Optional:** Transfer chicken to plate; keep warm. Add broth to skillet, heat and whisk to deglaze pan. Cook down. Pour over chicken.

Yield: 4 servings

Seasoning Ideas

Garlic powder, chili powder, cumin and oregano
OR Garlic powder, paprika and parsley
OR Garlic powder, basil and oregano

Start-to-Finish Quick-Fix Menu

Grilled Chicken Rub
Oven Fries (p. 76)
Roasted Asparagus (p. 46)

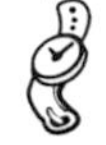

Meal Timing

1. Preheat oven—425°. Prepare and start oven fries.
2. Prepare asparagus; see recipe to know when to start.
3. Preheat skillet. Prepare and start chicken.
4. Turn fries, asparagus and chicken as needed.

Helpful Hints

Do-Ahead: Step 1 of Grilled Chicken Rubs can be done in advance, such as the night before, earlier in the day or on your Do-Ahead day and individually frozen in sandwich-sized bags.

Grilling Frozen Chicken: Seasoned breasts can be cooked straight from the freezer. Do not preheat skillet. Allow a few more minutes for cooking.

Sandwich Meal: Omit fries from the menu and serve chicken on whole-grain bread or buns with healthy sandwich garnishes, such as Pesto (p. 93), lettuce, arugula, tomato slices and/or onion slices.

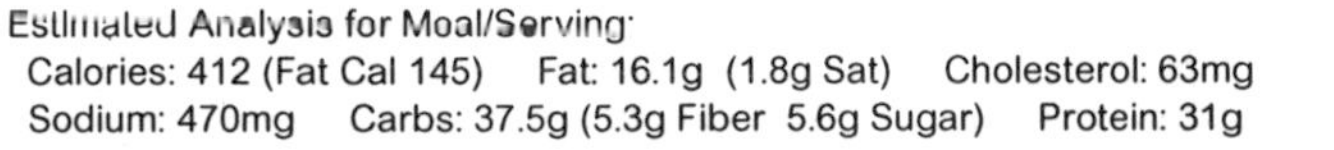
Estimated Analysis for Meal/Serving:
Calories: 412 (Fat Cal 145) Fat: 16.1g (1.8g Sat) Cholesterol: 63mg
Sodium: 470mg Carbs: 37.5g (5.3g Fiber 5.6g Sugar) Protein: 31g

Fancy Hamburgers

Mix and form patties: 20 minutes Photo on Front Cover

These hamburgers are full of flavor but not so fancy that they deter those who like things plain. When Dorie's son was four, he said, "Mommy, I don't like these. I LOVE 'em!"

This dinner can be prepared in 35 or40 minutes from start to finish. But if hamburgers are made in advance (chilled or frozen), this meal can be on the table in 20 minutes or less (see sidebar for outlined steps).

1/4 cup small diced red onion
1/4 cup small diced carrots
1/2 (15 oz.) can diced tomatoes (no salt added)
1 Tbsp. freshly squeezed lemon juice
2 lb. lean ground beef *or* venison
Seasoned garlic salt (p. 222)
Whole-grain bun (optional); see p. 191

1. Place onion and carrots in blender jar; pulse-**blend** until finely chopped. Add tomatoes and lemon juice; blend for several seconds to completely **puree**.
2. Pour mixture into large bowl; add meat. Use hands to **mix** thoroughly. Score into 8 equal portions. Using a hamburger press, **shape** into firm patties. (If no press, form into patties as firmly as possible. Refrigerating covered for a couple of hours will help them stay together if no press is used. Also, may freeze.)
3. **Preheat** skillet or grill pan on medium-low for a few minutes (too hot will quickly burn hamburgers). Gently add hamburgers, season and **cook** to desired doneness, turning only once so these juicy burgers hold together.

Garnish sandwich with lettuce, arugula, tomato, pesto, onion, etc.

Yield: 8 servings

Do-Ahead (*) Quick-Fix Menu

*Fancy Hamburgers
carrot sticks and/or
Green Beans (p. 62)

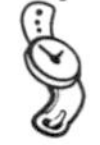

Meal Timing

1. Preheat skillet for hamburgers. (Do not preheat for frozen hamburgers.)
2. Steam green beans.
3. While hamburgers cook, sauté green beans, cut carrots and prepare sandwich garnishes.

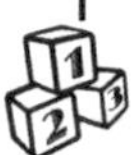

Variations

Southwestern: Add one or two chili peppers when blending carrots and onions. Sprinkle patties with chili powder before grilling. Serve with Black Bean Dip (p. 149) and/or pepper jack cheese.

Mushroom: Serve with sautéed sliced mushrooms and Monterey Jack cheese.

Onion: Top with Caramelized Onions (p. 72).

Low Carb – No Bun

This reduces calories, carbs and sodium but not flavor. Enjoy topping with one of the variations above.

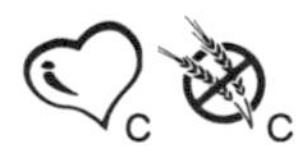

Analysis for Hamburger Patty/Estimate for Dinner:
Calories: 209/499 (Fat Cal 99/189) Fat: 11/21g (4.6/5.5g Sat) Cholesterol: 74mg
Sodium: 210/663 Carbs: 2.2/47g (0.4/11g Fiber 1.2/9g Sugar) Protein: 23/33g

Chicken Broccoli Mac 'n' Cheese

S→T: 25 minutes

This recipe was inspired by Rachael Ray's 30 Minute Meals program on Food Network.

8 oz. raw chicken chunks
1/2 med. onion, chopped (~1/2 cup)
1/2 tsp. paprika
1/8 tsp. cayenne
1 (10 oz.) pkg. frozen broccoli florets
6 oz. dry elbow *or* rotini macaroni
(100% whole wheat, blend, gluten-free; p. 137)
1 1/2 Tbsp. brown rice flour
1 cup chicken broth
1 tsp. Dijon-style mustard
1/2 cup milk (low-fat cow, unsweetened soy)
4 oz. shredded sharp cheddar cheese

1. Place chicken and onion in skillet. Season with paprika and cayenne and begin **sautéing** in water (p. 61).
2. Bring saucepan of water to a boil for pasta while cutting broccoli florets to make them bite-size. Stir chicken occasionally.
3. **Cook** macaroni without salt until al dente (p. 137). Drain. Return to pan and replace lid to keep warm.
4. While macaroni is cooking, **place** broccoli on top of chicken and onions and slide everything to side of skillet. **Add** flour and a small portion of broth to side of skillet, whisking together and cooking for about 1 minute.
5. Continue to **whisk** while slowly adding remaining broth, mustard, milk and cheese.
6. Stir in drained macaroni. **Heat** through. Remove from heat. Cover and allow to **set** for 5–10 minutes.

Yield: 4 servings 6 1/2 cups

Start-to-Finish Quick-Fix Menu

Chicken Broccoli Mac 'n' Cheese

Side Salad with Dijon Salad Dressing (p. 99)

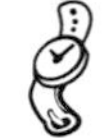

Meal Timing

1. Pull broccoli from freezer to allow it to thaw some.
2. Prepare a side salad.
3. If salad dressing is prepared in advance, set it out to allow it to come to room temperature.
4. Cut chicken and onions.
5. Follow steps in recipe.
6. While dish is setting, prepare salad dressing, if not prepared in advance.

Healthy Bites

Family Comfort Food: It can be difficult to make a macaroni and cheese dish that is healthy. By adding a vegetable, using a whole-grain pasta blend and using real cheese, we add fiber, protein and additional nutrients accompanied by lots of flavor. Better yet, preservatives and colorings are eliminated.

Broccoli has twice the amount of vitamin C found in an equal portion of orange.

Analysis/Serving: (Entrée/Meal)
Calories: 356/407 (Fat Cal 108/144) Fat: 12/16g (6/7g Sat) Cholesterol: 62mg
Sodium: 383/428mg Carbs: 35/39g (7/8.5g Fiber 3/5.8g Sugar) Protein: 27/28g

mustard

Do-Ahead (see Step 1)
Quick-Fix Menu

Venison Teriyaki
with pasta

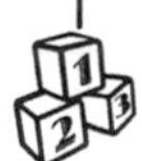

Vegetable Choices

Choose veggies to suit your tastes. Others to try include:

- Carrot matchsticks (add in Step 3 with meat)
- Cabbage, chopped
- French baby green beans (blanched or frozen)
- Broccoli (blanched or frozen)

Healthy Bite

It is important to boil the marinade (Step 4) to fully cook the meat juices.

Helpful Hints

Cutting Meat: Partially frozen meat is easier to cut into strips.

Venison Flavor: Wild game, such as venison, tastes better if allowed to soak in salt water. For this recipe, the soaking in the marinade accomplishes the same thing.

Honey: If only using 1 tablespoon of honey, you may desire to add more wine.

Beef Teriyaki: Substitute beef round steak.

Venison Teriyaki

Prep: 10 min. Marinate: 3 hrs. or longer Cook: 20 min.

Marinade Ingredients:

1–2 Tbsp. honey
3 Tbsp. liquid amino acids (*or* soy sauce, p. 232)
1/2 cup sulfite-free red wine
1/8 tsp. ground ginger (*or* a little less)

1/2 cup finely chopped shallot *or* onion
2 cloves garlic, minced
1 lb. venison round steak/chops

1 Tbsp. Medium-Heat oil
1 cup thinly sliced onions
2 tsp. cornstarch
1 (10 oz.) pkg. frozen asparagus
1 (10 oz.) pkg. frozen tri-color peppers
4 oz. whole-grain pasta (linguine *or* fettuccine)

Stainless steel skillet

1. **Do-ahead marinade:** Whisk marinade ingredients together. Chop shallot/onion and mince garlic, leaving both on cutting board. On a separate cutting board, cut meat into strips; place in a glass dish with lid. Lightly sprinkle with salt. Using your hands, work shallot/onion and garlic into the meat. Pour marinade over top, lifting pieces of meat so the marinade coats all sides. Cover. Place in refrigerator for 3–4 hours or overnight.
2. Begin water boiling for pasta
3. In skillet, **stir-fry** meat and sliced onions in oil, until browned and cooked through. Transfer to serving platter; keep warm.
4. **Stir** cornstarch into remaining marinade; add to skillet and bring to boil, cooking and stirring until **thickened**.
5. *Meanwhile*, **cook** pasta without adding salt to water until al dente; drain.

Analysis/Serving (includes pasta):
Calories: 391–407 (Fat Cal 52) Fat: 5.8g (1.2g Sat) Cholesterol: 73mg
Sodium: 575mg Carbs: 35–40g (5.6g Fiber 10–15g Sugar) Protein: 34g

6. Add asparagus and peppers to sauce in skillet. **Simmer** uncovered to desired doneness, stirring occasionally. (Simmer covered if a thinner consistency is desired.) Return meat to skillet; heat through. **Serve** over pasta.

Yield: 4 servings

Black Bean Dip

S→T: 10–15 minutes

High-Heat oil
2 cloves garlic, minced
1 small onion, chopped (1/4–1/2 cup)
1 jalapeño pepper, minced (seeding optional)
1 (15 oz.) can black beans, undrained (with added salt)
1 1/2 tsp. chili powder
1 1/2 tsp. ground cumin

1. In saucepan or skillet, **"Chop & Drop"** onion, garlic and pepper (use the seeds for increased spiciness; see pp. 74–75) in oil.
2. **Add** the bean liquid (this helps to create the right consistency and retain nutrients), half of the beans, chili powder and cumin. (Do not allow peppers to sit in pan too long before adding bean liquid, since the fumes can be powerful once they start cooking.)
3. Using a fork, **mash** the remaining beans in the can; add. **Simmer** about 10 minutes, or until the thickness of a stew, stirring occasionally. (Sauce will thicken further as it cools.)

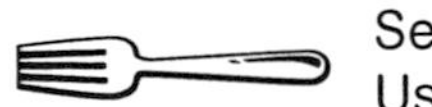

Serve warm or cold.
Use as a dip for raw vegetables.
Use as a spread on sandwiches, toast or crackers.
Use warm as a filling for tacos or burritos *or* as a sauce for Flat Bread Pizzas (see sidebar).

Yield: 21 (1 Tbsp.) servings   1 1/3 cups

Analysis for Black Bean Dip/Tablespoon:
Calories: 27 (Fat Cal 6)   Fat: 0.7g (0g Sat)   Cholesterol: 0mg
Sodium: 12   Carbs: 3.6g (0.8g Fiber 0.3g Sugar)   Protein: 1.2g

Start-to-Finish Quick-Fix Menu

Flat Bread Pizza
Side Salad (optional)

Spicy Flatbread Pizza

Create individual pizzas to suit each family member!

Whole-grain flatbread (or tortilla)
Bean dip (or salsa, pesto or tomato sauce)
Toppings
  With bean dip, we enjoy cooked chicken chunks, spinach and corn.
Shredded Cheese
  Our favorite with bean dip is a Monterey Jack and mozzarella blend.

Preheat oven—350°.

Place flatbreads in single layer on baking sheet. **Parbake** about 5 minutes while you gather toppings. **Remove** from oven. **Spread** bean dip (or salsa, pesto or tomato sauce) over flatbread, **add** toppings as desired and **sprinkle** with cheese. **Bake** 5–10 minutes, or until toppings are hot and cheese has melted.

Serve individuals whole pizzas, cut into halves to share, or into eighths for an appetizer.

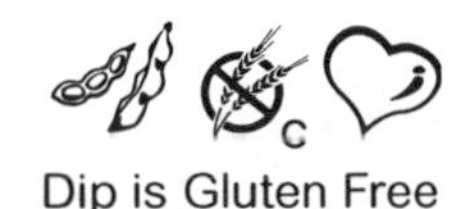

Dip is Gluten Free

Do-Ahead (*) Quick-Fix Menu

*Cabbage-Fish Bake
(prepare the night before or earlier in the day)
Roasted Asparagus (p. 46)

Helpful Hints

Do-Ahead: Poach and flake fish ahead of time. Store in fridge for one day or in freezer for one month.

Managing Oven Space: If you do not have two ovens and desire to serve Cabbage-Fish Bake with Roasted Asparagus (a delicious combination), we suggest baking the casserole at 375° and roasting the asparagus in the same oven, allowing about 5–7 minutes more roasting time.

Asparagus Healthy Bite & Tidbits

- The National Cancer Institutes says that asparagus has more glutathione (an anticarcinogen) than any other food.[1]
- An asparagus spear can grow ten inches a day!
- Asparagus dates back to the time of the dinosaurs. Tell your kids they're eating dino food!

Cabbage-Fish Bake

S→O: 25–30 minutes Bake: 10–15 minutes
Bake: 20–40 minutes when dish is cold

1 lb. fish fillets—sole, cod, pollack
1 Tbsp. freshly squeezed lemon juice
1 Tbsp. Medium-Heat oil
1 small fennel bulb, cored and sliced (1 cup)
1 cup sliced carrots
1/4 tsp. each: salt, pepper
1 tsp. dried dill
4 cups chopped cabbage
1 Tbsp. brown rice flour
1 cup vegetable broth
1/2 cup milk (low-fat cow)
3 Tbsp. Parmesan cheese (divided)
1/2 cup dry bread crumbs (p. 98; optional)

Preheat oven—350°. Two-quart baking dish

1. In skillet with lid, place ¼ cup water, followed by fish and lemon juice; **poach** while slicing fennel. When fish flakes easily with a fork, transfer to a plate, toss poaching water and wipe out upper portion of skillet with a cloth.
2. In same skillet, **sauté** fennel in oil for approximately 3–4 minutes while slicing carrots.
3. Add carrots, salt, pepper and dill. **Sauté** another 5–6 minutes while chopping cabbage.
4. Add cabbage. **Sauté** until it has "cooked down," about 3–4 minutes while flaking fish. (If pan gets dry, add a little water as needed.) **Stir** in fish. **Transfer** to baking dish.
5. **Add** 1–2 tablespoons of the broth to skillet and stir in flour. Allow flour to **cook** over medium heat for about a minute, stirring constantly with a whisk. Slowly **whisk** in remaining broth and milk. Bring to boil; reduce heat and **cook** until thickened. **Stir** in 2 tablespoons of the Parmesan cheese.

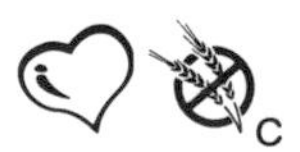

Analysis/Serving: (Entrée/Meal)
Calories: 242/337 (Fat Cal 72/117) Fat: 8/13g (2.5g Sat) Cholesterol: 64mg
Sodium: 510/649mg Carbs: 17/25g (4/7g Fiber 7/11 Sugar) Protein: 27/31g

6. **Pour** sauce over fish and vegetables.
7. In a bowl, drizzle ¼ teaspoon of oil over bread crumbs; stir in ¼ teaspoon of dried dill. Then stir in the remaining 1 tablespoon of Parmesan cheese. **Sprinkle** over fish mixture.
8. **Bake** in preheated oven 10–15 minutes, or until bubbly and vegetables reach desired doneness. (If refrigerated, allow extra time.)

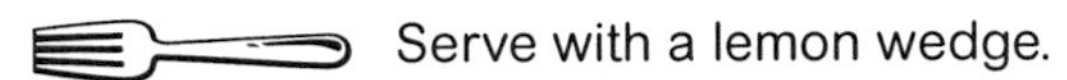
Serve with a lemon wedge.

Yield: 4 servings

Easy Baked Fish

S→O: 5 minutes Bake: 15–20 minutes

4 (~5 oz.) fish fillets—tilapia, orange roughy, flounder, cod, pollack

Seasoning Ideas—salt, pepper, parsley, paprika, garlic salt/powder, tarragon, and/or Dijon mustard (omit salt with Dijon mustard)

2–3 lemons

Preheat oven—375° to 400°.
Oil 9x13x2-inch baking dish.

1. Rinse fish fillets; lay in prepared baking dish. Add a little water to dish. If desired, spray High-Heat oil on fillets. Add your choice of fresh or dried seasonings. Thinly slice two lemons (8 slices); lay 2 slices on each fillet.
2. **Bake** for 15–20 minutes, or until fish flakes. (Time depends upon thickness of fillet, if using convection or conventional oven and oven temperature.) Remove from oven and garnish with flaxseed oil (or melted butter).

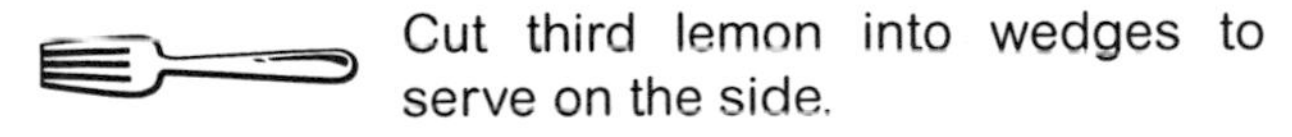
Cut third lemon into wedges to serve on the side.

Yield: 4 servings

Do-Ahead (*) Quick-Fix Menu

Easy Baked Fish
Glazed Carrots (p. 54)
Side Salad with Arugula
*Balsamic Vinaigrette Salad Dressing (p. 70)
*Cheese Biscuits (p. 183)
(Advance-prep the Cheese Biscuit Mix)

Meal Timing

1. Preheat oven to 400°. Set salad dressing out to allow it come to room temperature.
2. Prepare carrots for cooking, set aside.
3. Prepare fish for oven. If fish fillets are thin, hold for 5 minutes while you mix up and dip biscuits.
4. Slide fish and biscuits in oven; bake 10 minutes. Start carrots to cook.
5. Prepare salad, melt Seasoned Butter for biscuits and set out ingredients to glaze carrots.
6. Check biscuits for doneness and check to see if fish needs more water.
7. Brush butter on biscuits and keep warm in towel-lined basket. Glaze carrots. Check doneness of fish. Serve immediately, since fish cools quickly.

Estimated Analysis/Dinner:
Calories: 357 (Fat Cal 129) Fat: 14.3g (6.7g Sat) Cholesterol: 92mg
Sodium: 445mg Carbs: 25.8g (4.6g Fiber 7.5g Sugar) Protein: 34g

Start-to-Finish Quick-Fix Menu

Salmon & Pasta

Busy Moms

Chop vegetables, blanch fresh broccoli (or use frozen) and poach salmon earlier in the day, such as while child is napping. This eases the preparation stress at meal time. *Or*, on a **Do-Ahead Day**, poach salmon, flake, package in 1 cup portions and freeze.

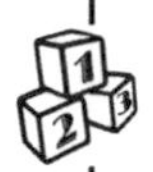

Summertime Variation

When summer squash varieties are plentiful, we enjoy this combination:

- 1 cup matchstick carrots
- 3/4 cup green beans
- 1 cup sliced red onion
- 1 1/4 cups sliced patty-pan or zucchini squash

Prepare according to recipe directions, sautéing carrots in place of fennel, steaming green beans in place of broccoli and adding squash and green beans with onions. We enjoy basil and oregano with this vegetable combo.

Salmon & Pasta

S→T: 30 minutes

8 oz. salmon fillets
1 Tbsp. freshly squeezed lemon juice
Fresh or dried dill
1 cup diced fennel (1 small fennel)
1 cup sliced red onions (*or* ½ cup sliced shallots)
2 cups fresh (*or* ~7oz. frozen) **broccoli florets** (cut to make bite-size)
2 tsp. Medium-Heat oil
1/4 tsp. each: salt, garlic powder
Freshly ground black pepper
2 tsp. brown rice flour
1–1 1/4 cups milk (low-fat cow, unsweetened soy)
2 oz. whole-grain fettuccine *or* noodles
2 cloves garlic, minced
1–2 Tbsp. freshly minced parsley

1. In large skillet with lid, place ¼ cup water, followed by salmon, lemon juice and dill; **poach** for 6–8 minutes while **preparing** vegetables.
2. In saucepan with small amount of water, **steam** fresh broccoli (seasoned lightly with salt and pepper) for 2–3 minutes. Remove broccoli and set aside. Add water; bring to **boil** for pasta.
3. When salmon flakes easily with a fork, transfer to a plate. Rinse out skillet.
4. In same skillet, **sauté** fennel in oil for 3 minutes while mincing garlic and parsley. Add onions, salt, garlic powder, pepper and more dill. **Sauté** for 3 additional minutes while flaking fish, adding a little water as needed.
5. **Cook pasta** without salt until al dente (p. 137). Drain; sprinkle lightly with salt.
6. If using frozen broccoli, add to skillet. Slide vegetables to side of skillet. Add 2 tablespoons of water; stir in flour; **cook** over medium heat for a minute, whisking constantly.

Analysis/Serving:
Calories: 454 (Fat Cal 127) Fat: 14.1g (2.6g Sat) Cholesterol: 51mg
Sodium: 421mg Carbs: 46g (8g Fiber 12g Sugar) Protein: 37g

7. Slowly **whisk** in milk; cook so sauce begins to **thicken**; **add** salmon and broccoli (if using fresh broccoli). Stir together and heat through. **Stir** in parsley and garlic. Taste and add lemon juice or sprinkle of salt as needed.
8. **Drain** pasta. **Serve** salmon and vegetables over pasta.

Yield: 2 servings   3 cups salmon mixture
Recipe can be easily doubled or cut in half.

Salsa Chicken Salad

1 lb. boneless, skinless chicken breasts
2 cups salsa (see below)
Romaine lettuce (3 cups/salad)
Low-fat shredded cheese (1/2 oz./salad)
Blue corn chips, broken (1/2 oz./salad)

Midsized or standard-sized slow cooker

1. **Place** chicken in slow cooker. If a "hotter" flavor is desired, stir green chili or chili paste into salsa. **Pour** salsa over chicken, lifting up chicken to get some underneath as well.
2. **Slow cook** on LOW for 3–4 hours, or until tender and easily pulls apart to shred.
3. **Serve:** Shred meat. Assemble individual salads (lettuce, chicken and cheese), using remaining salsa from slow cooker as dressing. Garnish with chips and dollop of sour cream.

Yield: 4 meal salads

Salsa: Choose a brand that has less than 100 mg. of sodium per 2 tablespoons. We love Peach Mango by Desert Pepper Trading Company or Green Mountain Gringo, adding diced frozen fruit (e.g., 8 peach slices and 8 large mango chunks for above recipe).

Tortilla Wrap: Pour only 1 cup of salsa on chicken (since do not need extra for dressing). Serve in whole-grain tortilla with lettuce and cheese.

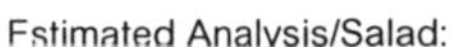
Estimated Analysis/Salad:
Calories: 326 (Fat Cal 84)   Fat: 9.3g (3g Sat)   Cholesterol: 71mg
Sodium: 332mg   Carbs: 31g (4.5g Fiber 14g Sugar)   Protein: 30g

Origin of the "Marathon"

The Greek word for fennel is "marathon." Back in 490 B.C., after a major victory of the Greeks over the Persians, a runner ran from the battlefield (in a field of fennel), twenty-six miles back to the town of Athens to report the good news. Ever since then, the marathon has been defined as a race of twenty-six miles.

Slow Cooker Quick-Fix Menu

Salsa Chicken Salad

Salad Helpful Hints

Slow Cooking Time depends upon amount of meat (if doubling the recipe or making 1–2 servings in small slow cooker), if meat is frozen and if cooking on low or high. Generally, a single serving on low takes 2–3 hours, and a couple of pounds (so have extras) takes 8 hours on LOW.

Variation: Use lean pork chops (boneless or bone-in) and pineapple salsa (or add crushed pineapple to slow cooker with salsa).

Start-to-Finish Quick-Fix Menu

Turkey Loaf Patties
Oven Fries (p. 76)
Steamed Broccoli (p. 52)

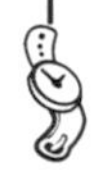

Meal Timing

1. Preheat oven.
2. Prepare and start Oven Fries.
3. Prepare and cook Turkey Loaf Patties, flipping occasionally.
4. Stir Oven Fries
5. Prepare and steam broccoli.

Serve and enjoy!

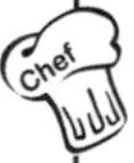

Do-Ahead

Turkey loaf patties can be mixed, shaped and refrigerated or frozen to cook later.

Mini Food Processor

To finely chop onions, etc., use a mini-sized processor, alternating between the chop and grind buttons.

Turkey Loaf Patties

Mix and patty: 15 minutes   Cook: 10–12 minutes

1 cup sliced carrots
1/2 cup chopped onions (optional)
1/2 cup quick oats
OR quinoa flakes
1/2 tsp. salt
1 lb. ground turkey breast meat
2–4 Tbsp. water

If using cast-iron skillet, **preheat** on medium-low.

1. In small food processor, finely **chop** carrots and onions (see equipment tip in sidebar). Add to a large bowl and **mix** with oats (or quinoa flakes) and salt. Add turkey and gently **combine** with your hands, adding water as needed to form mixture together.
2. Lightly **oil** skillet. **Shape** into 8 patties; place in skillet as shaped. Lightly oil tops of patties. **Cook** about 10–12 minutes, or until internal temperature is 160° (gently flip occasionally). **Optional Cooking Method:** Bake in oven as described on next page.

Meat Loaf: If desired, shape into 4 or 6 oval mini meat loaves. Bake in oven as directed in recipes on next page.

Dark Meat Turkey: Ground dark turkey meat can be used in place of ground breast meat; if so, do not oil the tops of patties.

Onions: The authors prefer red onions when using quinoa flakes.

Quinoa: This recipe is a tasty and easy way to introduce quinoa into your diet and it offers a gluten-free meat loaf.

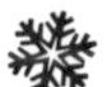 Extras may be frozen. Leftovers offer variety for breakfast.

Yield: 4–6 servings   8 patties

Analysis for Patty with Oats/Estimate for Meal with 2 Patties:
Calories: 101/387 (Fat Cal 29/101)   Fat: 3.2/11.2g (0.3/1g Sat)   Cholesterol: 30/60mg
Sodium: 168/579mg   Carbs: 5.8/45g (1.1/6.9g Fiber 1.3/4.7g Sugar)   Protein: 12.6/31g

Italian *or* Chili Meat Loaf Patties

Mix and patty: 15 minutes   Bake: 15–20 minutes

1 med. onion (1 cup coarsely chopped)
2 cloves garlic, cracked
3/4–1 cup quick oats (prefer 1 cup with beef)
1/2 (6 oz.) can tomato paste
1/2 tsp. salt
Freshly ground black pepper
Seasonings with beef
  2 tsp. Italian seasoning mix
    Or half the amount of seasonings below
Seasonings with venison
  2 tsp. chili powder
  1 tsp. ground cumin
  1 tsp. leaf oregano, crushed
  1/2 tsp. crushed red pepper
1 lb. lean ground—beef or venison

Preheat oven—400°. Lightly **oil** baking sheet with sides (e.g., jelly roll pan).

1. In small food processor, finely **chop** onions and garlic. Add to a large bowl and **mix** with oats, tomato paste, salt, pepper and seasonings. Add meat and gently **combine** with your hands.
2. **Shape** into 8 oval or round patties. Lay single layer on prepared baking sheet. Lightly oil top side with High-Heat oil. **Bake** in preheated (or preheating) oven for 10 minutes, flip and bake another 5–10 minutes, or until internal temperature is 160°. (Convection oven takes less time; venison patties take a little longer to cook.) If desired, after flipping spread on a thin layer of a healthier-choice ketchup.

Extras may be frozen. Leftovers are delicious cold or warm for a sandwich.

Yield: 4–6 servings   8 patties

Start-to-Finish Quick-Fix Menu

Italian *or* Chili Meat Loaf Patties
Green Beans (p. 62)
Side Salad
(use bagged mixed greens)
Salad Dressing (p. 70)

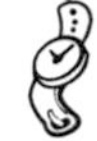

Meal Timing

1. Preheat oven; oil baking sheet. Prepare and start meat loaf patties.
2. Steam green beans, dice onion and begin Balsamic Vinaigrette Salad Dressing or other dressing of your choice.
3. Flip meat loaf patties.
4. Sauté green beans while finishing salad dressing and salad.

Serve and enjoy!

Helpful Hints

Do-Ahead: Meat loaf patties can be mixed, shaped and refrigerated or frozen to cook later.

Meat Loaf: If desired, shape into 4 or 6 oval mini meat loaves. Allow extra time to bake.

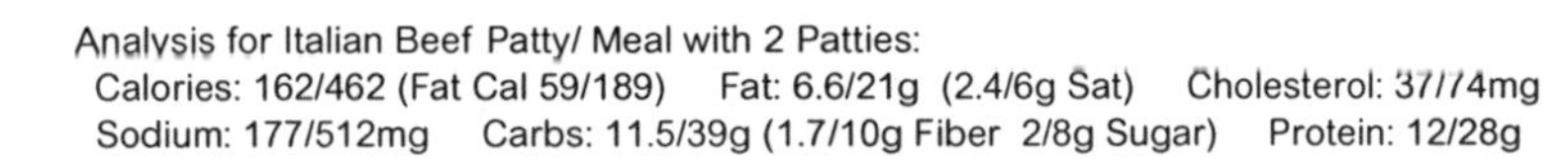
Analysis for Italian Beef Patty/ Meal with 2 Patties:
Calories: 162/462 (Fat Cal 59/189)   Fat: 6.6/21g (2.4/6g Sat)   Cholesterol: 37/74mg
Sodium: 177/512mg   Carbs: 11.5/39g (1.7/10g Fiber 2/8g Sugar)   Protein: 12/28g

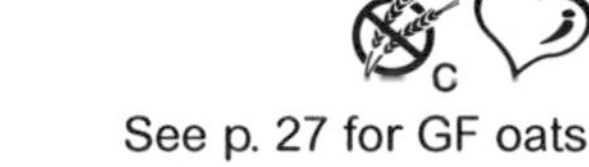

See p. 27 for GF oats

Slow Cooker Quick-Fix Menu

Slow Cooker Roast Pork
Spinach-Sweet Potato (p. 135; sidebar)
Sautéed Cabbage (p. 53)
applesauce

Meal Timing for both Dinners

Advanced Prep:

Start roast in slow cooker at the appropriate time.

Before Meal Prep:

1. Dice and cook potatoes.
2. Preheat skillet for vegetable side dish. Chop (and/or blanch) veggies.
3. Cut fresh fruit or set out applesauce.
4. Start stir-frying vegetables. Lay spinach on top of cooked potatoes.
5. Transfer roast to plate to rest for 5 minutes.
6. In between stirring vegetables, put broth in bowl to serve, if using; mash potatoes and slice meats.

Slow Cooker Quick-Fix Menu

Slow Cooker Roast Beef
Spinach-Red Potato (p. 135; sidebar)
Stir-Fry Vegetables (p. 38)
fresh fruit

Slow Cooker Pork Roast

Prep for slow cooker: 15 minutes Slow cook: 8–10 hours

3-4 small onions, cut in wedges (divided)
3/4 cup water (smaller roast needs more water)
2–3 pound pork loin roast
1/2 tsp dried sage
Fresh rosemary to taste (4–6 [6-inch] sprigs)

Standard-sized slow cooker

Place water and half of the onions in slow cooker. **Season** with salt and pepper. Add 1–2 sprigs of rosemary and roast. **Season** with salt, pepper, sage and sprig of coarsely minced rosemary. **Rub** in seasonings. **Flip** and repeat seasoning. Add remaining onions. **Cook** on LOW for 8–10 hrs. or on HIGH for 1 hr.; then on LOW for 7–9 hrs.

Optional: Approximately 2 hours before serving, lay a whole sprig of rosemary in slow cooker, gently crushing a few leaves to release the oils.

Serve sliced or shredded. Drizzle cooking liquid over pork, top with onions.

Slow Cooker Beef Roast

Prep for slow cooker: 10 minutes Slow cook: 3–8 hours

1/2 cup beef broth
1 lg. onion, cut in wedges (divided)
2 pound lean beef roast (arm, chuck)
1 tsp. Worcestershire sauce (optional)

Standard-sized slow cooker

Place broth and most of onions in slow cooker, followed by roast. **Rub** Worcestershire sauce into roast. Lightly **season** with salt, pepper and dried thyme. **Add** remaining onions on top of roast. **Cook** for 4–8 hours on LOW or for 3–5 hours on HIGH (time depends upon thickness).

Separate off the fat (see next page sidebar), using broth for gravy or use broth to heat leftover beef slices.

Slow Cooker Chicken & Veggies

Prep for slow cooker: 15 minutes   Slow cook: 2–6 hours

Large oval slow cooker

Pour 1 cup (or less) of low-sodium chicken broth or water in slow cooker. Thoroughly rinse whole chicken (~5 lb.). **Season** chicken, including underneath and inside cavity with salt and pepper (or seasoned garlic salt, p. 222). Place in slow cooker. **Layer** coarsely chopped/thick sliced vegetables (e.g., onions, potatoes, turnips, summer squash, carrots, celery, cabbage, colored bell peppers) around chicken (or some under). **Season** vegetables. Sprinkle top of chicken and vegetables with small diced fennel and/or fresh minced garlic. **Cook** on LOW for 5–6 hours or HIGH for 2–3 hours.

A turkey leg/thigh can be substituted for chicken.

Fresh Rosemary and Sage Variation: Place some sage leaves and 1–2 sprigs of rosemary under chicken. Tuck a few more into vegetables. (After cooking, remove stems and mix the leaves into vegetables.) Chop some sage and mince some rosemary to rub on chicken.

Extras: Debone chicken; combine chicken, vegetables and broth (see equipment tip) for a soup.

Great Meal for One or Two: Use bone-in chicken pieces instead of a whole chicken and cook in a small-sized slow cooker on LOW for 3–4 hours.

Chicken Cabbage Delight

Perfect Meal for One, Two or Family

Using the method described above, select chopped cabbage, thickly sliced celery and onions for the vegetables. Season with salt, pepper and fresh or dried dill.

Herbed Noodles: Cook pasta al dente (p. 137). Drain and season with salt, pepper and dill. Pour a little broth from the slow cooker over pasta; mix in vegetables. Serve.

Slow Cooker Quick-Fix Menu

Slow Cooker Chicken & Veggies
Hearty Homemade Bread

Meal Timing

Advanced Prep: Start bread (p. 190) in bread machine so that it completes the cycle 15 minutes before you will eat. Start chicken and vegetables in slow cooker at appropriate time.

At Serving Time: Remove chicken from slow cooker and allow to rest 5 minutes before slicing. Slice bread. Dish up vegetables.

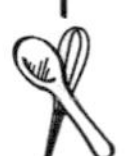

Broth-Fat Separator

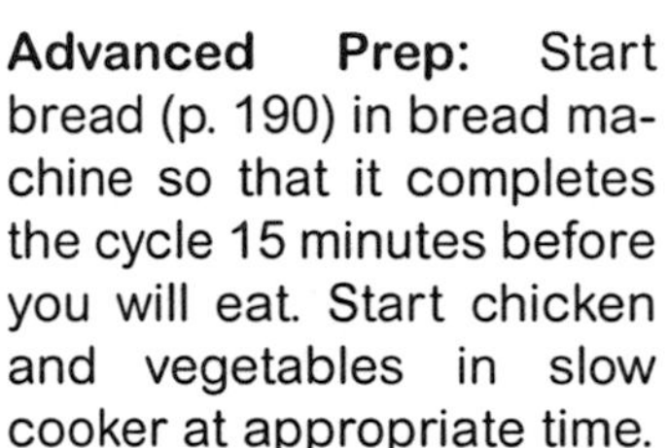

Pour broth into separator through a fine mesh strainer. Pour off fat. Toss. Pour broth off to use. Discard fat at the bottom. Some separators have a filter and so you do not need a strainer.

Slow Cooker Quick-Fix Menu

Chicken-Cabbage Delight
Herbed Noodles

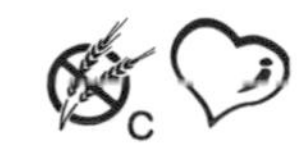

Start-to-Finish Quick-Fix Menu

Seared Tofu
Herbed Noodles
Seasoned Squash (p. 80)

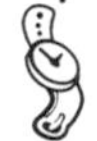

Meal Timing

1. Prepare squash to sauté.
2. Start water for pasta.
3. Coat/start sautéing tofu.
4. Preheat skillet for squash.
5. Begin pasta; do Step 3 of tofu; start squash.
6. Drain and season pasta.
7. Finish squash; serve.

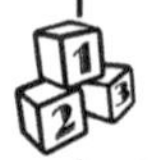

Variations

Cinnamon Blend: Great paired with Roasted Butternut Squash (p. 83):
1 tsp. each: onion powder, ground cinnamon
1/2 tsp. each: ground cumin, allspice, garlic powder
Freshly grated nutmeg and black pepper

Tofu Sandwich: Slice tofu approximately half-inch thick. Sprinkle and rub in seasonings. Follow Step 2 and 3 except flip tofu like a burger instead of stirring during cooking. Enjoy hot or cold on whole-grain bread with healthy sandwich garnishes (p. 145).

Seared Tofu

S→T: 20 minutes

Tofu has little flavor but accepts any you give it. Create your own blend, use those in this recipe, use the cinnamon blend in the sidebar or purchase a salt-free blend (e.g., Hickory Barbeque [p. 222], Sondra's favorite for Tofu Sandwich).

2 tsp. dried parsley flakes
1 tsp. garlic powder
1 tsp. onion powder
1 tsp. paprika
Freshly ground black pepper
6 oz. firm tofu, diced (1/2-inch) (~1 1/3 cups)
2 tsp. High-Heat oil
~1 Tbsp. water
2 tsp. liquid aminos (*or* tamari *or* soy sauce; be cautious of sodium)

Preheat cast-iron skillet on medium.

1. In bowl, **whisk** seasonings together. Add diced tofu (still moist from being packed in water). Gently **toss** to coat all sides.
2. Add oil to skillet; when warm add tofu. **Sauté** for 5 minutes to sear flavor into tofu; stir enough to keep it from burning but not so often that the tofu falls apart.
3. In bowl, stir water and liquid aminos together. Evenly pour over tofu, while stirring. Continue to stir often. **Sauté** to desired crispness. Best served immediately.

Yield: 2 servings (can be doubled or cut in half).

Herbed Noodles: Cook egg (or no-egg) whole-grain noodles until al dente. Drain; return to pan. Sprinkle lightly with salt and generously with dried parsley, garlic powder and paprika. Drizzle with flaxseed oil (for its buttery taste). Toss.

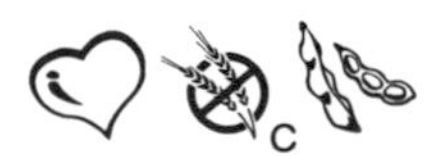

Analysis/Serving for Served Tofu/Estimate for Dinner:
Calories: 132/350 (Fat Cal 77/171) Fat: 8.6/19g (0.8/1.7g Sat) Cholesterol: 0mg
Sodium: 229/373mg Carbs: 5/31g (0.8/7g Fiber 0.8/4g Sugar) Protein: 8/15g

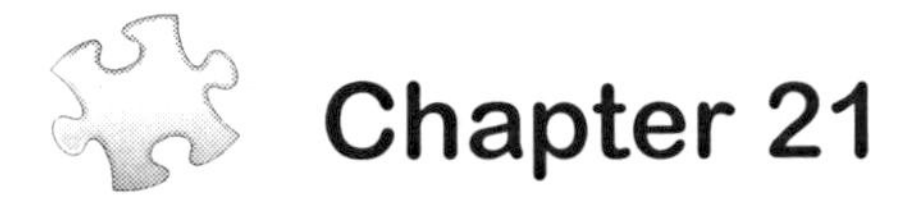

Chapter 21

Cooking for One or Two

It's hard to be motivated to cook for just one or two, and it's challenging to find recipes that don't create lots of hard-to-use leftovers. This chapter highlights three types of meals for one or two: (1) meals that can be prepared in small quantities without wasted ingredients, (2) meals with leftovers that can become future meals because they freeze easily and (3) meals using healthier convenience foods (see p. 143).*

Recipes and meals that are either written for two servings or can be prepared in small quantities
**Tips for preparing small portions are noted on the recipe or in the sidebar.*

20-Minute Stir Fry Dinner (p. 61)
Acorn Squash meals (pp. 82 and 160)
Asian Salmon Salad (p. 96)
*Barley Casserole (p. 180)
Basic Soup (p. 118)
*Biscuits (pp. 182–183)
*Breakfast Squares (p. 108)
Caramelized Onion Dinner (p. 72)
*Chicken/Pork Tortilla Wraps (p. 153)
*Chicken-Cabbage Delight (p. 157)
Chicken-Vegetable Spread (p. 160)
Collard Wraps (p. 57)
*Flatbread Pizzas (p. 149)
*Fruit Crisps (pp. 202–203)
*Grilled Chicken/Pork Rubs (p. 145)
Meal-in-a-Salad (p. 94)
Pea & Celery Salad (p. 74)
*Pecan Crusted Chicken Salad (p. 98)
Salmon & Pasta (p. 152)
*Salsa Chicken/Pork Salad (p. 153)
Chard & Balsamic Chicken (p. 56)
Seared Tofu (p. 158)
*Shortcakes (pp. 182 and 196)
*Slow Cooker Chicken Veggies (p. 157)
Smoothies (p. 106)
Stuffed Peppers (p. 75)
Vegetables Side Dishes
(pp. 38, 39, 43, 45, 46, 49–55, 58, 59, 62, 64, 66–72, 76, 80, 83, 86 and 88)
Wilted Spinach Salad (p. 101)

Recipes and meals that freeze well, using little space

Chili — several varieties (pp. 130–133)
Chunky Garden Spaghetti (p. 136)
Cookies (half batches or frozen logs) (pp. 85 and 197–199)
Fancy Hamburgers (p. 146)
Granola/Protein Bars (pp. 112–114)
Hearty Homemade Bread (p. 190)
Meat Loaf Patties (pp. 154–155)
Oven-Fried Chicken/Chunks (p. 144)
Pizzas (pp. 168–170)
Shepherd's Pie (p. 134)
Soups (pp. 120–127)
Sweet Potato Cakes (p. 89)
Tacos and Taco Salad (pp. 100–101)
Veggie Burgers (p. 78)

Do-Ahead Option

Squash can be roasted, blended, covered and refrigerated. Pull out of fridge when ready to begin Step 3.

Toaster Oven

A small countertop toaster-convection oven is handy for baking (and warming) meals for one or two people, especially when you're in a hurry.

Chicken-Vegetable Spread/Tortilla Wraps

1/2 cup cooked chicken
1/2 cup diced carrots
OR red bell pepper
2 Tbsp. walnuts
2 Tbsp. Pesto (p. 93) or
healthier-choice mayo

In small food chopper, grind all ingredients.
Serve as filling for tortilla wrap with lettuce, arugula, sliced tomatoes and/or sliced onions.
Or serve with lettuce and Arugula Pesto Dressing (p. 44) for an easy low-carb meal.

Vegetarian Spread

Use two Hard-Cooked Eggs in place of chicken; delicious with red pepper and arugula.

Makes a great travel lunch.

Yield: 1 cup

Acorn Squash with Pork Chops

S→T: 1 hour (Do-Ahead Option for 30-Minute Meal)

1 (1 lb.) acorn squash
1 tsp. Medium-Heat oil
1 cup sliced onions
2 (4–6 oz.) lean pork chops
(boneless/bone-in)
1 cup 100% apple juice

Preheat oven—400°, then 350°.
Oil baking dish.

1. Place whole squash in baking pan. **Roast** for approximately 30 minutes, or until squash gives a bit when gently pushed with the thumb. When done, remove from oven, cool slightly; lower oven temperature. Cut squash in half (vertically), remove seeds and **scoop** flesh out into bowl. Add a sprinkle of salt and allspice; **blend** with an immersion blender until creamy and smooth. Add to baking dish.
2. *Meanwhile*, in skillet, **sauté** onions in oil and sprinkle of salt for 5 minutes. **Rub** pork chops with oil, salt and allspice (see p. 145). **Cook** with onions until almost done. If skillet gets dry, add a little water.
3. Transfer pork and onions to a plate. Add apple juice to skillet; heat and whisk to **deglaze** pan. Pour half of this deglazed liquid over prepared squash; stir. Lay pork chops on top of squash; drizzle remaining liquid over meat.
4. **Bake** in 350° preheated oven 10–15 minutes, or until serving temperature.

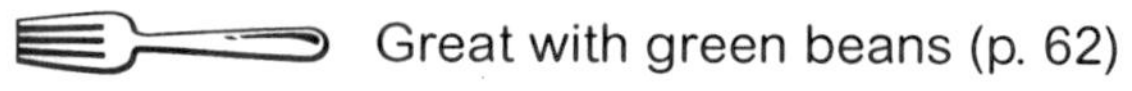
Great with green beans (p. 62)

Yield: 2 servings

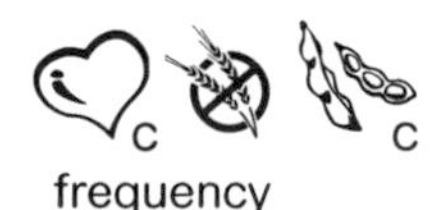

Estimated Analysis/Dinner:
Calories: 439 (Fat Cal 165) Fat: 18.3g (3.8g Sat) Cholesterol: 62mg
Sodium: 336mg Carbs: 41.6g (8.9g Fiber 22g Sugar) Protein: 30g

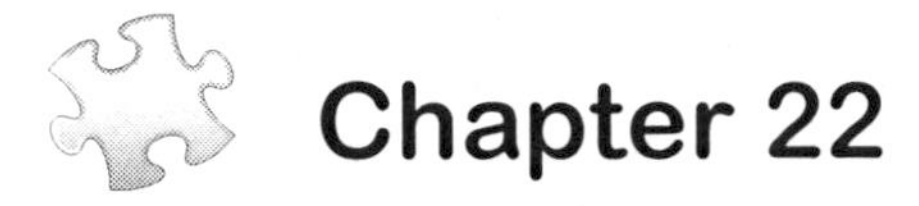

Chapter 22

Holiday Dinner Makeover

Holidays are a time when we enjoy meals with others, but that does not mean we must toss out healthier eating. These recipes can be used independently or as a complete meal.

Menu

Sparkling Apple Juice
Vegetables, Cheese, Crackers   Confetti Dip
Scarborough Fair Turkey Breast
Fruit Glazed Sweet Potatoes   Mixed Vegetables
Whole-Grain Bread or Dinner Rolls
Pie: Pumpkin or Pecan and/or Pumpkin Cheesecake
Whipped Topping (garnish for the desserts)

While guests arrive, have healthy appetizers and beverages available. Emphasize vegetables by providing a colorful variety (e.g., carrots, peppers, tomatoes, blanched fresh asparagus) along with Confetti Dip. Smaller amounts of low-fat cheese and whole-grain crackers make a nice accompaniment. Choose a (100% juice) sparkling apple juice or cider.

Recipes not in this chapter are:
Confetti Dip (p. 42)
Whole-Grain Bread (p. 190)
Dinner Rolls (p. 192)
Pumpkin Cheesecake (p. 201)

Timing: The easiest way to prepare a meal is to write out a plan. Start with reading the recipes, jotting down the estimated prep time, bake/cook time and whether things can be prepared in advance. Then complete a time line chart; working backward seems to be easier (e.g., turkey done at noon; start slow cooker at 9:30 a.m.; start prep at 9:10 a.m.).

Special Note: Do not forget to eat breakfast. We suggest Pumpkin Pie Smoothie (p. 106).

Increasing Fiber

Making your own whole- (or partially whole-) grain dinner rolls or bread increases fiber and typically reduces sodium and fats, along with avoiding harmful trans fats and preservatives.

Using a bread machine makes it quick and easy.

Scarborough Fair Turkey Breast

Prep: 20 minutes Cook: See Step 3

The seaside town of Scarborough, England, played host to an annual trading fair in late medieval times. The ballad known as "Scarborough Fair" has been written and revised in many different ways, including the popular version by Simon and Garfunkel recorded in 1966. The song tells the story of a young man offering to take back his love if she completes a series of impossible tasks. She counters with equally impossible tasks for him to perform. The refrain "parsley, sage, rosemary and thyme" is repeated in each stanza and refers to four virtues the lovers desired of each other. Parsley was to remove all bitterness; sage was a symbol of strength; rosemary was a symbol of love and faithfulness; and thyme was a depiction of courage.

This recipe was inspired by Rachael Ray's 60-minute Thanksgiving dinner (Food Network, 2005). It was only when typing up the list of herbs that Sondra was reminded of the song. Enjoy this easy turkey breast, "Scarborough Fair" style!

Fresh Herbs Amount to Purchase

The amount of fresh sage, rosemary and thyme used in this recipe is approximately half the amount found in a three-fourths ounce package of poultry mix.

Mini Food Processor

A mini-sized food processor is handy for chopping and blending small amounts of vegetables or herbs, such as with the herb mixture for this recipe.

Herb Mixture:

1/4 cup coarsely chopped onion
Small handful fresh parsley (1/4 cup packed)
6 fresh sage leaves
1/2 Tbsp. fresh rosemary leaves (stems removed)
1/2 Tbsp. fresh thyme leaves (stems removed)
1/4 tsp. salt
1 Tbsp. Medium-Heat oil

1 (~2 lb.) boneless turkey breast half, skin on OR turkey leg-thigh with bone and skin
Salt and freshly ground black pepper

Gravy:

1 Tbsp. raw apple cider vinegar (optional)
2 Tbsp. brown rice flour

Oil bottom/sides (up about 2 inches) of a large oval slow cooker crock. Add ¼ cup of water.

1. In mini food processor, **chop** onions, fresh herbs, salt and oil to create a coarse herb mixture.

2. Run your fingers between the skin and the flesh at one end of turkey breast to **create a pocket**, being careful not to pull skin completely off. **Stuff** herb mixture under the skin; spread evenly. **Season** underneath side of turkey breast with salt (~¼ tsp.) and pepper. Lay breast in slow cooker crock. Drizzle/brush **oil** onto skin. Season lightly with a little more salt and pepper.
3. **Slow cook** on HIGH for 2½ hours or LOW for 4–5 hours.
4. Remove to cutting board. Allow turkey breast to **set** for 5 minutes before slicing.
5. **Prepare gravy**: Transfer juices to small skillet. Add optional vinegar. Whisk a few tablespoons of water into flour; then whisk mixture into juices. Cook for 2 minutes. If needed, add broth or water. Simmer until thickened. Taste and season with salt and pepper if needed.
6. **Slice** the turkey breast on the diagonal.

Mixed Vegetables

Complement your healthy holiday dinner with a colorful array of lightly steamed fresh vegetables (e.g., broccoli and cauliflower florets with thick slices of carrots, celery, red peppers and zucchini).

The vegetables can be steamed together in the same pan. Just place the vegetables that take the longest to cook on the bottom (e.g. carrots, celery).

When transferring to serving bowl, lightly toss with flaxseed oil and garnish with freshly minced parsley or carrot tops.

Holiday Dinner Makeover continued on next page . . .

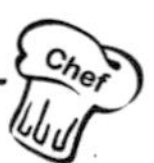

Serving Extras

Uneaten portions may be used in a variety of ways:

- sliced for sandwiches
- cut in strips for salads
- chunked for use in soups or casseroles (e.g., Pepper-Corn Chili on p. 130)

Decide how you are most likely to use the leftovers; cut accordingly and freeze in individual food freezer bags, in quantities required for recipes.

Ideas for Using Extra Herbs

- We often invite guests and therefore double the recipe, making two turkey breast halves in a large oval slow cooker.
- Add remaining herbs to a simple rice pilaf.

Optional Cooking Method

In uncovered roasting pan, roast turkey breast in a 375° oven for 1½ hours, or until 180° internal temperature. Baste approximately every 30 minutes with oil and/or turkey juices.

Enjoy the Natural Sweetness of Foods

Traditionally, sweet potatoes are served with syrups, sugars and marshmallows. Not only does this counter the healthful properties of sweet potatoes, but it also covers their natural sweetness.

A typical sweet potato side dish uses from three-quarters to one cup of brown sugar and two cups of marshmallows with four medium sweet potatoes. Consequently the sugar grams are as high as in a typical slice of pumpkin pie.

Instead of that, we complement the natural sweetness with 100% fruit juice and dried fruit, reducing the sugar carbs by 70 to 75 percent. The complete recipe makeover also significantly reduces calories (by 120 calories per serving) and carbohydrates (by 23 g. per serving).

Spiced Sweet Potatoes

Dice sweet potatoes, steam as you would white potatoes and mash, adding a splash of 100% apple juice (in place of milk) and spices such as cinnamon or allspice (instead of salt), enhancing the natural sweetness. Great paired with pork and green beans.

Fruit Glazed Sweet Potatoes

Prep (divided): 15 minutes   Bake: 45–60 minutes.

4 med. sweet potatoes, quartered
1 Tbsp. butter (melted) ***or* Medium-Heat oil**
1/2 cup 100% pineapple *or* apple juice
1 Tbsp. lemon juice
1/4 cup chopped walnuts *or* pecans
1/4 cup raisins *or* other dried fruit

Preheat oven—350°. Covered casserole dish.

1. **Pour** ¼ cup of water in casserole dish. **Add** sweet potatoes. Sprinkle lightly with salt (⅛ teaspoon). Cover and **bake** 30 minutes.
2. *Meanwhile,* **combine** butter and juices. **Pour** mixture evenly over potatoes. **Sprinkle** nuts and dried fruit over top.
4. **Bake** uncovered for 15–30 minutes, or until potatoes are tender and juice is mostly absorbed.

Yield: 8 servings

Pie Makeovers

Eating a rich dessert is a treat on special occasions. These pies are healthier versions of traditional pies; however, they still have significant amounts of carbohydrates and fats. Thus, portion size and other foods consumed during the day need to be taken into consideration.

Pumpkin: *This is a great recipe with which to begin the process of enjoying less sugar. Start by using one or two tablespoons less sugar than what is suggested on the can. Eventually move down to the half cup suggested here (or less).*

Pecan: *We use brown rice syrup instead of corn syrup, only a quarter cup of honey instead of a cup of sugar and increase the nut protein.*

Fruit Glazed Sweet Potatoes/Serving
Calories: 117 (Fat Cal 34)   Fat: 3.8g (1.0g Sat)   Cholesterol: 4mg
Sodium: 70mg   Carbs: 23.9g (2.5g Fiber 8g Sugar)   Protein: 1.8g

Pumpkin Pie

2 eggs, slightly beaten
1 (15 oz.) can pumpkin
1/2 cup sugar
1/4 tsp. salt
1 tsp. ground cinnamon
1/2 tsp. ground ginger
1/4 tsp. ground cloves
1 (12 oz.) can low-fat evaporated milk
1 (9-inch) whole-wheat unbaked pie shell*

Preheat oven—425°; then 350°.

In bowl, **whisk** eggs, pumpkin, sugar, salt and spices together. Gradually **stir** in milk. **Pour** into pie shell. **Bake** in preheated oven for 15 minutes; reduce heat to 350° and bake for an additional 40–50 minutes, or until knife inserted near center comes out clean.

Yield: 8 servings

Pecan Pie

3 eggs
1 cup brown rice syrup
1/4 cup honey
3 Tbsp. Medium-Heat oil
1 1/2 cup pecans, broken
1 (9-inch) whole-wheat unbaked pie shell*

Preheat oven—350°.

In bowl, **beat** eggs with whisk. **Stir** in rice syrup, honey and oil. **Stir** in pecans. **Pour** into pie shell. **Bake** in preheated oven for 50 minutes.

Yield: 10 servings

*For GF option, see p. 205.

Whipped Cream

Using heavy cream does not lower calories or fat, but it avoids the corn syrups and artificial ingredients found in prepared frozen whips.

1 cup heavy whipping cream
1–2 Tbsp. powdered sugar
1/2 tsp. vanilla

1. **Chill** mixer bowl and beater in freezer for 30 minutes.
2. In a cool area, beat cream on **low** speed in the chilled mixer bowl for a **minute**, or until small bubbles form.
3. Beat on **medium** speed for **30 seconds**.
4. Beat on **high** speed until it is **soft and billowy**.
5. Slowly **add** sugar and vanilla at the sides of the bowl while continuing to beat on **high**.
6. Continue beating on high until **stiff peaks** are formed. (Caution: overbeating creates butter.)

Cover tightly and chill until ready to serve.

Place a dollop on each piece of pie when serving.

Helpful Tip: We use powdered sugar instead of granulated sugar as it helps to keep the cream from separating for up to a week. If it separates, beat with whisk until cream is incorporated again.

Yield: 2 cups

Pumpkin Pie/Serving:
Calories: 218 (Fat Cal 71) Fat: 7.9g (1.4g Sat) Cholesterol: 61mg
Sodium: 248mg Carbs: 30.5g (3.4g Fiber 18.4g Sugar) Protein: 6.7g

Pecan Pie/Serving:
Calories: 380 (Fat Cal 166) Fat: 18.4g (6.4g Sat) Cholesterol: 80mg
Sodium: 140mg Carbs: 66g (0.9g Fiber 19.3g Sugar) Protein: 3.6g

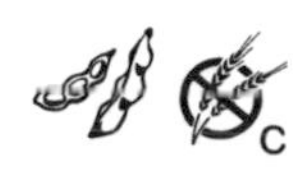

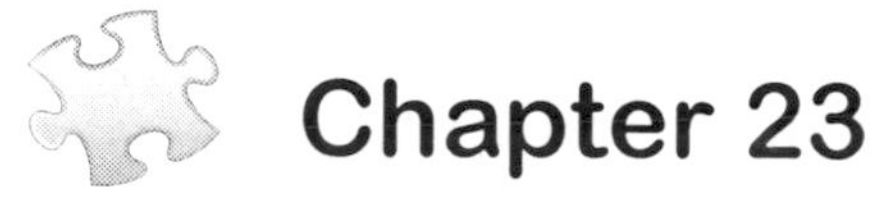

Chapter 23

Keep Snacking Healthy

Contrary to popular belief, healthy eating does not require the elimination of snacks. Certain types of snacks and certain snacking habits may need to be reduced or eliminated, but snacking itself can be quite healthy. Snacking can curb hunger, reducing binge eating and the desire for sugared drinks. It can also speed metabolism, making it easier to maintain bodyweight. And eating in small amounts throughout the day can reduce acid reflux and heartburn. See page 171 for a list of healthier snacking tips. Below is a list of quick and easy healthier snacks. (Some of our favorite products and brands are listed in the Healthier Choices Shopping Guide.)

Make it fun!
- Use "crinkled-edged knife" on veggies.
- Make faces/other shapes with foods.
- Serve with toothpicks.
- Eat off the bottom portion of a pretzel, creating a pair of "glasses"; use to play I Spy during the snack.

Vegetables:
- "Sticks": carrots, peppers, celery, cucumber, summer squashes.
- "Stuffed Celery Sticks": see page 55.
- "Chips" or "medallions": carrots, cucumber, summer squashes. (Kids like the carrot chips with little ripples!)

Fruits:
- Apples and bananas are easy to pack in a brief case or backpack.
- Keep grapes and berries washed and easy to grab – great finger foods!
- Drizzle apple, orange or lemon juice on apple slices to prevent browning.
- Choose whole fruits rather than most "fruit snacks," since they are primarily corn syrup and food dyes.

Include sweets wisely and sparingly.

Chips, pretzels and popcorn:
- Try blue corn chips (they are higher in nutrients than yellow corn chips).
- Choose pretzels without "extras" (e.g., corn syrups, high sodium). Our families (kids included) enjoy spelt pretzels – a great way to vary our grains.
- Popcorn (see p. 171).

Other grains, crackers and breads:
- Enjoy with guacamole/low-fat cheese.
- Spread with small amounts of healthier-choice peanut butter or bean dip.
- Pair with small amounts of sliced meat.

Instill good snacking habits:
- Snack in amounts to curb your hunger but not so much as to overdo.
- Take time to sit and enjoy your snack.
- Be intentional, portioning out your snack rather than eating out of a box.
- Use snacks to increase the day's nutrition, not hinder it.

Accessibility:
Keep snack foods on a designated shelf (fridge or cabinet) so kids can make choices within your desired parameters.

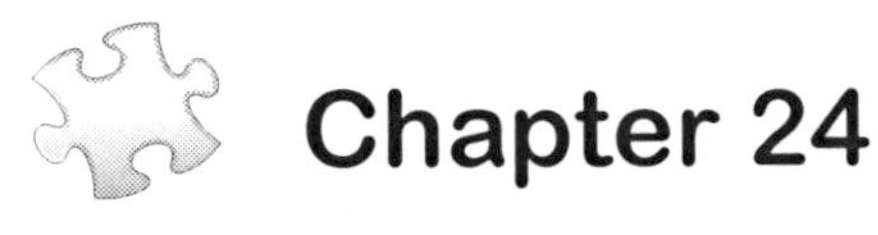

Chapter 24

Family Fun Nights

Games, movies, puzzles — whether you're spending time together as a family or inviting a "family" of friends over to hang out, fun nights are enhanced with appealing foods to eat at the table, on the floor or on the couch. This chapter highlights a variety of pizzas – the ultimate finger food that's both versatile and filling – as well as several munchies that can complete your meal and add to the fun.

Getting Started with Pizza

Pizza can be created to suit a variety of tastes and styles; the possibilities are endless. It can also be a healthy meal, incorporating all food groups, if appropriate choices are made. It's a great place to increase vegetable consumption and a good place to start increasing whole grains.

When designing your pizza, make the choice to:

- Incorporate whole grains into the crust.
- Use a variety of vegetables (mince a little pepper or onion and add to the sauce if family members resist having them on top).
- Select low-fat cheeses and limit to an appropriate amount of fat per serving (e.g., use less cheese with sausage).
- Select nitrate- and hormone-free meats/poultry.
- Limit the quantity of saturated fats by using small portions of meat and poultry.
- Use a sauce that is low in sugar. (Making your own is quick and easy — see p. 169.)

In addition to varying the toppings, you can:

- Vary the crust. Change the thickness, add seasonings or make personal-sized pizzas.
- Vary the sauce. Spice it up, try BBQ or experiment with pesto.

Anticipation Is Half the Fun

Let kids enjoy preparing the ingredients (chopping, dicing) earlier in the day so all is ready to go when the whole family gets home.

If you're inviting friends, ask them to each bring a favorite vegetable; the assembly of the pizzas becomes an activity in itself.

Beyond Pizza

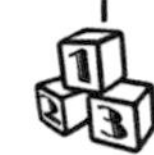

There are many other foods that can be served at fun nights. Consider burgers, other sandwiches, shish kebabs and wraps. If you want a break in the action, gathering around a table and assembling your own tacos or salads can be a fun group activity.

Spelt Pizza Crust

Use only 7/8 cup water
1 2/3 cups whole-grain spelt flour
3/4 cup white spelt flour

Helpful Hints

Flour: Best if flour is room temperature. Amounts of flour needed may vary, so start with slightly less.

Freezing crusts: Parbake crusts for 5 minutes, cool, wrap and freeze for up to a couple of months.

Using frozen crusts: Thaw; warm crust for 4 minutes in preheating oven so it melts the cheese, helping sauce and topping to stay on.

Purchased Crusts

Refrigerated pizza dough and prepared crusts often contain trans fats, preservatives and high levels of sodium, while being low in fiber.

Making this crust ahead — and freezing for later use, if desired (see above) — will likely save you 450 mg. of sodium per serving and offer up to 5 grams more fiber.

If purchasing crust, look for whole grains, low sodium and few preservatives.

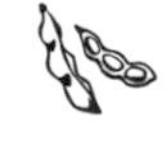

topping choices

Pizza Crust

1 cup water
1 pkg. rapid-rise dry yeast (2 1/4 tsp.)
1 tsp. honey
1 1/2 cups "white" whole-wheat flour
1 cup unbleached all-purpose flour
1 Tbsp. vital wheat gluten (p. 190)
1 tsp. salt
2 Tbsp. High-Heat oil

Oven Temperature—425°. Preheat at Step 4.

1. **Mix and proof dough:**
   - If using a **bread machine**, add ingredients in order recommended in owner's manual. (If dough is sticking to sides of gasket, add more flour. If dough is too stiff to be malleable when kneading, add a bit of water.) After completing dough cycle, allow dough to sit in bread machine for an additional 20–30 minutes.
   - If using a **stand mixer**:
     a. Heat water to lukewarm (110–115°); add to mixer bowl; stir in yeast and honey; allow to sit for 3–5 minutes.
     b. With whisk, beat in 1 cup flour, gluten, salt and oil for 30 seconds.
     c. Add remaining flour except a couple of tablespoons. With dough hook, stir in (knead speed).
     d. Continue on knead speed, gradually adding more flour until dough clings to hook and cleans sides of bowl.
     e. Knead on knead speed for 2 minutes.
     f. Form into dough ball; oil all sides. Flatten in bowl. Cover with moist cloth. Let rise in warm place, such as 100° oven, for 20–30 minutes, or until doubled.

Analysis for Crust Only/2 Pieces:
Calories: 187 (Fat Cal 34) Fat: 3.8g (0.5g Sat) Cholesterol: 0mg
Sodium: 133mg Carbs: 32.3g (3g Fiber 1.3g Sugar) Protein: 5.8g

2. **Shaping Crust:**
   a. Oil pan and sprinkle with cornmeal or line pan with parchment paper.
   b. With lightly oiled fingers, press or roll (with rolling pin) dough out from center, maintaining even thickness in all directions.
   c. If desired, push dough up on edge of pan.
3. **Proofing Crust:**
   Proof crust for 10–15 minutes in a warm place such as on range top while preheating oven.
4. **Dress & Parbake Crust:**
   a. Brush crust with small amount of oil (including the edges is optional).
   b. Sprinkle with pizza seasonings, garlic powder and/or fresh black pepper.
   c. With fork, pierce several holes in dough.
   d. Bake 5–7 minutes (called parbaking, the crust will not be completely baked).
5. **Sauce, Top & Bake Pizza:**
   a. Sprinkle hot crust with cheese.
   b. Spread sauce over melted cheese.
   c. Add toppings (see Pizza Topping ideas on next page).
   d. Sprinkle with cheese (we prefer to use frozen so it does not burn before crust and toppings are ready).
   e. Bake on bottom rack 15–20 minutes.

Yield: 16 pieces
Rectangular sizes: 1 (15x12-inch) without edges
1 (15x10-inch) with edges
Round sizes: 1 (14-inch), 2 (9-inch) or 4 (6-inch)

Simple Pizza Sauce

1 (8 oz.) can tomato sauce
2 tsp. Italian seasoning mix
1/4 tsp. garlic powder
2 pinches crushed red pepper (optional)

Stir seasoning directly into tomato sauce in can.

Yield: enough sauce for 1 (15x12 inch) pizza

Helpful Hints

Cheese: One (8 oz.) bag of shredded cheese (preferably low-fat) is enough for a 14-inch round or 15-by-12-inch rectangular pizza. Use approximately one-third of it under the sauce and the remainder on top.

Different Tastes: Portions of the pizza can be assembled differently to suit various tastes. Mark sections with colored toothpicks for ease of identification.

Baking: For best results, bake on bottom rack, using heavy-duty stainless steel pizza pans/baking sheets or pizza stones (below).

Pizza Stones Tips

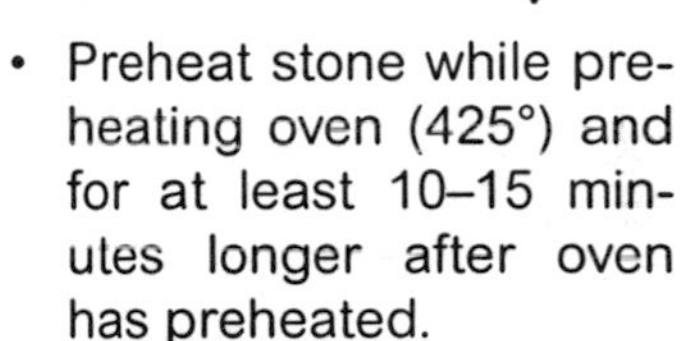

- Preheat stone while preheating oven (425°) and for at least 10–15 minutes longer after oven has preheated.
- Parbake crust 4 minutes.
- Add toppings and frozen cheese and bake only 6–8 minutes longer.
- Place stone on middle rack in oven.

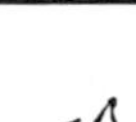

Vegetable Pizza

Assemble and bake similar to Hamburger Pizza, using any of the following as ideas to create your favorite combination of toppings.

- Mozzarella and/or Italian pizza blend cheese
- Pizza sauce
- Pesto (agugula and basil are our favorites)
- Thinly sliced red onions
- Sliced/diced bell peppers, any color
- Sliced yellow squash
- Sliced fresh mushrooms
- Chopped/torn arugula
- Ribbon-cut fresh spinach
- Sliced Kalamata olives
- Sun-dried tomatoes
- Italian seasoning mix
- Freshly minced garlic
- Ribbon-cut basil
- Crushed fresh oregano

English Muffin Pizza

Top a split whole-grain English muffin or whole-grain tortilla with pizza sauce, toppings and cheese. Bake for 5–10 minutes in 350° oven. Time depends upon how crispy you desire the "crust" and how thick the topping is.

Toppings for pizza are limited only by your imagination. Enjoy these or create your own combinations.

Hamburger Pizza

1/2 lb. lean ground beef
1/2 cup diced onions
1 tsp. Italian seasoning
1/4 tsp. salt
Additional vegetables, as desired

1. In skillet, **cook** all ingredients except additional vegetables until done, stirring often to brown evenly. Assemble:
   a. Sprinkle cheese over hot parbaked crust.
   b. Spread pizza sauce over melted cheese.
   c. Add meat mixture.
   d. Sprinkle with vegetables as desired (e.g., freshly minced garlic, thinly sliced red onions, sliced/diced any color bell peppers, sliced fresh mushrooms).
   e. Top with frozen shredded cheese.
2. Bake in preheated oven 15–20 minutes

Yield: 16 pieces 1 (15x12-inch) Pizza

Sausage-Pepper Pizza

Assemble and bake as above recipe, using half recipe of Sausage-Pepper-Onion Mix (p. 110).

Taco Pizza

Assemble/bake like Hamburger Pizza except:

a. Sprinkle garlic powder, dried leaf oregano, crushed red pepper and black pepper on crust before baking.
b. Use Tacos recipe for meat mixture. Top with Monterey Jack and/or mild cheddar cheese and garnish cooked pizza as you would tacos (see ideas on p. 100).

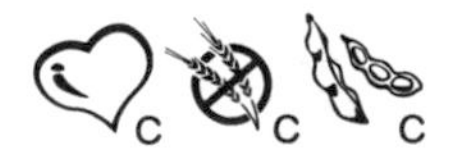

GF - see our websites (p. 242) for tips on using gluten-free pizza mixes with these recipes.

Healthier Family Fun Snacking Tips

Playing games and watching movies are natural times for snacks. All the munchies can add up to lots of sodium, lots of fat and lots of calories. However, they can just as easily be a healthy addition to your evening. The trick comes with being intentional about choices. When choosing munchies, make the choice to:

- Plan ahead – deciding ahead of time what you will serve helps to ensure that healthy options are ready and accessible.
- Include raw vegetables for a nice crunch and a convenient finger food. Add a moderate amount of a healthy dip to increase their appeal (pp. 42, 49, 79 and 149).
- Use vegetables to enhance other snacks. Sliced avocadoes, guacamole and healthy salsas are great ways to increase vegetable consumption.
- Offer "whole" fruits (as opposed to juice). Apple slices (with the peel) are a great source of fiber; berries and grapes are good finger foods; citrus fruit offers a bit of "zest." Serving fruit also helps to curb the urge for sugared drinks.
- Offer water instead of sugared beverages.
- If sugared beverages are served, chose those with natural forms of sugar (e.g., 100% fruit juice) and serve in limited quantities.
- Choose whole-grain and/or whole-grain blends for crackers, pretzels and chips.
- Include foods with fiber and protein, reducing sugar spikes and allowing your body to fill "full" sooner. Try whole grains, bean dips, vegetables and fruits.
- Purchase healthier-choice prepared products lower in sodium and lower in sugars.
- Avoid products with high-fructose corn syrup.
- Offer the snacks with the most nutrients first before everyone fills up on the foods with less "efficient" calories.
- Be intentional about bringing out and putting away snacks. Conscious decisions to eat are generally healthier than arbitrary eating.
- Avoid eating during the first and last 30 minutes of a movie or TV show. (We often train our bodies to "think" that being in front of TV means it's time to eat.)

Keeping Popcorn Healthy: Popcorn is a healthy, fun and tasty treat that can quickly become unhealthy. If you make your own, we suggest using an air popper. Use oil or melted butter and salt sparingly. (Flaxseed oil is a healthy buttery-flavored alternative.) Place popped popcorn in a container with a lid, drizzle with oil, sprinkle with salt, cover and shake, allowing the popcorn to get evenly flavored.

If you purchase popcorn already popped, choose brands that use healthier fats, no chemicals and a minimum amount of oil and salt. Our favorite brand (Vic's "Lite Half-salt") has three ingredients (including the corn) and 88 calories, 5 g. of fat, 3 g. of fiber and 37 mg. of sodium per 2½-cup serving. Compare that with an unhealthy brand that has twelve ingredients, 190 calories, 15 g. of fat, 325 mg. of sodium and 2 g. of sugar for the same size serving.

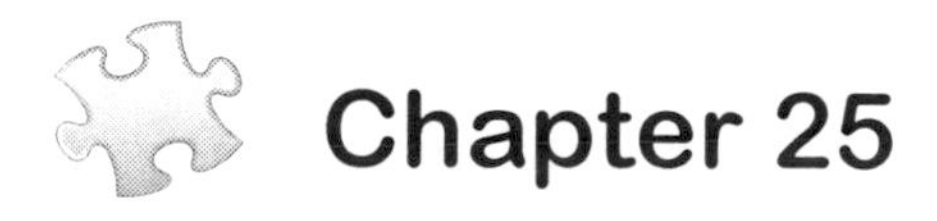

Chapter 25

Beverages

Beverages are an important part of our daily lives. We drink to quench thirst, to wake up, to keep warm, to cool down, to be social. ... This chapter looks at how beverages fit into the equation of healthier eating.

We need water in order to live. It is involved in every function of our body, from delivering nutrients to our cells to regulating body temperature. How much water we need varies according to our bodies (gender, weight, health status, activity level, pregnant or breastfeeding) and our environment (humidity, temperature, altitude). We lose several cups of water every day through perspiration, excretion and breathing. When we don't replenish it, we begin to dehydrate. Often dehydration is minimal and we don't notice the effects or we fail to associate them with a need for water. Thirst, headaches, fatigue, muscle weakness, lightheadedness and dizziness are signs of potential dehydration.[1]

The best source of water is water itself. It's a great idea to start the day with a glass of water, giving your body the fluid it needs to function as you begin your many activities. Keep water close at hand, drinking as you can, before you get thirsty.

Food, especially fruits and vegetables, provides some of our water as well. And, of course, there are numerous other beverages that contain varying amounts of water. Along with the water, however, they contain many other things, some good, some okay in moderation and some worth limiting or avoiding.

Here are some things to consider as you make your beverage selections:

- **Nutritional Benefit:** there are many drinks, such as fruit and vegetable juices and teas, that have nutritional benefit.

  Dark juices, such as grape, cranberry, blueberry and pomegranate, are typically rich in antioxidants. (Incidentally, these are often the fruits that are harder to find year-round in their whole form. So drinking the juice is a good alternative.) Even 100% fruit juices should be limited in quantity, however, and it's always a good choice to go with the whole fruit when you can.

  There are herbal teas (made from various herbs and flowers) and "true" teas (made from the leaves of an actual tea tree). While both kinds of tea can have various healing properties, there is extensive research available on the health benefits of true tea. **Green tea**, the least refined of true teas, has received special attention in recent years for its numerous healthful properties. Keep in mind that these studies refer to the tea itself; many companies have produced prepared "green tea" beverages that contain some green tea but are mainly water and corn syrup. Drinking these may not provide many health benefits and can drastically increase calorie consumption.

- **Calories:** most beverages contain calories. It is easy to consume 500 to 1000 calories a day in drinks alone – even if you only drink 100% juice. Since most of us should limit our total caloric intake to about 2,000 calories (see p. 4), that doesn't leave much room for food! A typical 32-ounce glass of sweetened tea from a popular fast food restaurant will add over 300 calories to your intake for the day. A large orange juice (21 ounces) from the same chain contains 250 calories.
- **Sweeteners:** Many drinks, including flavored water and energy drinks, are sweetened; most use high-fructose corn syrup. Even drinks that are considered "healthy" are often produced with corn syrup. Companies depend on customers to see the "health value" in the name and to ignore the label. "No sugar added" juices often contain artificial sweeteners and are not really 100% juice.
- **Sodium:** Many drinks contain sodium. The most notable are sports drinks. While they can be helpful to replace sodium lost during intense perspiration, they were never intended to be used by people in sedentary activities.
- **Caffeine:** While there have been some proven health benefits to caffeine, there are many reasons to curb caffeine consumption. Most agree that caffeine consumed in small amounts is not harmful, but large quantities can create many complications. Some people are more sensitive to caffeine than others – and sensitivity can increase with stress (when many to turn to caffeine).[2] Some caffeinated beverages, such as green tea, contain nutrients that lessen the effect of caffeine.[3]
- **Other Fillers:** As with other foods, producing beverages made from whole ingredients is costly, and companies often avoid doing so. A popular brand of orange juice contains twenty different ingredients, including high-fructose corn syrup, two different food dyes and two different preservatives.
- **Quantity:** A typical "juice glass" is six ounces and provides a good frame of reference when pouring a glass of something other than water. Even 100% juice contains 20 to 30 grams of sugar per six- to eight-ounce glass. It's natural sugar, paired with great nutrients, but it's also calories that fill and fatten us up if we drink in excess.
- **Timing:** Right before a meal is not the best time to down a glass of juice; your body will feel full and you won't consume the nutrients you need. This is especially important for kids who eat smaller portions of food.

Diet Drinks: Many diet and "no sugar added" drinks (sodas, lemonade, juices) use artificial sweeteners. As mentioned before, there is a lot of controversy about these. It is our belief that chemically based artificial sweeteners are seriously damaging our health, with effects ranging from neurological disorders to infertility and depression.

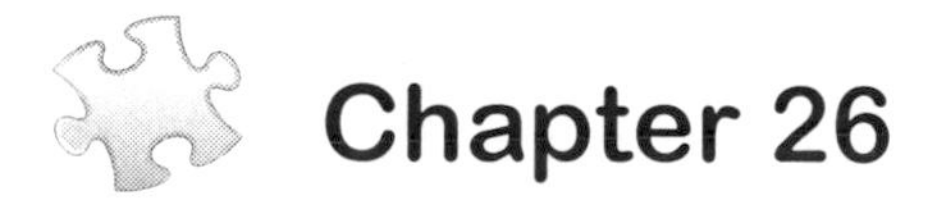

Chapter 26

Breads and Grains

Whole grains have been staple foods for thousands of years. They are a common source of carbohydrates and an inexpensive form of protein. Whole grains provide a rich array of nutrients (e.g., fiber, complex carbohydrates, minerals, vitamins, protein). Refined grains are not as nutrient rich because most of their nutrients have been stripped in the refining process. Finding ways to integrate whole grains into our snacks and meals is an important part of healthier eating.

What are whole grains? Whole grains are seeds with three natural components: (1) **bran**, the tough protective coating that is rich in fiber and nutrients; (2) **germ**, which contains vitamin E, essential fatty acids and proteins that provide food for the plant seed to sprout; and (3) **endosperm**, or the starchy bulk layer of the grain (rich in complex carbohydrates and protein) that nourishes seedlings before leaves begin photosynthesis. Examples include whole wheat, brown rice, oats, corn, whole spelt and hulled barley.

What are refined grains? Refined grains have been degermed or polished, which removes the germ and the bran layers and lowers the nutritional content. For example, white "all-purpose" flour is a wheat flour that has been refined, removing 80 percent of its nutrients. Even though these products are "enriched," more than twenty nutrients have been removed and only four have been added back (thiamin, niacin, riboflavin and iron.)

Making the transition: When working to include whole grains in snacks and meals, consider mixing them with refined grains. As your taste buds adjust, increase the amount of whole grain. You will likely find this is easier in some foods than in others, and that's okay. We love the whole-grain coffee cake, but we prefer a blend with the pizza dough.

In a movement toward eating more whole grains, make the choice to:

- use blended pastas or combine whole-grain pasta with refined pasta (whole grains are often more "acceptable" inside casseroles, where their taste is camouflaged)
- use brown rice (great taste, awesome aroma!) or mix white rice with brown rice
- use whole-grain flours in baking (starting with half; p. 181)
- use oats and oat bran in baking
- experiment with new grains (barley and quinoa are worth trying!)
- make or purchase whole-grain or partially whole-grain breads
- use brown rice flour for sauces (p. 177)
- look for whole-grain, or partially whole-grain, crackers and cereal

Wheat

There are three main categories of wheat: hard wheat, soft wheat and durum wheat. Hard wheat is higher in protein (gluten) and is best for breads and foods that use yeast as a leavening agent. Soft wheat has less gluten, is higher in carbohydrates and works better for crackers, pastries and foods using baking powder as a leavening agent. Durum wheat is ideal for pastas. The refined form of durum wheat is semolina.

Hard Wheat: High in gluten (protein); good for yeasted breads

There is hard **red** wheat and hard **white** wheat. In our book, "white whole wheat" refers to a hard white variety. Generally, the hard red wheat has a more rustic look and a more hearty taste. The hard white wheat is closer in texture and flavor to the refined white flour many are used to consuming. That makes it a good choice for making the transition to whole grains.

In addition to the color variations, there are spring and winter varieties of hard wheat. Spring wheat is higher in protein and is ideal for breads. Winter wheat (which has "wintered over") is higher in mineral content. Many packages of flour will identify the wheat as being "hard white spring wheat" or the like.

Spelt

Spelt is an ancient grain related to wheat. It has a broader spectrum of nutrients than most other types of wheat and its "particular combination of nutrients ... may make it a particularly helpful food for persons with migraine headache, atherosclerosis, or diabetes."[1] Spelt flour is available as **whole grain spelt** and **white spelt** (the refined version). The whole spelt flour is often tolerated by those who are otherwise sensitive to wheat.

Types of Wheat Flour Used in This Cookbook

Whole-Wheat Flours: made from whole hard wheat berries (can be "red" or "white"). All of the forty-plus nutrients found in wheat are retained during processing, making it the richest form of wheat flour in nutrients and the heartiest in taste. In this book, we regularly use **"white" whole wheat,** which has the softer and lighter texture of the two.

Whole-Wheat Pastry Flour: made from whole soft wheat berries. The whole-grain counterpart to cake flour, it is a good choice when baking pastries that do not rely on yeast as the leavening agent. We use it in our Baking Mix (p. 181).

Unbleached All-Purpose Flour: made from a blend of hard and soft wheat. Bran and germ have been removed. It is less nutritious than whole-grain varieties, but when combined with whole grains, it provides a lighter taste and texture that helps with the transition. It is "enriched" (four of the many vitamins removed during processing are put back in) by law, but it is processed with far less than the thirty chemicals used to process its bleached counterpart.

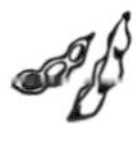

Rice

Nutrition:

Whole-grain rice (brown rice) is a great source of B vitamins and fiber.

History:

Rice originated in India, Southeast Asia and China around 4000 B.C. Today it is grown in many parts of the world, including the United States.

Cooking with Rice:

Rice has a rather plain flavor that provides an excellent canvas waiting to be colored with other foods and spices. The only limiting factor is the imagination of the cook.

Play to Learn

Kids love to pour! Give your child some measuring cups or spoons and some rice or beans. Allow him to scoop and pour, possibly measuring quantities, maybe just feeling the grains on his hands. A funnel or kitchen scale can add to the fun. He'll be entertained while you're cooking, and one day your budding chef will be able to do all of your measuring for you!

Rice

Rice is a gluten-free grain and the second-most-produced food in the world. Brown rice is available in many forms, including whole grain, flour, puffed, rice cakes, pastas and creamy hot cereal. Brown rice flour has a drier consistency than wheat flour but is great for making roux and thickening sauce.

Basic Rice

S→T: 30 (or more) minutes (mostly inactive)

The smell of brown basmati rice cooking is like that of popcorn. It is an irresistible draw to the dinner table, making it our favorite.

1 cup dry basmati brown rice
2 1/4 cups water (*or* use some broth; often we use 1 cup of low-sodium broth)
Scant 1/4 tsp. salt (optional)

1. Place rice in fine mesh strainer and **rinse** under running water.
2. In saucepan, combine ingredients. (To save time, begin bringing liquids to boil while rinsing rice.) Cover and **simmer** until liquid is absorbed and rice is al dente. Test for doneness (see below). (Packages often indicate to cook brown rice for 50 minutes; we rarely cook it longer than 25–30 minutes.)
3. Remove from heat and allow to **set** for approximately 5 minutes. Stir to fluff.

Test for Doneness: When cooking grains, it is best not to uncover or stir. So to test for doneness, remove lid, remove a small bite from the surface and quickly return lid. This minimizes loss of steam and does not disrupt the even cooking of the grain.

Yield: 6 servings 3 cups

Analysis/Serving:
Calories: 107 (Fat Cal 10) Fat: 1.1g (0g Sat) Cholesterol: 0mg
Sodium: 89mg Carbs: 23g (1.3g Fiber 0.7g Sugar) Protein: 2.7g

Roasted Rice Pilaf Dinner

S→T: 45-Minute Meal

1 cup basmati brown rice
4 cups low-sodium chicken broth (divided)
1/4 cup water
1 Tbsp. dehydrated onion flakes
1 tsp. each: dried parsley, oregano
1/2 tsp. each: dried basil, garlic powder
1/4 tsp. salt
1 cup frozen Gardener's Blend vegetables
1/2 cup diced peppers (fresh or frozen)
1/4 cup slivered almonds
6 (4 oz.) boneless lean pork chops
2 Tbsp. brown rice flour

1. **Preheat** skillet on medium-high while rinsing rice; add. **Roast** rice 5 minutes, stirring often while bringing 2 cups of the broth, water and seasonings to boil. Add rice. Reduce heat; cover; **simmer** for 20 minutes
2. *Meanwhile*, reduce heat of skillet to low, **toast** almonds for a few minutes until fragrant, stirring often; pour into a bowl.
3. **Rub** oil, salt and garlic powder on meat (p. 145). **Cook** in skillet until done while preparing side salad and dressing.
4. When rice has cooked for 20 minutes, quickly **add** vegetables and a light sprinkle of salt on top of rice. Recover pan and **simmer** for 5–10 minutes, or until rice is done. Remove from heat; set for 5 minutes. Stir in almonds
5. When meat is done, transfer to a plate; keep warm. Add flour and a small portion of remaining broth in skillet, whisking together and cooking for about 1 minute. Then continue to whisk while slowly adding remaining broth to **deglaze** the "drippings" and **thicken** the gravy.

Serve meat on bed of pilaf. Drizzle with gravy. Serve with side salad.

Yield: 6 servings ~4 cups Pilaf

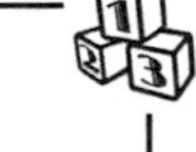

Variations

- Use boneless, skinless chicken breast.
- Try dill and paprika with chicken.
- Try frozen broccoli (bite-size), sautéed onions (omit onion flakes), sautéed celery and/or ribbon-cut spinach.

Healthy Bites

Brown Rice Flour: Brown rice flour does not clump as easily as refined wheat flour when making a gravy or roux, and it is a great way to begin incorporating whole grains in your cooking. Plus, it offers a gluten-free option.

Pilaf Box Mixes: Our pilaf is lower in calories, fat and saturated fat than the boxed varieties and offers 70 to 80 percent less sodium while adding more fiber and protein. If you are cooking meat anyway, making this pilaf from scratch doesn't dirty any more dishes and adds only a few minutes to preparation.

Analysis Pilaf/Est. Dinner per Serving:
Calories: 159/440 (Fat Cal 30/171)
Fat: 3/19g (0.2/3g Sat)
Cholesterol: 0/62mg
Sodium: 143/318mg Protein: 5/32g
Carbs: 28/35 (3/5g Fiber 3/5g Sugar)

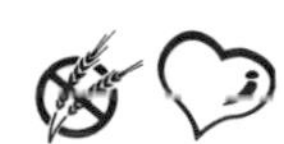

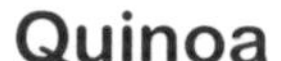

Quinoa

Quinoa (pronounced keen-wah) is a quick-cooking, gluten-free grain-like food.

History:

Quinoa has been cultivated in the Andes Mountains of South America since 3000 B.C. It was named "the mother grain" by the Inca Indians for its life-giving properties. Young plants supplied deep, green, leafy vegetables. The seeds were their staple nourishment. The stalks were used for fuel in high-altitude areas where wood was unavailable. In 1982, Steve Gorad, founding president of the Quinoa Corporation, traded an Andean farmer the shirt off his back for quinoa seeds. This launched the Colorado quinoa growing program under the supervision of Colorado State University.

Saponin Coating:

Quinoa seeds have a coating called saponin, which functions as a natural repellent to insects and birds and protects the seed from the high intensity of the altiplano sun.

To remove this unharmful, but bitter, saponin coating so the seed can be ground into flour, the Quinoa Corporation developed a system of belts that jostle the whole seeds. This method, called *pearling*, uses friction rather than chemicals to buff off the saponin.

Rinsing Quinoa Before Cooking:

Before cooking the seeds, place them in a fine mesh strainer and thoroughly rinse under running water to remove the saponin coating.

Interestingly, the Incas saved the foam from washing quinoa to use as shampoo.

Quinoa

Nutrition:

Quinoa is high in vitamin E, B vitamins, calcium, phosphorus and iron. It is a complete protein source, containing all eight essential amino acids, and is high in lysine. The National Academy of Sciences has called quinoa "one of the best sources of vegetable protein in the vegetable kingdom." The essential amino acid balance is close to the ideal set by the United Nations Food and Agriculture Organization.[2] Quinoa protein is equal in quality to that of dried milk and close to that of mother's milk.

Recipes Using:

- Quinoa Pilaf
- Turkey Loaf Patties
- Stuffed Peppers

Other Facts:

The Incas encouraged pregnant and lactating mothers to eat quinoa every day for healthy babies and an adequate milk supply.

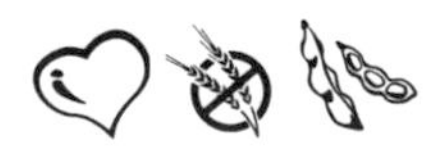

Quinoa Pilaf

S→T: 30 minutes (20 minutes inactive)

1/2 cup dry quinoa grain
1/2 cup + 2 Tbsp. water
1/2 cup broth—vegetable, chicken
1/4 cup finely chopped onion
OR sliced scallions
1 sm. carrot, shaved or shredded
1/2 med. red pepper, chopped (1/2 cup)
2 Tbsp. walnuts, chopped
1/8 tsp. salt
2 med. chard leaves, ribbon-cut
OR 2 cups baby spinach leaves (loosely packed)

1. Place quinoa in a fine mesh strainer and thoroughly **rinse** under running water.
2. In saucepan, begin heating quinoa, water and broth while preparing and adding the remaining ingredients. Lay chard/spinach on the top.
3. Cover and **simmer** 15 minutes, or until quinoa is done.
4. Remove from heat. Allow to **set** 3–5 minutes. Stir to fluff before serving.

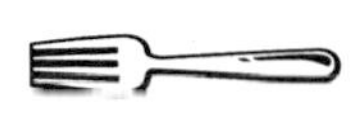

Delicious served with grilled chicken breast and raw veggie platter.

Extras are great as stuffing for green peppers. Mix the pilaf with cooked chicken chunks and shredded mozzarella cheese (also see p. 75).

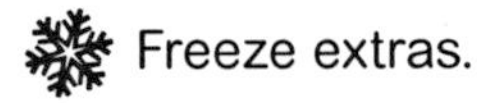

Freeze extras.

Yield: 4 servings 2 1/2 cups

Basil Quinoa Pilaf

When fresh basil is in season, we enjoy following the above recipe, replacing the red pepper with ~¼ oz. of ribbon-cut fresh basil (~2½ Tbsp.).

Quinoa
(continued)

Whole Grain:

Quinoa can be considered a fast food within whole-grain cookery since the seeds cook quickly. As the whole quinoa cooks, the germ (outside of the grain) unfolds, disclosing a glistening translucent partial spiral. Quinoa is an excellent food for infants and toddlers.

Cooking with Quinoa:

Quinoa's flavor can easily be enhanced with vegetables, fruits, meats and so on. The subtle, nutty taste makes it a great side dish with almost any meal.

Quinoa also comes in the form of flakes and can be served as a hot cereal (similar to oatmeal). These flakes can also be used in meat loaf (p. 154) and stuffings to offer extra nutrition and a gluten-free option.

Analysis/Serving:
Calories: 120 (Fat Cal 29) Fat: 3.2g (0.2g Sat) Cholesterol: 0mg
Sodium: 194mg Carbs: 18g (2.6g Fiber 2.6g Sugar) Protein: 3.8g

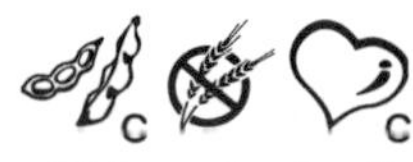

HH - paired with

Barley

With a nutty, earthy flavor, the appearance of puffy rice and the texture of pasta, barley is a healthy, homey addition to many meals. If served with meat, such as in this Barley Casserole, you can reduce the quantity of meat (thus reducing saturated fat) and still have a reasonable serving of protein. High in fiber and selenium, barley also contains important trace minerals.

Two Forms of Barley:

Hulled: only the outermost hull is removed. Most nutrients remain. This form requires more soaking and cooking. It has a chewier taste (used in Beef Barley Soup, p. 121).

Pearled: parts of the grain have been removed to varying degrees. Regular pearled barley has lost the fewest nutrients, followed by medium, fine and baby pearled barley. A great way to introduce your family to this rich grain.

Serving Suggestions:

- Breakfast cereal
- Add to soups or stews with long simmering time
- Create a pilaf

Barley Casserole

S→O: 25 minutes Cook: see Step 4

Roasting barley speeds the cooking process but most importantly enhances its delightfully nutty taste.

3/4 cup dry medium pearled barley, rinsed
9 oz. hot Italian fully cooked chicken/turkey sausage links, diced (p. 232)
1 1/2 cups chopped onion
1 cup sliced leeks
2 cups chopped cabbage
OR 1 cup diced fennel
1 (10 oz.) pkg. frozen tri-color peppers
1/2 (10 oz.) pkg. frozen green beans (1 1/4 cups)
2–3 cups low-sodium chicken broth

Oven temperature—350°. 9x13x2-inch baking dish or standard-sized slow cooker

1. Place barley in skillet. Spray with oil. **Roast** over medium-low heat for about 5 minutes, stirring occasionally. Add sausage and onions and **sauté** while preparing other vegetables. Add a little water if skillet gets dry.
2. **Layer** ingredients in baking dish or slow cooker as follows: barley mixture, leeks, cabbage (or fennel), peppers, green beans.
3. **Oven:** pour 3 cups of broth over mixture. Cover and refrigerate overnight, or for at least 3–4 hours. **Slow cooker**: cover and refrigerate until ready to cook. Add 2 cups of broth just before cooking (third cup not needed).
4. **Bake** uncovered for 60 minutes. Press food into liquid. Bake 15 minutes longer, or until liquid is absorbed and barley is tender. **Set** 5 minutes. Or **slow-cook** for 4–5 hours on LOW. Gently stir before serving.

Yield: 4 complete meal servings
Can be cut in half; bake in 8x8x2-inch baking dish.

Analysis/Serving:
Calories: 300 (Fat Cal 50) Fat: 5.5g (1.2g Sat) Cholesterol: 49mg
Sodium: 426–444mg Carbs: 47g (8.6g Fiber 8g Sugar) Protein: 19g

Converting to Whole Grains

Converting to whole grains in baking can be a challenge, especially when our taste buds are used to the more refined grains. However, even small additions of whole grain can add nutritional benefit to the diet. This baking mix provides one way to move toward the use of whole grains without challenging taste buds too much. Once a taste for this flour combination has developed, people often find they can move more easily to increased amounts of whole grain in their baking.

Baking Mix

Prepare: < 3 minutes

1 cup whole-wheat pastry flour
1 cup unbleached all-purpose flour
4 tsp. baking powder
1/4 tsp. salt

Triple Batch of Baking Mix

Prepare: < 5 minutes

3 cups whole-wheat pastry flour
3 cups unbleached all-purpose flour
4 Tbsp. baking powder
3/4 tsp. salt

Measure ingredients into a "storage jar." It is easy to use a quart jar for small batches and a short ½ gallon jar for a triple batch. To mix, rock jar back and forth for several times.

To save time mixing, alternate ingredients when measuring into jar.

Yield (triple batch): ~7 cups

Time Saver

Preparing this baking mix ahead of time saves the steps of measuring several ingredients when you are ready to bake. Adding a few additional ingredients makes great cookies, biscuits and coffee cakes.

Little Chefs

Measuring and mixing are wonderful teaching activities. Kids learn not only cooking skills but also fine motor skills and even math skills. As you measure the flour together, discuss the measurements. Instead of putting in a whole cup of flour, ask them to put in two half cups or three third cups.

The best part comes at the end when they get to rock the jar. Feel free to put on some music and create your own baking mix dance!

Healthy Bite

Potlucks and family gatherings are often places where people resist choosing whole grains, because there are many refined options available. Preparing foods with only half whole grain (such as using this baking mix) introduces whole grains to their diet in a more acceptable fashion.

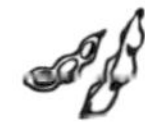

Helpful Gadgets

Pastry Blender (p. 202)

Dipper: A dipper is an easy way to drop biscuits or dip muffins and cupcakes.

Handy Measure: A one-fourth cup angled-style liquid measure (p. 230) is handy to measure one to three tablespoons of liquid without spilling.

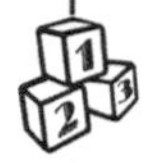

Whole-Grain Biscuits

Replace Baking Mix with the following:

2 cups whole-wheat pastry flour *or* whole-grain spelt flour
4 tsp. baking powder
1/4 tsp. salt

Healthy Bite

Refrigerated biscuit dough often contains trans fats, corn syrup and high levels of fat, sodium and sugar. Our biscuit mix is made with whole foods and is lower in calories, fat, sodium and sugar than even the reduced fat brands available. It is also higher in fiber. What a winner!

Biscuit/Shortcake Mix

This recipe is very versatile. Biscuits are a quick and easy addition to any meal that you would typically serve with bread. If desired, brush warm biscuits with melted butter or serve with all-fruit jam or jelly. For a garlic flavor, brush warm biscuits with melted Garlic Butter (see next page sidebar). For a fun dessert, serve with fruit as individual shortcakes (p. 196).

Do-Ahead Mix:

2 cups Baking Mix (p. 181)
2 Tbsp. sugar
1/4 cup unsalted butter

In bowl, **whisk** Baking Mix and sugar together. Using a pastry blender, **cut** in butter to evenly distribute. **Store** in freezer or refrigerator.

# of biscuits	1	4	12
Amount of Do-Ahead Mix (above)	1/4 cup	1 cup	3 cups (entire mix)
Milk (low-fat cow, unsweetened soy)	~4 tsp.	~1/3 cup	~1 cup

Preheat oven—425°. Lightly **oil** baking sheet.

1. **Stir** mix before measuring out portion needed.
2. Gradually **add** milk to mix while stirring until it forms a soft, cohesive batter.
3. With a number 24 dipper (sidebar), **drop** on prepared baking sheet about 1 inch apart. If desired, slightly flatten with back of dipper.
4. **Bake** in preheated oven for 8–10 minutes, or until golden brown and toothpick comes out clean. Keep warm in towel-lined basket until ready to serve.

Biscuits are best within a few hours of baking.

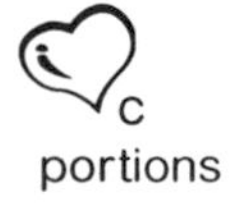

portions

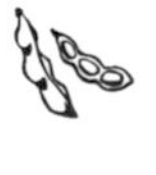

Analysis/Biscuit:
Calories: 115 (Fat Cal 37) Fat: 4.1 (2.5g Sat) Cholesterol: 11mg
Sodium: 172mg Carbs: 17g (1g Fiber 3.4g Sugar) Protein: 3g

Cheese Biscuit Mix

Do-Ahead Mix:

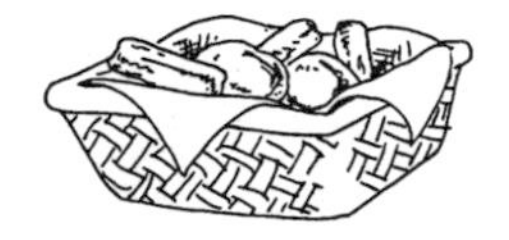

2 cups Baking Mix (p. 181)
1/2 tsp. garlic powder
1 Tbsp. sugar
1/4 cup unsalted butter
4 oz. shredded sharp cheddar cheese

In bowl, **whisk** Baking Mix, garlic powder and sugar together. Using a pastry blender, **cut** in butter to evenly distribute. **Stir** in cheese. **Store** in freezer. Biscuits brown better if mix is used directly from freezer.

# of biscuits	1	4	14
Amount of Do-Ahead Mix	1/4 cup	1 cup	3 1/2 cups (entire mix)
Milk (low-fat cow, unsweetened soy)	1 Tbsp.	1/4 cup	7/8 cup

Preheat oven—400–425°. Lightly **oil** baking sheet.

For Drop Biscuits, mix by following Steps 1–3 of recipe on previous page. **Bake** in preheated oven for 10–12 minutes, or until golden brown. *Meanwhile*, melt appropriate amount of Garlic Butter (sidebar). **Brush** on warm biscuits.

For Rolled Biscuits (photo on front cover), prepare mix as directed above, using slightly less milk. On floured surface, **knead** dough with short gentle strokes, adding small amounts of Baking Mix or flour until dough is not sticky. **Pat** out to ½-inch thickness. **Cut** with biscuit cutter. Lay on prepared baking sheet. Lightly **brush** biscuit tops with melted Garlic Butter (sidebar). **Bake** as described above; may take longer (depends on size).

Biscuits are best within a few hours of baking.

Garlic Butter

1/4 cup unsalted butter, softened
1/4 tsp. seasoned garlic salt (p. 222)

Stir garlic salt in butter. Spoon onto waxed paper. Form into a log. Wrap. Store in refrigerator. Slice and melt as needed.

Yield: coats 36 biscuits.

Whole-Grain Biscuits

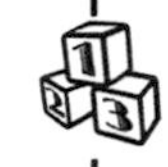

Replace Baking Mix with the following:

2 cups whole-wheat pastry flour *or* whole-grain spelt flour
4 tsp. baking powder
1/4 tsp. salt

These whole-grain biscuits usually require one teaspoon more milk per biscuit.

Healthy Bite

Several people have duplicated a popular restaurant chain's cheese biscuit. We compared our recipe with one that seemed to have captured the biscuit as well. Yet our version has 35% less fat calories, offers over 100 mg. less sodium and doubles the fiber.

Analysis/Drop Cheese Biscuit: (includes estimate for Garlic Butter)
Calories: 126 (Fat Cal 54) Fat: 6g (3.8g Sat) Cholesterol: 18mg
Sodium: 195mg Carbs: 13.7g (1g Fiber 2g Sugar) Protein: 4.3g

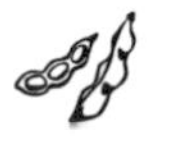

portions; paired with

Healthy Bites

Sweet Tooth: The topping on these coffee cakes gives an immediate sweet satisfaction without using high amounts of sugar.

Transitioning: Begin with gradually cutting the sugar in the batter from 4 to 2 tablespoons. Then gradually cut the sugar in the topping from 2 to 1 tablespoon.

Recipe Makeover: The original recipe used:

- Shortening. We use oil to cut the saturated fat. We use 44% less fat overall.
- 1 cup sugar. We cut overall sugar by 18–35% and refined sugar by 75–87%, adding honey and fruits for sweetness, flavor and additional nutrition.
- Buttermilk. We use applesauce to lower fat content.
- All-purpose flour. We use half whole-grain flour for additional nutrition.

By doing these things, we:

- tripled the amount of fiber

and reduced

- fat by 30%,
- saturated fat by 30%,
- sugars by 18 to 35% and
- calories by 22 to 43 per serving.

Overnight Blueberry Coffee Cake

S→O: 15 minutes Bake: 25–30 minutes

This is a great recipe for transitioning your sweet tooth.

1 cup + 2 Tbsp. Baking Mix (p. 181)
1/4 tsp. baking soda
1/2–1 tsp. ground cinnamon
1/8 tsp. ground nutmeg
1 egg, slightly beaten
3 Tbsp. Medium-Heat oil
2–4 Tbsp. brown sugar
1/4 cup light honey
1 tsp. vanilla extract
1/2 cup unsweetened applesauce
3/4–1 cup frozen blueberries (divided)

Topping Ingredients:
1–2 Tbsp. brown sugar
1/4 cup walnuts, chopped
1/4–1/2 tsp. ground cinnamon
1/8 tsp. ground nutmeg

Oven temperature—350°
Oil an 8x8x2-inch glass baking dish.

1. In bowl, **whisk** together Baking Mix, baking soda, cinnamon and nutmeg; set aside. In larger bowl, **whisk** together egg, oil, sugar, honey, vanilla and applesauce to dissolve sugar. Add dry ingredients to egg mixture. **Stir** gently to moisten all ingredients.
2. Gently **fold** in three-fourths of fruit (straight from freezer). **Pour** into baking dish; **spread** evenly. **Sprinkle** remaining fruit over batter.
3. **Mix** topping and **sprinkle** evenly over batter.
4. **Bake** in preheated oven for 25–30 minutes. *Or* cover and refrigerate up to 12 hours. Bake straight from the refrigerator in preheated oven.

Yield: 12 servings (cut 4x3)

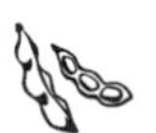

Analysis/Serving:
Calories: 132–143 (Fat Cal 50) Fat: 5.6g (0.5g Sat) Cholesterol: 18mg
Sodium: 126 Carbs: 19–22g (1.5g Fiber 11–14g Sugar) Protein: 2g

Whole-Grain Heart-Healthy Blueberry Coffee Cake

S→O: 15 minutes Bake: 25–30 minutes

This is a great recipe to make when beginning to try all whole-grain flour. It does not have an overwhelming grain taste.

1 cup "white" whole-wheat flour
2 tsp. baking powder
1/4 tsp. baking soda
1/8 tsp. salt
1/2–1 tsp. ground cinnamon
1/8 tsp. ground nutmeg
1 egg, slightly beaten
3 Tbsp. Medium-Heat oil
2–4 Tbsp. brown sugar *or* maple granules
1/4 cup honey *or* agave nectar
1 tsp. vanilla extract
2/3 cup unsweetened applesauce
1 cup frozen blueberries (divided)

Topping Ingredients:
1–2 Tbsp. brown sugar *or* maple granules
1/4–1/2 tsp. ground cinnamon
1/8 tsp. ground nutmeg
1/4 cup walnuts, chopped

Blueberries

When using frozen blueberries, select berries from a company that freezes berries soon after picking, retaining flavor and nutrients as much as possible. We enjoy wild blueberries from Maine – the small, tender berries are bursting with flavor.

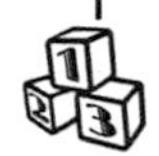

Variations

1 cup of whole-grain spelt flour can be used in place of "white" whole-wheat flour. Use only 1/2 cup of applesauce.

Diced frozen strawberries can be used in place of blueberries in these coffee cakes.

Oven temperature—350°
Oil an 8x8x2-inch glass baking dish.

1. In bowl, **whisk** together flour, baking powder, baking soda, salt, cinnamon and nutmeg; set aside. In larger bowl, **whisk** together egg, oil, sugar, honey, vanilla and applesauce to dissolve sugar. Add dry ingredients to egg mixture. **Stir** gently to moisten all ingredients.
2. Gently **fold** in three-fourths of fruit (straight from freezer). **Pour** into baking dish; **spread** evenly. **Sprinkle** remaining fruit over batter.
3. **Mix** topping and **sprinkle** evenly over batter.
4. **Bake** in preheated oven for 25–30 minutes.
   Or cover and refrigerate up to 12 hours. Bake straight from the refrigerator in preheated oven.

Yield: 12 servings (cut 4x3) 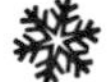 May be frozen for a couple of weeks. Wrap tightly.

Analysis/Serving:
Calories: 138–149 (Fat Cal 50) Fat: 5.6g (0.5g Sat) Cholesterol: 18mg
Sodium: 130mg Carbs: 20–23g (2.3g Fiber 11–14g Sugar) Protein: 2.2g

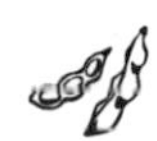

Oat

Unlike many grains, oats are processed in a way that does not dramatically reduce their nutritional value. Oats contain a specific type of fiber that helps to lower cholesterol more than most fibers, strengthens the immune system and stabilizes blood sugars, making it an excellent breakfast food! Oats have a combination of antioxidants found in no other food. Great for preventing and managing cardiovascular disease.

Forms of oats:

Groats: kernels that have not been rolled flat.

Steel-cut/Irish/Scottish: kernel has been sliced; chewy.

Old-fashioned: kernels have been steamed and rolled into thick flakes.

Quick-cooking: kernels are cut before rolling flat. Nutrition is not lost.

"Instant" oatmeal: very thin flakes. Often sugar, salt and other ingredients are added.

Oat bran: outer layer of grain. The bran is present in all forms of oats. It may be purchased separately.

Serving Suggestions:

Oats can be added to muffins, pancakes, cookies and breads.

Honey-Applesauce Bran Muffins

S→O: 20 minutes   Bake: 20–22 minutes

Wheat Bran Version

1/4–1/2 cup raisins *or* dates
OR 1/2 cup dried cranberries
1 1/4 cups "white" whole-wheat flour
1 cup wheat bran
2 tsp. baking powder
1/8 tsp. salt
1/4 tsp. baking soda
1/4 tsp. allspice

2 eggs, slightly beaten
1 cup unsweetened applesauce
1 cup milk (low-fat cow, unsweetened soy, unsweetened almond)
1/4 cup High-Heat oil
1/4 cup honey
1 tsp. vanilla

Oat Bran Version

1/4–1/2 cup raisins *or* dates
OR 1/2 cup dried cranberries
1 cup "white" whole-wheat flour
1 cup oat bran
2 tsp. baking powder
1/8 tsp. salt
1/4 tsp. baking soda
1 tsp. ground cinnamon

2 eggs, slightly beaten
1 cup unsweetened applesauce
3/4 cup milk (low-fat cow, unsweetened soy, unsweetened almond)
1/4 cup High-Heat oil
1/4 cup honey
1 tsp. vanilla

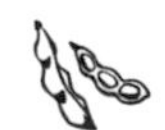

Analysis/Wheat Bran Muffin: (based on 12 muffins)
Calories: 164–175 (Fat Cal 54)   Fat: 6g (0.7g Sat)   Cholesterol: 36mg
Sodium: 141mg   Carbs: 25–27g (4g Fiber 11–13g Sugar)   Protein: 4g

Analysis/Oat Bran Muffin: (based on 12 muffins)
Calories: 172–183 (Fat Cal 55)   Fat: 6.1g (0.8g Sat)   Cholesterol: 36mg
Sodium: 145mg   Carbs: 25–27g (3g Fiber 11–13g Sugar)   Protein: 4g

Spelt Oat Bran Version

1/4–1/2 cup raisins *or* dates
OR 1/2 cup dried cranberries
3/4 cup whole-grain spelt flour
1/4 cup white spelt flour
1 cup oat bran
2 tsp. baking powder
1/8 tsp. salt
1/4 tsp. baking soda
1 tsp. ground cinnamon

2 eggs, slightly beaten
1 cup unsweetened applesauce
3/4 cup milk (low-fat cow, unsweetened soy, unsweetened almond)
1/4 cup High-Heat oil
1/4 cup honey
1 tsp. vanilla

Preheat oven—400°.
Line muffin cups with paper liners.

1. In food processor, **chop** dried fruit with approximately ¼ cup of the flour.
2. In large mixing bowl, **whisk** fruit mixture, flour, bran, salt, baking powder, baking soda and allspice or cinnamon together.
3. In separate bowl, **whisk** together eggs, applesauce, milk, oil, honey and vanilla. Add to dry ingredients and **stir** just until flour is moistened.
4. **Portion** into muffin cups (they will be almost to the top of the paper liner). **Bake** in preheated oven for 20–22 minutes, or until toothpick clean. (Mini-sized muffins bake in about 17 minutes.)

Keep muffins warm in cloth-lined basket.

Yield: 12–14 muffins or 48 mini muffins

Tips on Storage and Reheating

Store leftover muffins in tightly sealed container.

Best served within 2 days.

If the tops become moist from storing in sealed container, warm in a preheating oven (150–200°) for a few minutes. This removes the extra moisture as well as makes the muffins smell and taste freshly baked.

Muffins may be frozen (tightly wrapped) for a couple of weeks.

Variations

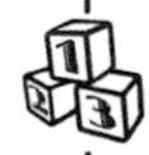

Blueberry: Gently stir in 3/4 cup of frozen blueberries after most of the flour is moistened.

Cranberry-Pecan: Gently stir in 1 cup diced frozen cranberries and 1/2 cup chopped pecans after most of the flour is moistened.

Preparation Hint: It is best to measure out (and dice, if needed) the frozen fruit before starting muffin preparation so the fruit thaws a little.

Baking: Bake 1–3 minutes longer than muffins without frozen fruit.

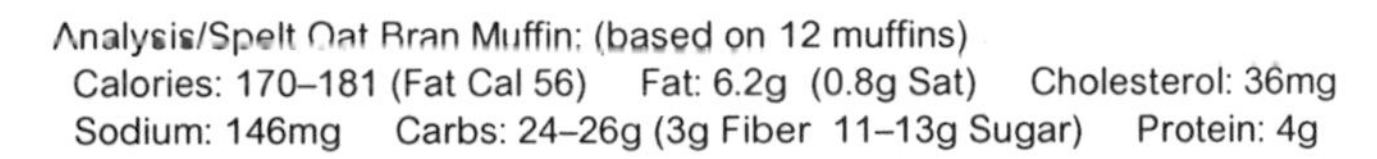
Analysis/Spelt Oat Bran Muffin: (based on 12 muffins)
Calories: 170–181 (Fat Cal 56) Fat: 6.2g (0.8g Sat) Cholesterol: 36mg
Sodium: 146mg Carbs: 24–26g (3g Fiber 11–13g Sugar) Protein: 4g

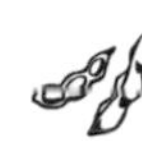

Healthier Pancake Toppings

- Warm apple slices/chunks
- Applesauce or blends (e.g., apricot-applesauce)
- Fruit Pancake Syrup (below)
- Pure 100% maple syrup (small amounts)

Fruit Pancake Syrup

S→T: 15 minutes (10 minutes inactive)

Authors' favorite is blueberry with agave nectar.

Photo on Front Cover (on pancakes).

1 (10 oz.) pkg. frozen fruit (e.g., blueberries, strawberries, raspberries)
2 Tbsp. cornstarch
1–2 Tbsp. sweetener—agave nectar, brown rice syrup, honey
1 cup water

In saucepan, **combine** ingredients. **Cook** over medium heat until thickened, stirring often to prevent sticking/burning.

Chill or serve warm as topping for pancakes, *or* use only 1/2 cup water and serve as "jelly" on biscuits, muffins and/or toast.

Refrigerate extra for several days. May also freeze.

Analysis for 2 Tablespoons
Calories: 19–24; Sugar: 3–4g; Fiber: 0.6g

Yield: 1 2/3 cups

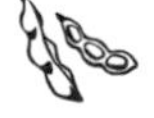

High-Fiber Oat Spice Pancakes

Mix: 5 minutes

1 cup whole-wheat pastry flour
1 cup unbleached all-purpose flour
4 tsp. baking powder
1/2 tsp. salt
1 Tbsp. sugar (optional)
3/4 cup quick oats
1/4 cup oat bran (optional)
3/4–1 tsp. ground cinnamon
1/4–1/2 tsp. nutmeg
1/4–1/2 tsp. ginger
3 cups milk (tested with almond, soy; both sweetened and unsweetened)
1/2 tsp. vanilla
2 Tbsp. High-Heat oil

Variation: Sprinkle cranberries on top of batter soon after pouring onto griddle.

Preheat griddle. Lightly **oil** after preheating.

Mix: Whisk dry ingredients together. Add wet ingredients and stir until just mixed (batter will be lumpy; do not overmix or pancakes will be tough). Batter is very thin. Cook according to cooking directions on next page.

Pumpkin Pancakes

Photo on Front Cover

Mix: 6 minutes

1 cup whole-wheat pastry flour
1 cup unbleached all-purpose flour
2 Tbsp. sugar
4 tsp. baking powder
1 tsp. salt
1 tsp. ground cinnamon
Pinch of nutmeg
1/2 (15 oz.) can pumpkin (~1 cup)
2 1/2 cups milk (tested with almond, soy; both sweetened or unsweetened) (use more/less milk as needed)

Variation: Sprinkle 3–4 dark chocolate chips on each pancake soon after pouring onto griddle.

Preheat griddle. Lightly **oil** after preheating.

Mix: Whisk dry ingredients together. Stir in pumpkin. Stir in milk to desired consistency (do not overmix or pancakes will be tough). The batter needs to be fairly thick but pourable. Cook according to directions below.

Pumpkin Deluxe Pancakes

Photo on Front Cover

Mix: 6 minutes

2 cups "white" whole-wheat flour
2 Tbsp. sugar (optional)
2 Tbsp. flaxseed meal
4 tsp. baking powder
1 tsp. salt
1 tsp. ground cinnamon
1 egg, slightly beaten
1/2 (15 oz.) can pumpkin (~1 cup)
2 1/2 cups unsweetened soy milk
1/2 cup pecans, broken (optional)

Preheat griddle. Lightly **oil** after preheating.

Mix: Whisk dry ingredients together. Stir in egg and pumpkin. Stir in milk to desired consistency (do not overmix or pancakes will be tough). Allow batter to set a few minutes; stir in pecans. The batter needs to be fairly thick but pourable. Cook according to directions below.

Cooking Directions for Pancakes: Lightly oil preheated griddle, using High-Heat oil. Pour batter on griddle in desired shapes/sizes. Cook on first side until edge turns opaque in color and the bubbles on top begin to pop. Flip. Cook until done.

Each Recipe Yields: ~20–24 (4-inch) pancakes.

SPECIAL NOTE: We developed these pancake recipes to taste great with less topping. If using a lot of topping, cut salt in half.

Soy Deluxe Pancakes

Mix: 6 minutes

2 cups flour (choose one)
whole-wheat flour
OR "white" whole-wheat flour
OR whole-grain spelt flour
1/2 cup soy protein isolate (p. 89)
2 Tbsp. sugar (optional)
2 Tbsp. flaxseed meal
4 tsp. baking powder
1 tsp. salt
1 egg (slightly beaten)
2 Tbsp. High-Heat oil
2 1/2–3 cups water (lower amount with spelt)
1/2 cup pecans, broken (optional)

Preheat griddle.
Lightly **oil** after preheating.

Mix: Whisk dry ingredients together. Mix in egg, oil and water (do not overmix or pancakes will be tough). Allow batter to set a few minutes; stir in pecans. Batter is fairly thick but pourable. Cook according to cooking directions at left.

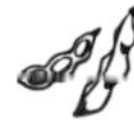

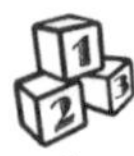

Blended Whole-Wheat Bread

If you and your family are not ready for 100% whole-grain bread, try a blend of flours. We have successfully tested the following combination:

2 1/4 cups "white" whole-wheat flour
1 1/2 cup unbleached all-purpose flour
Use only 2 teaspoons of vital wheat gluten.

Vital Wheat Gluten

Adding gluten to whole grains increases the ability of the dough to rise, improving the texture of the bread. The higher the percentage of whole grain, the more gluten needed.

Hearty Homemade Bread *for* Bread Machines (large loaf)

1 cup water
1/2 cup + 2 Tbsp. milk (unsweetened almond, rice or soy milk; low-fat cow)
1 1/2 tsp. salt
2 Tbsp. Medium-Heat oil
1 Tbsp. honey
2 Tbsp. sugar
3 3/4 cup "white" whole-wheat flour (best at room temperature)
1 Tbsp. vital wheat gluten
1 Tbsp. active dry bread machine yeast

1. Place ingredients in bread machine in order suggested by manufacturer's manual.
2. Process on whole-wheat bread cycle.
3. Remove loaf from pan and allow to rest for 10–15 minutes before slicing.

Slice thick pieces for dinner (see next page sidebar) or thin slices for sandwiches. Slices may be frozen.

Nutritional analysis on next page.

Yield: 22 (1.5 oz.) half slices

Seasoned Croutons

Prepare: 5 minutes Bake: 6–10 minutes

4 cups bread cubes (~5 slices) (Ezekiel *or* whole grain)
High-Heat spray oil
Seasonings, as desired
Sondra's favorite combo is:
Light sprinkle of salt
1/4 tsp. paprika
1/4 tsp. garlic powder

Preheat oven—400°.
Baking sheet with sides

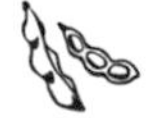

1. Place cubes single layer on baking sheet. **Spray** oil with Kitchen Spritzer (p. 144) while tossing to lightly coat cubes with oil. Lightly **toss** while evenly sprinkling with seasonings of your choice.
2. **Bake** 6–10 minutes, or until dry (time depends upon size of cubes and heaviness of bread), stirring midway through. **Cool**.

Yield: 16 (1/4-cup) servings

Why Bother with Homemade Bread?

There is nothing quite like the smell of homemade bread. And when you make it, you control the ingredients.

Bread machines make it easier to try bread making at home. All ingredients are combined in the machine, and the machine runs automatically, mixing, kneading and proofing the dough. If you want to shape your own rolls or pizza crust, you can do this and bake it on your own. If you simply want a loaf of bread, the machine will bake it for you – and keep it warm until you are ready to eat! Most machines have a timer on them; you can prepare the ingredients early in the day and set the machine to have your bread done whenever you plan to eat. (Or put ingredients together before bed ... and the smells of freshly baked bread will help you get up in the morning!) Not only are the smells and tastes of homemade bread delightful, but you save money and the nutrition is superior to that of most bread on the market.

Purchasing Bread (loaves of bread, dinner rolls, English muffins, tortillas, flatbreads, sandwich buns)

Many breads come packaged with preservatives and sweetened with corn syrup. Companies often attempt to appeal to the buyer's desire for a healthy product and give their bread names like "all natural," "multigrain" or "whole wheat." These names are often misleading; check the ingredient list and nutritional panel to determine a wise choice. Two companies that make breads we enjoy using are *Rudi's Organic Bakery* (loaves and buns) and *Food For Life* (Ezekiel bread, buns, tortillas and English muffins).

Analysis/Slice for 100% Whole-Wheat Bread:
Calories: 102 (Fat Cal 15) Fat: 1.7g (0.1g Sat) Cholesterol: 0mg
Sodium: 150mg Carbs: 18g (2.8g Fiber 1.9g Sugar) Protein: 3g

Analysis/Slice for Blended Whole-Wheat Bread:
Calories: 99 (Fat Cal 14) Fat: 1.6g (0.1g Sat) Cholesterol: 0mg
Sodium: 150mg Carbs: 18 (1.7g Fiber 2.2g Sugar) Protein: 2.6g

Estimated Analysis for Ezekiel Bread Croutons/Serving:
Calories: 30 (Fat Cal 6) Fat: 0.7g (0g Sat) Cholesterol: 0mg
Sodium: 32mg Carbs: 4.7g (1g Fiber 0g Sugar) Protein: 1.3g

Bread Machine Tips

- Every bread machine is different. The first few times you use a recipe, do so while you are home so you can watch during the first mixing cycle. The dough should form into a cohesive ball. If it is hard and lumpy, add water a teaspoon or two at a time. If it seems too mushy and sticky, add a bit of flour. You will soon know how to adjust the recipe for your machine.
- Do not use cow's milk if you are using the timer (milk will spoil before it is mixed up).
- Use bread machine or fast-rising yeast.

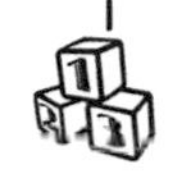

Bread with Olive Oil

Slice Hearty Homemade Bread into thick slices, then cut each slice in half. Serve with olive oil seasoned with garlic powder or garlic salt, freshly ground black pepper and Parmesan cheese. Especially delicious with Italian dishes.

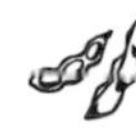

Spelt Dinner Rolls

Use only 2/3 cup water with the following flours instead of the wheat flours:
~2 1/8 cups whole-grain spelt flour
1 cup white spelt flour

Healthy Bites

"Good" Fats: In five minutes you can prepare a butter spread (Omega Butter) that increases the consumption of "good" fats (omega fatty acids, polyunsaturated fat, monounsaturated fats) while cutting saturated fat in half.

Omega Butter: Whisk together a stick of softened unsalted butter and 1/2 cup of flaxseed oil for a cup of spread. Store covered in refrigerator. At room temperature it softens quickly, so it is also convenient as a "margarine."

Purchase or Prepare: It is hard to find healthy choices for purchased frozen and refrigerated dough. Our rolls contain half the sodium and half the fat calories, eliminate preservatives and unhealthy oils and add fiber in comparison with most prepared doughs.

Whole-Grain Dinner Rolls

Prep Time: varies   Bake: 10–12 minutes.

3/4 cup water
1 Tbsp. rapid-rise dry yeast
1/2 cup milk
(we prefer sweetened almond milk)
2 Tbsp. High-Heat oil
2 Tbsp. sweetener—honey or agave nectar
1 tsp. salt
1 cup unbleached all-purpose flour
~2 1/8 cups "white" whole-wheat flour
1 Tbsp. vital wheat gluten (p. 190)

Oven temperature—425°
Preheat and oil baking sheets at Step 4.

1. **Mix and proof dough:**
   - If using a **bread machine**, add ingredients in order recommended in owner's manual. (If dough is sticking to sides of gasket, add more flour. If dough is too stiff to be malleable when kneading, add a bit of water.) After completing dough cycle, allow dough to sit in bread machine for an additional 20–30 minutes.
   - If using a **stand mixer**:
     a. Heat water to lukewarm (110–115°); stir in yeast to dissolve; allow to set for 5 minutes in mixer bowl.
     b. Heat milk to lukewarm; add oil, sweetener and salt; stir.
     c. To mixer bowl, add milk mixture; followed by 1 cup of the flour and gluten. Beat with whisk for 30 seconds.
     d. Add remaining flour except a couple of tablespoons. With dough hook, stir in (knead speed). Continuing on knead speed, gradually add more flour until

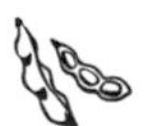

Analysis/Dinner Roll:
Calories: 81 (Fat Cal 12) Fat: 1.3g (0.1g Sat) Cholesterol: 0mg
Sodium: 91mg Carbs: 14.6g (1.4g Fiber 1.8g Sugar) Protein: 2.4g

dough clings to hook and cleans sides of bowl.

e. Knead on knead speed for 2 minutes.

f. Form into dough ball; oil all sides. Flatten in bowl. Cover with moist cloth. Let rise in warm place, such as a 100° oven, for 20–30 minutes, or until doubled.

3. **Shape:** Shape your favorite way or see our favorite ways below.
4. **Preheat** oven and **oil** baking sheets.
5. **Proof:** Cover with dry cloth. Proof in warm place, such as on range top while oven is preheating, for about 20 minutes, or until doubled (do this proofing step even if you have used a bread machine).
6. **Bake** in preheated oven for 10–12 minutes.

Yield: 24 dinner rolls

Shaping Dinner Rolls

Round: Shape dough into 2-inch balls. Place on baking sheet or 9-inch round pan about 1/2 inch apart.

Crescents: Divide dough in half. On lightly floured surface, roll out each portion into a 14-inch circle. Lightly brush with melted butter. Cut into 12 wedges. Roll up, beginning at rounded edge. With point underneath, place on baking sheet 1 inch apart.

"Buttery" Rolls: If desired, brush tops with melted unsalted butter or healthier-choice margarine (1) before proofing, (2) approximately 8 minutes into baking time or (3) immediately after baking.

Hamburger Buns: Shape into 10 hamburger buns. Sprinkle tops with wheat bran or sesame seeds. Press bran/seeds into bun. Proof and bake. Split buns after baking. Freeze extras.

Breadsticks: Shape into 12 (or more) breadsticks. Proof and bake. For garlic breadsticks, stir a little garlic powder or garlic salt into melted unsalted butter. Brush breadsticks as described above.

Do-Ahead

Shaped rolls may be stored on a baking sheet and covered in the refrigerator for several hours or overnight. Then allow them to rise in a warm place for two hours, or until doubled.

Shaped rolls may also be frozen. Place on lined baking sheet. Freeze for about one hour and then transfer to food storage bag. Allow about three hours to thaw before proofing as described to the right.

Stuffed Crescents

When Dorie was a child, her mother often made "surprise rolls" on Christmas Eve. These were typical dinner rolls with a bite of "something" inside – a piece of ham, a piece of cheese, an olive, or some other treat. Kids can help roll a surprise into these crescents ... or simply enjoy the surprise at the dinner table. They can even help decide what the surprise will be. For a fancy twist, consider spreading the dough with pesto and rolling up an asparagus spear. Have fun and be creative!

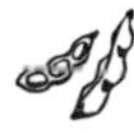

Low-Sugar Cinnamon Rolls

Prep: varies Bake: 15 minutes.

$1\frac{3}{4}$ cups water
4 tsp. rapid-rise dry yeast
$\frac{3}{4}$ cup regular *or* quick oats
$1\frac{1}{2}$ tsp. salt
2 Tbsp. Medium-Heat oil
$\frac{1}{4}$ cup honey, maple syrup *or* agave nectar
$2\frac{1}{4}$ cups whole-wheat flour
$1\frac{1}{2}$ cups unbleached all-purpose flour
1 Tbsp. vital wheat gluten (p. 190)

Filling Ingredients:
- **$\frac{1}{4}$ cup unsalted butter**
- **$\frac{1}{4}$ cup light brown sugar *or* maple sugar**
- **2 tsp. ground cinnamon**
- **1 cup chopped pecans** (optional)
- **1 cup raisins *or* dried cranberries** (optional)

Glaze Ingredients:
$\frac{2}{3}$ cup powdered sugar with ~1 Tbsp. water

Oven Temperature—375°. **Preheat** at Step 4.
Oil baking sheets.

1. **Mix and proof dough**:
   - If using a **bread machine**, add ingredients in order recommended in owner's manual. (If dough is sticking to sides of gasket, add more flour. If dough is too stiff to be malleable when kneading, add a bit of water.) After completing dough cycle, allow dough to sit in bread machine for an additional 20–30 minutes.
   - If using a **stand mixer**:
     a. Heat water to lukewarm (110–115°); stir in yeast; allow to sit for 5 minutes.
     b. To mixer bowl, add oats, salt, oil and sweetener. Add yeast mixture; followed by 1 cup of the flour and gluten. Beat with whisk for 30 seconds.
     c. Add remaining flour except a couple of tablespoons. With dough hook, stir in (knead speed).

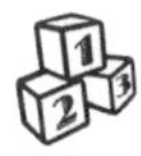

Other Flour Options

Wheat: Use the following wheat flours in place of those listed in the recipe:

- $2\frac{1}{2}$ cups "white" whole-wheat flour
- $1\frac{1}{2}$ cups unbleached, all-purpose flour

Spelt: Use $1\frac{1}{2}$ cups water with the following flours instead of the wheat flours:
~$2\frac{1}{2}$ cups whole-grain spelt flour
1 cup white spelt flour

Healthy Bite

A typical cinnamon roll made from purchased tubes of dough has almost twice the fat, three times the sodium and about half the fiber as ours. Plus, it contains over thirty ingredients, including hydrogenated oils (trans fats), corn syrup and food dyes.

Freezing Rolls

Unproofed rolls may be frozen for up to two weeks (see Do-Ahead tips on p. 193). Place on prepared baking sheet. Allow about three hours to thaw, then proof and bake as usual.

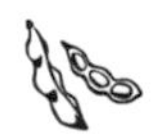

d. Continuing on knead speed, gradually adding more flour until dough clings to hook and cleans sides of bowl.
e. Knead on knead speed for 2 minutes.
f. Form into dough ball; oil all sides. Flatten in bowl. Cover with moist cloth. Let rise in warm place, such as a 100° oven, for 20–30 min., or until doubled.

2. **Prepare Filling:** In saucepan, melt butter. Stir in sugar and cinnamon. (We mix half the filling mixture at a time, so we know how much to spread on each portion in Step 3b.)
3. **Shape Rolls:**
   a. Divide dough in half. On lightly floured surface, roll out each portion into approximately 15x11-inch rectangular.
   b. Pour cinnamon mixture on dough. Using a rubber spatula, spread mixture evenly on dough surface, leaving about ¼ inch on one of the 15-inch edges plain. Evenly sprinkle pecans and dried fruit on dough.
   c. Beginning with the coated 15-inch edge, roll dough into a log. Slice about 1 inch thick with bench knife (sidebar). Lay flat on prepared baking sheet 1 inch apart.
4. **Preheat** oven and **oil** baking sheets.
5. **Proof:** Cover rolls with dry cloth. Proof in a warm place, such as on range top while oven is preheating, for 20–30 minutes, or until doubled.
6. **Bake** in preheated oven for 15 minutes. Transfer to cooling rack.
7. **Glaze:** Gradually add water to powdered sugar, stirring until smooth and desired consistency. Drizzle in a circle on each roll.

Yield: 30 (3–3½-inch) rolls.

Do-Ahead

Shaped rolls may be stored on baking sheet, covered in refrigerator for several hours or overnight. Then allow to rise in warm place for two or three hours, or until doubled.

Bench Knife

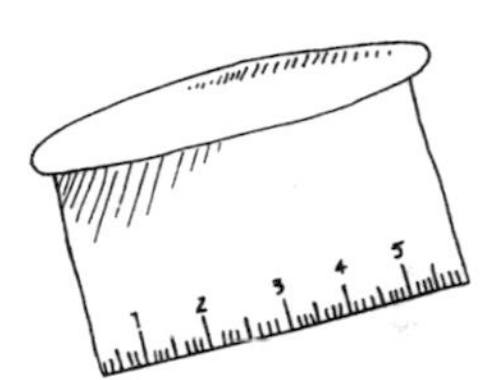

Bench knives (dough scrapers) are designed to slice dough. Some have a ruler printed on the blade for measuring the width of whatever is being sliced. It is a great tool for slicing these cinnamon rolls. Other cool uses for these knives include the following:

- scraping crumbs and other food from counter
- carrying prepared vegetables to the skillet from cutting board
- slicing cucumbers and summer squash
- slicing soft cheeses
- slicing logs of refrigerated cookie dough (Pumpkin Cookies, p. 85)
- cutting brownies or bars

Analysis/Cinnamon Roll (without/with raisins and pecans)
Calories: 116/156 (Fat Cal 24/45) Fat: 2.7/5g (1.5/1.7g Sat) Cholesterol: 4mg
Sodium: 108mg Carbs: 21/25g (1.5/2g Fiber 7/10.7g Sugar) Protein: 2.6/3g

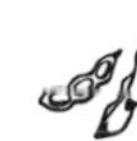

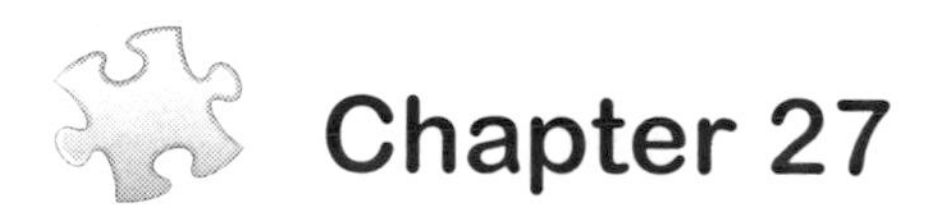

Chapter 27

Desserts

Transitions are a process; this is just as true with desserts as with anything else. And we want the transition to be a positive experience. If foods become taboo and we focus on what we can't have, eating becomes a chore instead of a healthy part of life. This chapter is dedicated to looking at small changes in our desserts that can make a big difference in our health. In part, this involves how we prepare our desserts. But it also involves how we serve our desserts.

Moving toward a healthier consumption of treats, make the choice to:

- **Increase nutrition:** use more fruits and vegetables, whole grains and better sugars
- **Increase protein and fiber:** reduces sugar spikes
- **Change fats and sugars:** use healthier fats and sugars
- **Reduce sugar and fat calories**: reduces empty calories and bad fats
- **Reduce serving size:** e.g., smaller cookies, smaller slices of pie, less fruit crisp when accompanied by ice cream, mini-sized cupcakes/muffins
- **Include more fruit:** serve fruit alongside small cookies or cupcakes; or incorporate fruit within the dessert (e.g., shortcake, frozen yogurt, fruit crisps)

Shortcake

Use biscuits (p. 182), flattening dough slightly (Step 3). Slice biscuit horizontally. Lay bottom half in bowl; top with lightly sweetened fresh or frozen (thawed) fruit (e.g., strawberries, peaches, blueberries, mangos). Lay top biscuit on the fruit; top with more fruit. If desired, top with a dollop of Whipped Cream (p. 165) and a few chopped nuts.

Frozen Yogurt

Frozen yogurt can be an easy, fun family snack to create. With the right equipment and a variety of ingredients, the combinations are endless. Many ideas in the bullet list above can be incorporated to make this a healthier treat.

Use an ice cream and frozen yogurt maker. Follow directions included with equipment. Choose plain or vanilla yogurt. Choose fresh or frozen fruit over canned fruit. As you transition your taste buds, gradually use less sugar and/or switch to other sweeteners (e.g., fruits, honey, agave nectar, brown rice syrup). Have fun!

Chocolate Chip Cookie Makeover

Original Recipe	Alteration	Benefit
all-purpose flour	use half whole-grain flour	increases fiber, protein and other nutrients
1 cup of butter	reduce by one-third	reduces saturated fat
$1^1/_2$ cups sugar	reduce by one-third	decreases calories and sugar content
2 cups chocolate chips	cut in half	decreases calories and reduces fat and sugar content

Chocolate Chip Cookies

Mix: 15 minutes

2/3 cup unsalted butter, softened
OR healthier-choice margarine
1/2 cup granulated (white) sugar
1/2 cup brown sugar
2 eggs
OR "egg substitute" (p. 206)
2 tsp. vanilla extract
2 1/2 cups Baking Mix (p. 181)
1 cup semi-sweet chocolate chips

Preheat oven—350°. **Oil** cookie sheets.

With mixer, **cream** butter and sugars. **Beat** in vanilla and eggs (or substitute). **Stir** in Baking Mix. Stir in chips. **Drop** by spoonfuls or small dipper onto cookie sheet. Using back of spoon or fork, **flatten** dough slightly. **Bake** 10–12 minutes. (Cookies made with the egg substitute may take longer to bake.) Transfer to cooling rack.

Store cookies in airtight container for two or three days. Freeze extra. To eliminate "unintentional snacking," bake less; freeze unbaked batter (simply thaw, dip and bring to room temperature while preheating oven).

Yield: 3 1/2 dozen

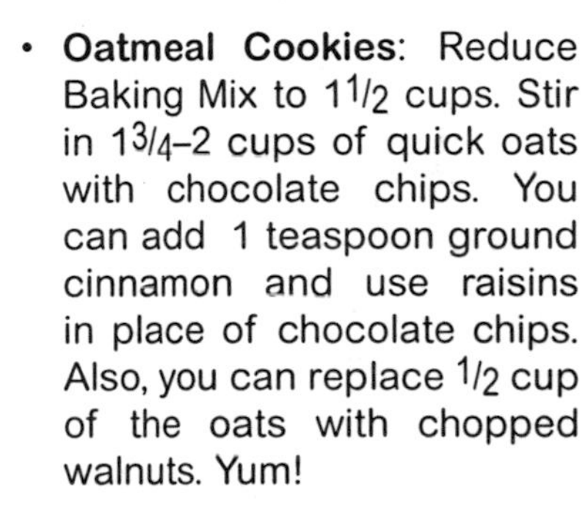

Variations

- **Oatmeal Cookies**: Reduce Baking Mix to 1 1/2 cups. Stir in 1 3/4–2 cups of quick oats with chocolate chips. You can add 1 teaspoon ground cinnamon and use raisins in place of chocolate chips. Also, you can replace 1/2 cup of the oats with chopped walnuts. Yum!
- **Sugar Cookies:** Use all granulated sugar instead of half brown sugar. Omit chocolate chips. Lightly sprinkle cookies with sugar before baking.
- **Rum-Pecan Sugar Cookies:** Substitute rum extract for vanilla and stir in 1 cup of chopped pecans.
- **Gluten-Free Chocolate Chip Cookies:** Replace Baking Mix with same amount of Gluten-Free Flour Mix (p. 27) plus 4 teaspoons baking powder and 1/4 teaspoon salt.

Analysis/Cookie:
Calories: 94 (Fat Cal 40) Fat: 4.4g (2.6g Sat) Cholesterol: 19mg
Sodium: 62mg Carbs: 12.5g (0.4g Fiber 7.1g Sugar) Protein: 1.3g

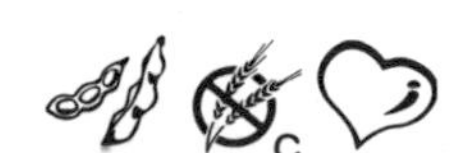

flour mix, vanilla, chocolate chips

Gingerbread Cookie Makeover

Original Recipe	Alternation	Benefit
1 cup salted butter	cut in half, use unsalted	reduces saturated fat reduces sodium
¾ cup brown sugar	reduce by one-third	decreases calories/sugar carbs
¼ tsp. salt	cut in half	reduces sodium
½ tsp. baking soda	cut in half	reduces sodium
½ cup molasses	reduce by one-third	decreases calories/sugar carbs
all-purpose flour	use mostly whole grain	increases fiber

Recipe Makeover

Increases fiber by 225%

and at the same time it reduces

calories by 30%

fat by 50%

cholesterol by 34%

sodium by 62%

sugars by 32%.

And still tastes great! Some said it was the best Gingerbread Cookie ever.

Wow!

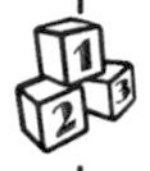

Gluten-Free Cookies

Replace both wheat flours with 2 3/4 cups of Gluten-Free (GF) Flour Mix (p. 27). Use rice flour for rolling; roll out slightly thicker.

Gingerbread Cookies

Mix: 15 minutes

1/2 cup unsalted butter, softened
OR healthier-choice margarine
1/2 cup brown sugar
1/8 tsp. salt
1/4 tsp. baking soda
2 tsp. ground ginger
1 tsp. ground cinnamon
1/4 tsp. ground nutmeg
1/4 tsp. ground cloves
1 egg
1/3 cup molasses *or* honey
1 3/4 cups "white" whole-wheat flour
3/4 cup unbleached all-purpose flour

Oven temperature—350° (preheat at Step 3).
Cookie sheets

1. With mixer, **beat** softened butter and sugar on high until creamy. Beat in salt, baking soda and spices. Beat in egg and molasses on medium. **Mix** in flours on low until well blended. If dough does not form a cohesive ball, mix in a few drops of water. Scrape sides and bottom as needed. (Use flat beater with stand mixer.)

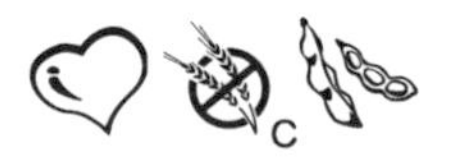

Analysis/Cookie without frosting:
Calories: 174 (Fat Cal 52) Fat: 5.8g (3.4g Sat) Cholesterol: 27mg
Sodium: 38mg Carbs: 24.8g (1.8g Fiber 9g Sugar) Protein: 2.8g

2. **Divide** dough into thirds, flatten each into disc-like portions and wrap in plastic wrap. **Chill** 1 hour.
3. **Preheat** oven—350°. **Roll** out one portion of dough to desired thickness (yield is based on 1/8 to 1/4 inch) on a lightly floured board. **Cut** with a cookie cutter and transfer to unoiled cookie sheet. Repeat with remaining dough.
4. **Bake** in preheated oven for 8 minutes, or until done. As soon as possible, transfer cookies to wire cooling rack to cool.
5. **Decorate** cooled cookies, if desired. Mix a spoonful of powdered sugar with a few drops of water to make a fairly stiff icing. Place icing in baggie. Cut off one of the bottom corners of the baggie, making a small hole. Gently squeeze out a small amount of icing to make eyes, mouth and buttons.

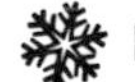 Freeze extra.

Yield: 17 (5-inch) shaped cookies

Shaped Sugar Cookies

1/2 cup unsalted butter, softened
OR healthier-choice margarine
1/2 cup granulated sugar
1/8 tsp. salt
1/4 tsp. baking soda
3/4 tsp. vanilla extract
1 egg
1/3 cup honey
1 3/4 cups "white" whole-wheat flour
3/4 cup unbleached all-purpose flour

Prepare and bake same as Gingerbread Cookies except roll out slightly thicker or bake less time.

Decorate with naturally colored icing. Natural food colorings can be purchased, or create your own using spices, fruit juices and vegetable juices. See sidebar for a few ideas to get started. Also, see our websites (p. 242). Enjoy experimenting.

Little Chefs

Enjoy baking and decorating cookies as a family.

Some foods that make natural colorings are the following:

- 100% grape juice or the juice of blueberries for purple/blue
- 100% cranberry juice or the juice from beets or other berries for pink/red
- Spinach broth for green
- Ground cinnamon for brown

Be aware that some sources of colors (especially 100% fruit juices) will add subtle flavors to your icing. This can be quite a classy touch, but you want to make sure it goes with the flavor of the cookie or cake.

Using two tablespoons of powdered sugar adds approximately 0.9 grams of sugar to each cookie.

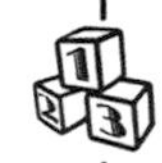

Gluten-Free Cookies

Do the same as Gingerbread Cookies and use cookie cutters without a lot of detail. Also, choose a gluten-free vanilla.

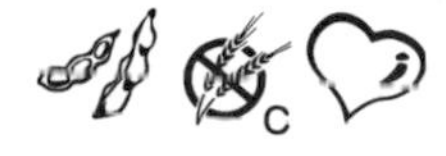

Spice Cake Makeover

Original Recipe	Alternation	Benefit
⅓ cup butter	use oil; reduce by half	reduces saturated fat
¾ cup sugar	reduce by one-sixth	decreases calories/sugar carbs
all-purpose flour	use whole grain	increases fiber
NONE	added carrots	increases nutrition, sweetness

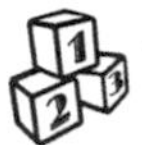

Creating!

Dorie's son is allergic to eggs, so this recipe makeover started out in an attempt to make an egg-free birthday cake. The cake is muffinlike in density and taste, so it really needs no frosting. If frosting is desired, we recommend a sugar-water glaze (oil-based frostings seep into the cake) or use Cream Cheese Frosting (p. 207).

Egg-Free: Use below ingredients with method to right; bake 5–10 minutes longer.

1 1/2 cups "white" whole-wheat flour
2/3 cup sugar
1/8 tsp. salt
1 1/2 tsp. ground cinnamon
1/2 tsp. ground nutmeg
3/4 cup water
8 oz. baby carrots
1/3 cup High-Heat oil
1/2 cup applesauce
4 tsp. baking powder
1/2 tsp. baking soda

Spice "Muffin" Cake

S→O: 15 minutes Bake: 35 minutes

1 1/2 cups "white" whole-wheat flour
2/3 cup sugar
1/4 tsp. salt
1 1/2 tsp. ground cinnamon
1/2 tsp. ground nutmeg
1/3 cup water
2 eggs
8 oz. baby carrots (~1 1/2 cups sliced)
2 Tbsp. Medium-Heat oil
1/2 cup applesauce
2 tsp. baking powder
1/2 tsp. baking soda

Preheat oven—350°. **Line** a 7x11x2-inch baking dish with parchment paper.

1. In large bowl, **whisk** flour, sugar, salt, cinnamon and nutmeg together. Set aside.
2. **Place** water in blender, followed by eggs (if using), carrots and oil. **Blend** for a minute, until mixture becomes uniform in color and well blended. **Add** applesauce, baking powder and baking soda. **Blend** for a few seconds.
3. Add carrot mixture to dry ingredients and **stir** until just combined. **Spread** evenly in baking dish. **Bake** in preheated oven for 35 minutes, or until toothpick comes out clean.

Yield: 12 servings. For cupcakes, bake in 12 paper-lined muffin cups for 30 minutes. Freezes well.

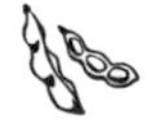

Analysis/Serving:
Calories: 146 (Fat Cal 30) Fat: 3.3g (0.4g Sat) Cholesterol: 35mg
Sodium: 197mg Carbs: 26g (2.9g Fiber 12.6g Sugar) Protein: 3.3g

Pumpkin Cheesecake

S→O: 20 minutes Bake: 55–60 minutes

This cheesecake is light and fluffy compared to the traditional rich and heavy cheesecake.

1/2 cup pecans
4 whole-grain graham crackers
2 Tbsp. unsalted butter

16 oz. Neufchâtel cheese, softened (p. 43)
1/4 cup sugar
2 tsp. ground cinnamon
1/2 tsp. ground ginger
1/2 tsp. mace
Freshly grated nutmeg
2 eggs
1/4 cup honey
2 tsp. vanilla
1–2 Tbsp. cornstarch
(depends upon consistency of canned pumpkin)
1 (15 oz.) can pumpkin

Preheat oven—350°. **Line** bottom of 9-inch springform pan with nonbleached parchment paper.

1. Finely **chop** pecans and crackers in small food processor. Melt butter and **drizzle** evenly over crumbs; **process** to mix. Transfer to prepared pan and firmly **press** to form bottom crust.
2. With electric mixer **beat** Neufchâtel cheese, sugar and spices on medium-high speed until light and fluffy. **Add** remaining ingredients; mix on medium until combined thoroughly. Scrape mixer bowl as needed.
3. Pour into prepared pan. **Bake** in preheated oven for 65–70 minutes, or until knife comes out almost clean when inserted in the center. **Cool** on wire rack for 30 minutes. Cover and **chill** thoroughly in refrigerator.

Yield: 16 servings

Helpful Hint

You may cut the recipe in half and bake in a 6-inch springform pan for about 10 minutes less time.

Gluten-Free

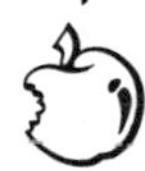

Use a half batch of the Gluten-Free version of Stir & Press Pie Crust (p. 205) and use a gluten-free vanilla.

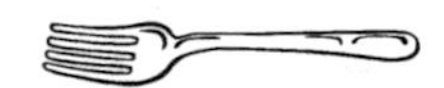

Best if prepared a day before serving. Garnish with a dollop of Whipped Cream (p. 165).

Recipe Makeover

The original recipe called for twice the butter in the crust, extra egg yolks, one and half times more cream cheese and very little pumpkin. The recipe makeover is 134 calories less for the same size piece. It also reduces:

Fat by 50%
Saturated fat by 57%
Sugars by 47%
while increasing nutrients by using more pumpkin.

Delicious!

Analysis/Serving:
Calories: 172 (Fat Cal 91) Fat: 10.1g (5.3g Sat) Cholesterol: 55mg
Sodium: 139mg Carbs: 14.5g (1.5g Fiber 9.7g Sugar) Protein: 3.6g

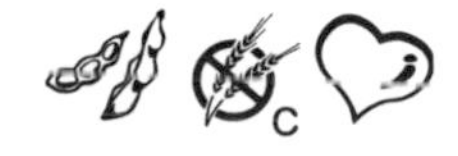

Pastry Blender

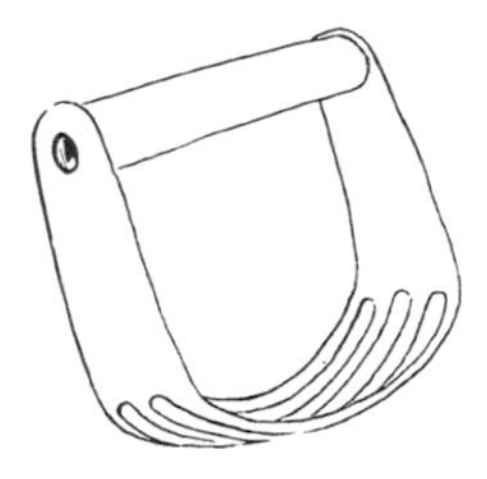

A pastry blender offers a fast way to evenly distribute butter into a batter.

Gluten-Free Crisp Topping

Mix: < 10 minutes

1/2 cup brown rice flour
3 Tbsp. brown sugar
1/8 tsp. salt
1 tsp. ground cinnamon
Dash ground nutmeg
2 Tbsp. butter *or* healthier-choice margarine
2–3 Tbsp. ice-cold water

In bowl, **whisk** dry ingredients together. **Cut** in butter using pastry blender. **Drizzle** water gradually while lightly and quickly blending with fork to create moist balls of dough. Refrigerate until ready to bake.

Yield: Topping for 1 pie/crisp

Oat Crisp Topping

Mix: < 10 minutes

1/4 cup flour— "white" whole-wheat flour
OR whole-wheat flour
OR whole-grain spelt flour
1/4 cup oat bran
1 cup quick oats
1/3 cup brown sugar
1 tsp. ground cinnamon
1/8 tsp. nutmeg
1/4 cup butter *or* healthier-choice margarine
OR 3 Tbsp. High-Heat oil

In bowl, **whisk** all ingredients except butter (or margarine or oil) together. **Cut** in butter using pastry blender or gradually add oil while stirring with fork. Refrigerate until ready to bake.

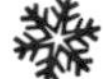 Extra may be frozen.

Yield: 2 cups; enough topping for 2 pies/crisps

Strawberry-Rhubarb Crisp

S→O: 15 minutes Bake: 35 minutes

2 cups sliced fresh rhubarb
2 cups sliced fresh strawberries
1/3 cup honey *or* 1/4 cup + 2 Tbsp. sugar
2 Tbsp. cornstarch
1/8 tsp. salt
1/2 recipe Crisp Topping (above or sidebar)

Preheat oven—400°. **Oil** 9-inch deep pie pan.

1. **Place** fruit in pie pan. In bowl, combine sweetener, cornstarch and salt. **Pour** evenly over fruit. **Stir**.
2. Prepare topping. Evenly **sprinkle** over fruit. **Bake** 35 minutes, or until fruit is tender and topping is golden brown.

Yield: 8 servings

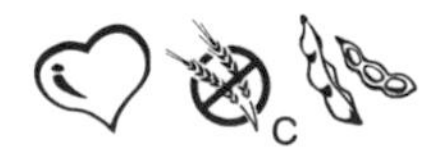

Analysis for Strawberry-Rhubarb Crisp with Oat Topping/Serving:
Calories: 140 (Fat Cal 30) Fat: 3.3g (1.8g Sat) Cholesterol: 8mg
Sodium: 36mg Carbs: 27.5g (2.6g Fiber 18g Sugar) Protein: 2g

Peach/Mango-Blueberry Crisp

S→O: 15 minutes   Bake: 20 minutes

1 (10 oz.) pkg. frozen peaches *or* mangos
1 cup frozen blueberries
2 Tbsp. honey
1/2 tsp. cornstarch
1/2 recipe Crisp Topping (p. 202)

Preheat oven—375°. **Oil** 9-inch deep pie pan.

1. **Place** fruit in pie pan. Put in preheating oven for about 10 minutes to thaw fruit.
2. *Meanwhile*, prepare topping.
3. **Drizzle** honey evenly over fruit. **Stir** in cornstarch. **Sprinkle** with topping. **Bake** in preheated oven for 20 minutes, or until fruit is tender and topping is golden brown.

Yield: 6 servings

Single Servings

Crisp is an easy dessert to make for one or two.

- Prepare crisp topping; keep in the freezer.
- Choose a fruit or fruit combo (apples or frozen fruit works great).
- Thaw frozen fruit or slice apples while preheating a convection-toaster oven (p. 160).
- Drizzle on a little honey (or sprinkle with sugar), adding a few spices to the fruit.
- Sprinkle on the topping and bake.

Quick and easy!

Apple Crisp

S→O: 10 minutes   Bake: 25–35 minutes

2–3 Tbsp. sugar
1/2 tsp. cinnamon
Shake of nutmeg
3 1/2 cups diced apples, with peel
1/2 recipe Crisp Topping (p. 202)

Preheat oven—375°.
8x8x2-inch baking dish/pan

1. In small bowl, **stir** together sugar, cinnamon and nutmeg.
2. Place apples in medium-sized bowl. **Shake** sugar mixture over apples. **Stir** thoroughly to evenly coat apples. **Transfer** to baking pan; sprinkle with topping.
3. **Bake** 25–35 minutes,* or until apples are fork tender and crisp is golden brown.

Yield: 4 servings
(6 servings if serving with ice cream)

*Varies depending upon size of apple pieces and preference of doneness

Analysis for Peach-Blueberry Crisp with Oat Topping/Serving:
Calories: 144 (Fat Cal 40) Fat: 4.4g (2.4g Sat) Cholesterol: 10mg
Sodium: 0mg Carbs: 26g (3g Fiber 16.8g Sugar) Protein: 2.2g

Analysis for Apple Crisp with Oat Topping/Serving:
Calories: 203–224 (Fat Cal 61) Fat: 6.8g (3.7g Sat) Cholesterol: 15mg
Sodium: 1mg Carbs: 30–33g (3.3g Fiber 17.6–20.6g Sugar) Protein: 2.3g

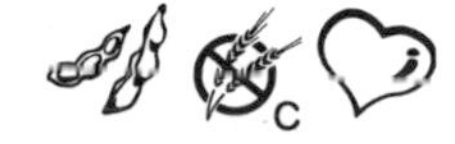

Apples

Using a combination of sweet-tart eating apples or tart-sweet baking apples, especially when in season, requires much less sugar. One day Sondra used Granny Smith apples for a pie and needed 1/2 cup sugar with the apple juice concentrate for the same low-sugar pie taste. Her Mom said, "Do not make another one with those green apples." Traditional apple pies use 1–1 1/2 cups of sugar and far fewer apples than our pies. Leaving the peels on adds both beautiful color and fiber.

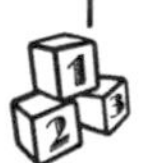

Apple Suggestions

Sweet-tart eating apples:

- Braeburn
- Jonagold
- Golden Supreme

Tart-sweet baking apples:

- Cortland
- Burgundy
- Paula Red

Little Chefs

When making a pie or crisp, or when having a snack, allow children to enjoy slicing apples using an apple peeler-corer-slicer.

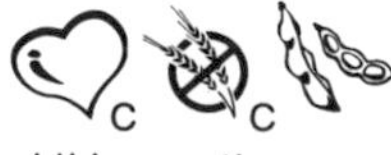

HH - portions

Apple Crisp Pie

Prep filling and assemble pie: 15 minutes

1/2 cup sugar
3/4 tsp. ground cinnamon
1/4 tsp. ground nutmeg
4 1/2 cups sliced apples (1 1/2 lbs.) (see sidebar)
1/2 recipe Crisp Topping (p. 202)
1 (9-inch) unbaked whole-grain pie shell

Preheat oven—375°.

1. In bowl, **whisk** sugar and spices together.
2. Using an apple peeler-slicer, **slice** and core apples (we do not peel). Quarter the slices.
3. Add apples to sugar mixture and **stir** to coat. **Transfer** to pie shell; spread evenly. **Sprinkle** crisp topping evenly over filling.
4. **Bake** 55 minutes, or until apples are fork tender.

Yield: 8 servings   1 (9-inch) pie

Saucy Apple Pie

Prep filling and assemble pie: 20 minutes + chilling time

6 cups sliced apples (2 lb.) (see sidebar)
3/4 cup unsweetened apple juice concentrate
2 Tbsp. sugar
2 Tbsp. cornstarch
1 tsp. ground cinnamon
2 (9-inch) unbaked whole-grain pie shell
OR 1 Stir & Press Pie Crust
with 1/2 recipe Crisp Topping (p. 202)

Oven temperature—425°; then 350°

1. Prepare apples (see Step 2 in above recipe).

Analysis/Serving: Apple Crisp Pie with purchased crust + Oat Crisp Top:
Calories: 248 (Fat Cal 80) Fat: 8.9g (2.8g Sat) Cholesterol: 8mg
Sodium: 110mg Carbs: 35g (3.8g Fiber 18g Sugar) Protein: 3.3g

Analysis/Serving: Saucy Apple Pie w/ Stir & Press Crust + Oat Crisp Top:
Calories: 282 (Fat Cal 92) Fat: 10.2g (2.3 Sat) Cholesterol: 8mg
Sodium: 34mg Carbs: 45.6g (4.8g Fiber 25.8g Sugar) Protein: 3.2g

2. In saucepan, **simmer** apples for 5 minutes in ½ cup of the juice concentrate. In bowl, **whisk** remaining ¼ cup juice, sugar, cornstarch and cinnamon together. Add to apples and **heat** until thickens, stirring often. **Chill.** (Using hot filling causes finished pie crust to be soggy.)
3. See sidebar to assemble a 2-Pie Crust.
   For crisp-topped: Sprinkle crisp topping evenly over filling.
4. **Bake** 20 minutes at 425°; then for 40–45 minutes at 350°, or until apples are fork tender.

Yield: 8 servings   1 (9-inch) pie

Stir & Press Pie Crust

Prepare: 10 minutes + chilling time

1/4 cup ice-cold water
1/8 tsp. salt
1/4 cup High-Heat oil
Flour Choices: (choose one; best if chilled)
3/4 cup whole-wheat pastry flour
OR 3/4 cup "white" whole-wheat flour
OR 7/8 cup whole-grain spelt flour
OR 3/4 cup Bob's Red Mill brand All-Purpose Gluten-Free Baking Flour

1. Chill bowl for approximately 30 minutes.
2. In chilled bowl, **add** water and salt. Gradually add oil while **whisking**. Continue to whisk until mixture is thick and opaque. **Stir** in flour to form a moist ball of dough. Sometimes 1 or 2 more tablespoons of flour is needed to get dough to hold together; see tips in sidebar.
2. Transfer and **press** dough into bottom and up the sides of pie pan as evenly as possible. **Chill** until ready to use

Yield: 1 (9-inch) bottom pie crust

Prepared Pie Crusts

When purchasing frozen whole-grain crusts, transfer crusts from aluminum pan to glass pie dish to avoid heating the aluminum (see p. 228 for explanation).

Assembling Two-Crust Pie

- Allow frozen crust for the top to thaw. Carefully lay it out flat. Gently fold it into fourths.
- Add filling to bottom crust in pie pan.
- With fingertips, moisten lip of bottom pie crust with ice-cold water.
- Lay center tip of top crust in center of pie.
- Unfold and press around crust lip to seal crusts together. Crimp crusts, forming ridge. Flute.
- Cut four steam vents in top crust (one at each quarter of pie) from near center to near edge.

Pie Crust Tips

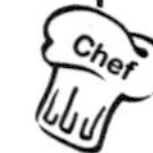

When making Stir & Press Pie Crust, note that too much flour will make crust tough; too little flour will be difficult to press into shape.

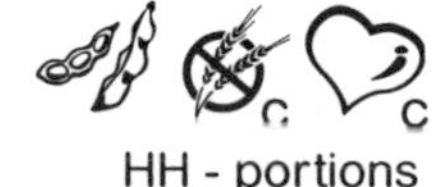

HH - portions

Egg-Free Version

Use same ingredients as recipe to the right, except use the 2-egg substitute below for eggs. Follow directions to right except use a handheld electric mixer in Step 4, beating for approximately 2 minutes. Stop as needed to scrape sides.

2 Egg Substitute

3 Tbsp. Medium-Heat oil
3 Tbsp. water
2 tsp. baking powder

In small bowl, whisk together oil, water and baking powder until frothy. Immediately add to batter, usually right before baking.

Kitchen Scales

To measure out one-fourth of a can of pumpkin, use kitchen scales (it is easier to weigh the portions in grams). Or portion into four same-sized containers.

Extra Pumpkin

Use remaining pumpkin for more cupcakes/cake, Pumpkin Pancakes (pp. 188–189) or Pumpkin Pie Smoothie (p. 106). Freeze pumpkin that is not used in two to three days.

Pumpkin Cupcakes

S→O: 20 minutes Bake: 30 minutes

2 oz. unsweetened baking chocolate
$^{2}/_{3}$ cup sugar
$1^{1}/_{3}$ cups Baking Mix (p. 181)
$^{1}/_{4}$ cup Medium-Heat oil
$^{1}/_{2}$ cup water
$^{1}/_{4}$ (15 oz.) can pumpkin (~$^{1}/_{2}$ cup)
2 eggs

Preheat oven—350°.
Line 12 muffin cups with paper liners.

1. **Melt** chocolate over very low heat. Remove from heat source.
2. In bowl, **whisk** together sugar and Baking Mix.
3. **Whisk** oil, water, pumpkin and eggs into melted chocolate. Stir into flour mixture.
4. **Beat** with rubber spoonula/spatula for approximately 30 seconds, or until creamy (cake-like batter). It is best not to over mix.
5. Fill muffin cups three-fourths full. **Bake** in preheated oven for 30 minutes, or until toothpick comes out clean when inserted in the center. Cool.
6. If desired, frost (see next page). We prefer Cocoa Frosting prepared with almond oil.

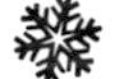 Freeze extra.

Yield: 12 cupcakes

Analysis/Cupcake without/with Almond Cocoa Frosting:
Calories: 164/212 (Fat Cal 72/81) Fat: 8/9g (2.1/2.3g Sat) Cholesterol: 35mg
Sodium: 121mg Carbs: 22/31 (1.8/2g Fiber 11/19g Sugar) Protein: 3/3.4g

Cocoa Frosting

1 Tbsp. oil—almond, safflower or coconut
1/4 cup unsweetened baking cocoa
1 tsp. vanilla extract
3/4 cup powdered sugar
4 tsp. milk (soy, rice, nut or low-fat cow)

If using, **melt** coconut oil over low heat; cool. **Mix** cocoa and vanilla into oil. **Stir** in powdered sugar. Gradually add milk and **beat** until creamy, fluffy and spreadable.

Yield: 1/2 cup   Enough for 12 cupcakes

Analysis/Amount for 1 Cupcake:
Calories: 48 (Fat Cal 12) Fat: 1.3g (0.1g Sat) Cholesterol: 0mg
Sodium: 0mg Carbs: 8.6g (0.3g Fiber 7.5g Sugar) Protein: 0.4g

Vanilla Frosting

1 Tbsp. oil—almond, safflower or coconut
1 tsp. vanilla extract
3/4 cup powdered sugar
1 1/2 tsp. milk (soy, rice, nut or low-fat cow)

Follow directions as above, omitting cocoa. See page 197 for ideas for coloring frosting.

Yield: 1/3 cup   Enough for 12 cupcakes

Analysis/Amount for 1 Cupcake:
Calories: 40 (Fat Cal 10) Fat: 1.1g (0.1g Sat) Cholesterol: 0mg
Sodium: 0mg Carbs: 7.6g (0g Fiber 7.5g Sugar) Protein: 0g

Peanut Butter Frosting

3 Tbsp. healthier-choice peanut butter
1/2 tsp. cornstarch
1 tsp. vanilla extract
3/4 cup powdered sugar
~4 tsp. milk (soy, rice, nut or low-fat cow)

Mix peanut butter, cornstarch and vanilla together. **Stir** in powdered sugar. Gradually add milk and **beat** until creamy, fluffy and spreadable.

Yield: 1/2 cup   Enough for 12 cupcakes

Analysis/Amount for 1 Cupcake:
Calories: 56 (Fat Cal 18) Fat: 2g (0.4g Sat) Cholesterol: 0mg
Sodium: 2mg Carbs: 8.8g (0.4g Fiber 7.7g Sugar) Protein: 1.2g

Cream Cheese Frosting

4 oz. Neufchâtel cheese, softened (p. 43; sidebar)
4 Tbsp. unsalted butter, softened
1/4 cup soy protein isolate (p. 89)
1 tsp. vanilla extract
1/4 cup honey

Stir all ingredients together until smooth. Yield: 1 cup

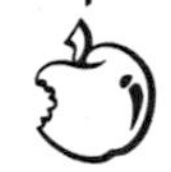

The Icing on the Cake!

Frosting adds a special touch. The trick is to use a reasonable amount and to avoid artificial ingredients. Purchased frostings often contain hydrogenated oils and artificial flavors and colors (even the white ones). In contrast, these recipes have the consistency of canned varieties without the junk; thick enough to be creamy and thin enough to spread easily. This ensures easy coverage on the cupcake without using an overabundance.

The Extras: Store extras in the fridge or freezer. When ready to use them, set them out to warm slightly and stir. If frosting becomes stiff, stir in a few drops of water or milk when ready to use.

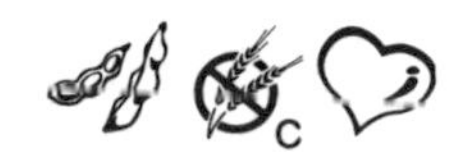

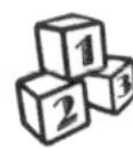

Spelt Option

Use whole-grain spelt flour in place of wheat flour.

Choosing an Ice Cream

There are a great variety of commercially prepared frozen treats. They vary tremendously in both flavor and nutrition. Make an effort to avoid products with high-fructose corn syrup as well as those with artificial colors and flavors. Frozen yogurt is generally lower in fat than ice cream; frozen custard is usually higher in fat. Soy and rice varieties offer an alternative to dairy products and often have fewer preservatives, but they rarely have fewer calories. Reading labels and being an informed shopper is the key!

Another fun option is to make your own ice cream. An ice cream maker is a small appliance worth considering – you get to choose what goes in and everyone can get in on the process!

Granola

S→0: 10 minutes Bake: 35–40 minutes

1 1/2 cups regular oats (prefer extra thick)
1/2 cup "white" whole-wheat flour
1/2 cup wheat germ (optional)
1 Tbsp. brown sugar (*or* maple sugar granules)
1/4 tsp. each: salt, ground cinnamon
2 Tbsp. Medium-Heat oil
2 Tbsp. sweetener—100% pure maple syrup, honey, agave nectar
2–4 Tbsp. water (higher amount with wheat germ)

Preheat oven—275°.
Baking sheet with sides (e.g., jelly roll pan)

1. In bowl, **combine** oats, flour, wheat germ, sugar, salt and cinnamon. In small bowl **whisk** oil, sweetener and water together. Add to oat mixture and stir to **coat**. Transfer to baking sheet.
2. **Bake** for approximately 35–40 minutes, stirring every 10 minutes.

Serve as cereal, adding fruit if desired. Use as topping on fruit for a dessert. Use in Trail Mix (p. 117) or recipe below.

❄ Cool and store in air tight container.

Yield: 12 (¼ cup) servings 3 cups

Red, White and Blue Sundaes

Dress It Up for the Holidays

Top vanilla frozen yogurt or ice cream with blueberries, strawberries and/or raspberries for a patriotic sundae. Sprinkle with Granola.

For an elegant look, fill a wine glass, alternating fruit, ice cream and Granola. Add a dollop of real whipped cream (p. 165). A classy touch for celebrating patriotic holidays.

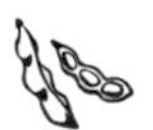

Analysis for Granola Topping/Serving (with wheat germ):
Calories: 104 (Fat Cal 30) Fat: 3.3g (0.3g Sat) Cholesterol: 0mg
Sodium: 44 Carbs: 16g (2g Fiber 4.5g Sugar) Protein: 3g

Squash Apple Bake

S→O: 15 minutes Bake: 45–50 minutes

Assemble this recipe while dinner is cooking. Then bake while you are enjoying dinner with guests. Wow! A healthy, warm dessert to round out the evening. (And no one needs to know they're eating vegetables for dessert.)

3 cups sliced butternut squash
1 lg. eating apple, sliced (1 1/2–2 cups)
1/2 cup raisins
1/2 cup walnuts, chopped
2 Tbsp. Medium-Heat oil
2 Tbsp. pure maple syrup
1 tsp. vanilla
1 1/2–2 tsp. ground cinnamon
Sprinkle of salt
1/2 cup water

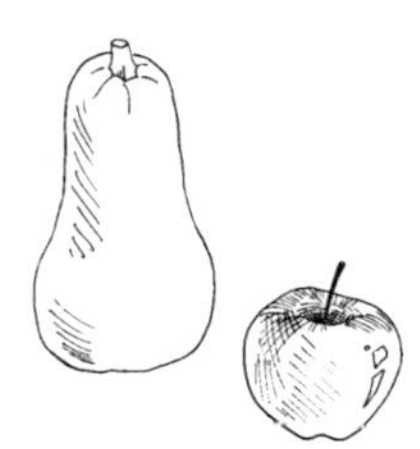

Preheat oven—350°.
Oil a two-quart covered casserole dish.

In prepared casserole dish, evenly **layer** all ingredients in order listed. **Stir**. **Cover** and **bake** for 45–50 minutes, or until apples and squash are tender.

Best served warm. **Drizzle** topping (see below) on individual servings.

Yield: 8 servings

Topping Ideas:

- Combine:
  1/2 cup unsweetened, low-fat plain yogurt
  1–2 Tbsp. pure maple syrup
  1 tsp. vanilla

Or use one of the following:
- Vanilla yogurt
- Maple yogurt
- Low-fat milk
- Soy milk
- Half and half

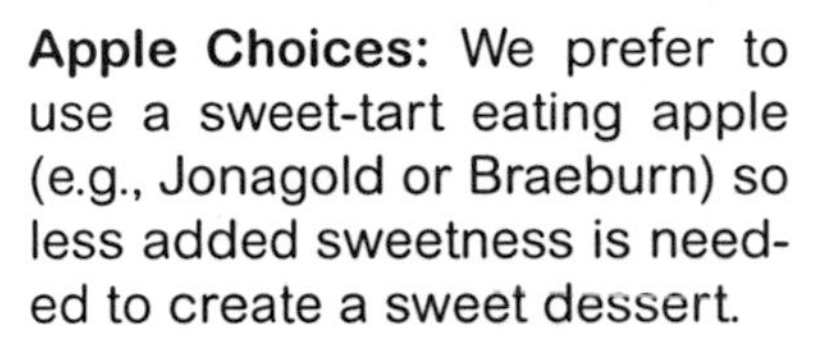

Healthy Bites

Apple Choices: We prefer to use a sweet-tart eating apple (e.g., Jonagold or Braeburn) so less added sweetness is needed to create a sweet dessert.

Adding Nutrition: For added nutrition (fiber as well as vitamins and minerals) and additional flavor, we do not peel the butternut squash or the apples. This also makes preparation go much faster!

Eating in Season: Though we are spoiled by having most foods available to us at any time of the year, our bodies often benefit when we can follow the variety the seasons naturally bring. Also, fruits and vegetables are generally much richer (in both taste and nutrients) when they are in season. This dessert is a great one for the fall and early winter months, when butternut squash is fresh and at its peak ... and when warm desserts on a cold night warm both body and soul.

Little Chefs

Kids love to chop soft nuts, such as walnuts, by placing them in a zip-top plastic bag and crushing them with the bottom of a measuring cup.

Analysis/Serving:
Calories: 160 (Fat Cal 74) Fat: 8.2g (1g Sat) Cholesterol: 0mg
Sodium: 14 Carbs: 21g (2.8g Fiber 13.7g Sugar) Protein: 2g

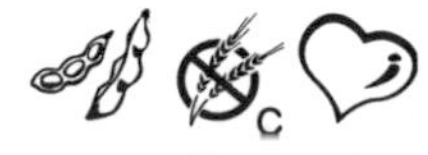

vanilla, raisins

Part Three
The Extras

Notes

Chapter 1

1. Andrew Weil, *Eight Weeks to Optimum Health* (New York: Alfred A Knopf, 1997), 37.

Chapter 2

1. Tabulated using calculator tool provided at www.mypyramid.gov.
2. Harvard School of Public Health, "Fats and Cholesterol," 2007. Retrieved February 2008 from http://www.hsph.harvard.edu/nutritionsource/fats.html.
3. U.S. Department of Health and Human Services and U.S. Department of Agriculture, "Fats," in Dietary GuidelinesforAmericans,6thed.(Washington,DC:U.S.GovernmentPrintingOffice,January2005).Retrieved February 2008 from http://www.health.gov/dietaryguidelines/dga2005/document/html/chapter8.htm.
4. American Heart Association, "Cholesterol: AHA Scientific Position." Retrieved February 2008 from http://www.americanheart.org/presenter.jhtml?identifier=4488.
5. American Heart Association, "Sodium: AHA Recommendation." Retrieved February 2008 from http://www.americanheart.org/presenter.jhtml?identifier=4708.
6. Harvard School of Public Health, "Protein: Moving Closer to Center Stage," 2007. Retrieved February 2008 from http://www.hsph.harvard.edu/nutritionsource/protein.html.
7. Center for Science in the Public Interest, "Food Additives." Retrieved February 2008 from http://www.cspinet.org/reports/chemcuisine.htm.
8. Elson M. Haas, "Food Additives and Human Health." Retrieved February 2008 from http://www.healthychild.com/food-additives.htm.

Chapter 3

1. F. B. Hu, J. E. Manson and W. C. Willett, "Types of Dietary Fat and Risk of Coronary Heart Disease: A Critical Review," *Journal of the American College of Nutrition* 20 (2001): 5-19.
2. School of Public Health, "Fats & Cholesterol." Retrieved February 2008 from http://www.hsph.harvard.edu/nutritionsource/fats.html.
3. Mayo Foundation for Medical Education and Research, "Dietary Fats: Know Which Types to Choose," January 31, 2007. Retrieved February 2008 from http://www.mayoclinic.com/health/fat/NU00262.
4. R. P. Mensink et al., "Effects of Dietary Fatty Acids and Carbohydrates on the Ratio of Serum Total to HDL Cholesterol and on Serum Lipids and Apolipoproteins: A Meta-Analysis of 60 Controlled Trials," *American Journal of Clinical Nutrition* 77 (2003): 1146-55.
5. American Heart Association, "Know Your Fats." Retrieved February 2008 from http://www.americanheart.org/presenter.jhtml?identifier=532.
6. Harvard School of Public Health, "Fats & Cholesterol."
7. American Heart Association, "Fat." Retrieved February 2008 from http://www.americanheart.org/presenter.jhtml?identifier=4582.

8. Mayo Foundation for Medical Education and Research, "Trans Fat: Avoid This Cholesterol Double Whammy," December 21, 2006. Retrieved February 2008 from http://www.mayoclinic.com.
9. Harvard School of Public Health, "Fats & Cholesterol."
10. American Heart Association (February 22, 2008), "Obesity Linked to Stroke Increase Among Middle-aged Women," ScienceDaily. Retrieved February 2008, from http://www.sciencedaily.com¬/releases/2008/02/080221080606.htm.
11. Mayo Foundation for Medical Education and Research, "Obesity," May 9, 2007. Retrieved from http://www.mayoclinic.com/health/obesity/DS00314#.
12. Harvard School of Public Health, "Fats & Cholesterol."
13. Mayo Foundation for Medical Education and Research, "Butter v. Margarine: Which Is Better for My Heart?" June 2, 2006. Retrieved February 2008 from http://www.mayoclinic.com/health/butter-vs-margarine/AN00835.

Chapter 4

1. American Heart Association, "Factors That Contribute to High Blood Pressure." Retrieved February 2008 from http://www.americanheart.org/presenter.jhtml?identifier=4650
2. "Salt Raises Stomach Cancer Risk," BBC News, January 7, 2004. Retrieved February 2008 from http://news.bbc.co.uk/2/hi/health/3370141.stm.
3. Mayo Foundation for Medical Education and Research, "Sodium: Are You Getting Too Much?" December 7, 2007. Retrieved February 2008 from http://www.mayoclinic.com/health/sodium/NU00284.
4. American Heart Association, "Sodium." Retrieved February 2008 from http://www.americanheart.org/presenter.jhtml?identifier=4708.
5. U.S. Department of Health and Human Services and U.S. Department of Agriculture, "Sodium and Potassium," in *Dietary Guidelines for Americans*, 6th ed. (Washington, DC: U.S. Government Printing Office, January 2005). Retrieved February 2008 from http://www.health.gov/dietaryguidelines/dga2005/document/html/chapter8.htm.
6. American Medical Association, "AMA Urges Immediate FDA Action to Reduce Excess Salt in Food," November 29, 2007. Retrieved February 2008 from http://www.ama-assn.org/ama/pub/category/18178.html.
7. Heart and Stroke Foundation of Canada, "Reductions Needed in the Sodium Added to Foods," October 25, 2007. Retrieved February 2008 from http://ww2.heartandstroke.ca/Page.asp?PageID=33&ArticleID=6567&Src=news&From=Category.
8. J. Anderson et al., "Sodium in the Diet," Food and Nutrition Series, no. 9.345, Colorado State University Extension, May 2007. Retrieved February 2008 from http://www.ext.colostate.edu/pubs/foodnut/09354.pdf.
9. American Heart Association, "High Blood Pressure." Retrieved February 2008 from http://www.americanheart.org/presenter.jhtml?identifier=2114.

Chapter 5

1. Harvard School of Public Health, "Fiber." Retrieved February 2008 from http://www.hsph.harvard.edu/nutritionsource/fiber.html.
2. Ruth Papazian, "Bulking Up Fiber's Healthful Reputation," U.S. Food and Drug Administration, September 1998. Retrieved February 2008 from http://www.fda.gov/fdac/features/1997/597_fiber.html.
3. Joslin Diabetes Center, "How Does Fiber Affect Blood Glucose Levels?" Retrieved February 2008 from http://www.joslin.org/managing_your_diabetes_697.asp.
4. U.S. Department of Health and Human Services and U.S. Department of Agriculture, "Carbohydrates," in *Dietary Guidelines for Americans*, 6th ed. (Washington, DC: U.S. Government Printing Office, January 2005). Retrieved February 2008 from http://www.health.gov/dietaryguidelines/dga2005/document/html/chapter7.htm

Chapter 6

1. "Diet and Lifestyle Recommendations revision 2006: A Scientific Statement for the American Heart Association Nutrition Committee," *Journal of the American Heart Association* 114 (2006): 82–96. Retrieved February 2008 from http://circ.ahajournals.org/cgi/reprint/CIRCULATIONAHA.106.176158.
2. American Dental Association Division of Communications, "Diet and Tooth Decay," *Journal of the American Dental Association* 133 (April 2002). Retrieved February 2008 from http://www.ada.org/prof/resources/pubs/jada/patient/patient_13.pdf.
3. J. Bernstein et al., "Depression of Lymphocyte Transformation Following Oral Glucose Ingestion," *American Journal of Clinical Nutrition* 30 (1997): 613.
4. There are many theories about the relationship between sugar consumption and a variety of health conditions; we have named just a few. Evidence is not yet conclusive. If you are interested in considering a possible connection, try conducting an Internet search for the latest research, or consult with your health provider.
5. Mayo Foundation for Medical Education and Research, "High-Fructose Corn Syrup: Why Is It So Bad for Me?" April 5, 2007. Retrieved from http://www.mayoclinic.com/health/high-fructose-corn-syrup/AN01588
6. George A. Bray, Samara Joy Nielsen and Barry M. Popkin, "Consumption of High-Fructose Corn Syrup in Beverages May Play a Role in the Epidemic of Obesity," American Journal of Clinical Nutrition 79, no. 4 (April 2004): 537-43. Retrieved February 2008 from http://www.ajcn.org/cgi/gca?allch=&SEARCHID=1&FULLTEXT=corn+syrup&FIRSTINDEX=0&hits=10&RESULTFORMAT=&gca=ajcn%3B79%2F4%2F537&allchb=.
7. Mayo Foundation, "High-Fructose Corn Syrup."
8. Sarah R. Stender, George A. Burghen, and Johanna T. Mallare, "The Role of Health Care Providers in the Prevention of Overweight and Type 2 Diabetes in Children and Adolescents," *Diabetes Spectrum* 18 (2005): 240-48. Retrieved February 2008 from http://spectrum.diabetesjournals.org/cgi/content/full/18/4/240.
9. George A. Bray, Samara Joy Nielsen and Barry M. Popkin, "Consumption of High-Fructose Corn Syrup in Beverages May Play a Role in the Epidemic of Obesity," *American Journal of Clinical Nutrition* 79: 537-543.
10. Andrew Weil, "7 Substitutes for Sugar," *Self Healing*, June 2006, 3.

Chapter 7

1. Harvard School of Public Health, "Protein: Moving Closer to Center Stage." Retrieved February 2008 from http://www.hsph.harvard.edu/nutritionsource/protein.html.
2. Ibid.
3. JAMA and Archives Journals (January 19, 2006), "Higher Intake of Vegetable Protein Associated with Lower Blood Pressure Levels," ScienceDaily. Retrieved February 2008 from http://www.sciencedaily.com¬/releases/2006/01/060118100742.htm.
4. Loren Cordain and Joe Friel, *The Paleo Diet for Athletes* (Emmaus: Rodale, 2005) p. 201.

Chapter 8

1. American Heart Association, "Heart Disease and Stroke Statistics — 2008 Update." Retrieved February 2008 from http://www.americanheart.org/downloadable/heart/1200082005246HS_Stats%202008.final.pdf.
2. American Heart Association, "Carbohydrates and Sugars." Retrieved February 2008 from http://www.americanheart.org/presenter.jhtml?identifier=4471.
3. Mayo Foundation for Medical Education and Research, "Dietary Fiber: An Essential Part of a Healthy Diet," November 2007. Retrieved February 2008 from http://www.mayoclinic.com/health/fiber/NU00033#.
4. H. C. Bucher et al., "N-3 Polyunsaturated Fatty Acids in Coronary Heart Disease: A Meta-Analysis of Randomized Controlled Trials," *American Journal of Medicine* 112 (2002): 298–304.
6. Harvard School of Public Health, "Fats & Cholesterol." Retrieved February 2008 from http://www.hsph.harvard.edu/nutritionsource/fats.html.

7. Heather I. Katcher et al., "The Effects of a Whole Grain–Enriched Hypocaloric Diet on Cardiovascular Disease Risk Factors in Men and Women with Metabolic Syndrome," *American Journal of Clinical Nutrition* 87, no. 1 (January 2008): 79-90.
8. American Dietetic Association, nutrition fact sheet, "Eat 5 to 9 a Day for Better Health," 2003. Retrieved February 2008 from http://extension.usu.edu/fsne/files/uploads/lessons/Fruits%20and%20Vegetables/5%20to%209%20A%20Day.pdf.
9. Harvard School of Public Health, "Fats & Cholesterol."

Chapter 9

1. American Diabetes Association, "How to Prevent or Delay Diabetes." Retrieved February 2008 from http://www.diabetes.org/diabetes-prevention/how-to-prevent-diabetes.jsp.
2. American Diabetes Association, "Make the Link: Diabetes, Heart Disease and Stroke." Retrieved February 2008 from http://www.diabetes.org/heart-disease-stroke.jsp.
3. American Diabetes Association, "All About diabetes." Retrieved February 2008 from http://www.diabetes.org/about-diabetes.jsp.
4. Ibid.
5. Ibid.
6. American Diabetes Association, "How to Prevent or Delay Diabetes."
7. American Diabetes Association, "Complications of Diabetes in the United States." Retrieved February 2008 from http://www.diabetes.org/diabetes-statistics/complications.jsp.
8. American Diabetes Association, "Direct and Indirect Costs of Diabetes in the United States." Retrieved February 2008 from http://www.diabetes.org/diabetes-statistics/cost-of-diabetes-in-us.jsp.
9. Ibid.
10. National Institutes of Health, "Study Will Identify Best Treatment for Type 2 Diabetes in Youth," *NIH News*, March 15, 2004. Retrieved February 2008 from http://www.nih.gov/news/pr/mar2004/niddk-15.htm.
11. Per Serving, "Connections Between Heart & Health: Diabetes." Retrieved February 2008 from http://www.per-serving.org/connections.asp

Chapter 10

1. Celiac Disease Foundation, "The Face of Celiac Disease," 2007. Retrieved February 2008 from http://www.celiac.org/downloads/Face-of-Celiac-Brochure.pdf.
2. Ibid.
3. Celiac Disease Foundation, "Treatment of Celiac Disease." Retrieved February 2008 from http://www.celiac.org/cd-treatment.php.
4. Stefano Guandalini and Michelle Melin-Rogovin, "Celiac Disease: Myths and Facts," University of Chicago Celiac Disease Program. Retrieved February 2008 from http://www.uchospitals.edu/pdf/uch_002799.pdf.

Chapter 11

1. CUESA, "How Far Does Food Travel to Get to Your Plate?" 2006. Retrieved February 2008 from http://www.cuesa.org/sustainable_ag/issues/foodtravel.php.

Chapter 12

1. Robert H. Fletcher and Kathleen M. Fairfield, "Vitamins for Chronic Disease Prevention in Adults," *Journal of the American Medical Association* 287, no. 23 (June 19, 2002).
2. Donald R. Davis, Melvin D. Epp and Hugh D. Riordan, "Changes in USDA Food Composition Data for 43 Garden Crops, 1950 to 1999," *Journal of the American College of Nutrition* 23, no. 6 (2004): 669-82.

Chapter 13

1. Partnership for Food Safety Education, "Safe Food Handling." Retrieved February 2008 from http://www.fightbac.org/content/view/6/11/.
2. Partnership for Food Safety Education, "Heat it Up Chart." Retrieved February 2008 from http://www.fightbac.org/content/view/172/2/;
   Mary Schroepfer, "Keep Venison Safe from Field to Table." October 2004. Retrieved February 2008 from http://extension.missouri.edu/stcharles/qfk/oct04/venison.html. February 2008.
3. Clemson Extension, Home & Garden Information Center, "Food Storage: Refrigerator and Freezer," May 1999. Retrieved February 2008 from http://hgic.clemson.edu/factsheets/HGIC3522.htm, "Food Storage: Refrigerator and Freezer."

Chapter 14

1. Fred Hutchinson Cancer Research Center, "Veggies Help Reduce Prostate-Cancer Risk," Center New Weekly, July 30, 2007. Retrieved February 2008 from http://www.fhcrc.org/about/pubs/center_news/weekly/2007_0730_br3_veggies.html.
2. George Mateljan Foundation, "Asparagus." Retrieved February 2008 from http://www.whfoods.com/genpage.php?tname=foodspice&dbid=12.
3. M. C. Morris et al., "Associations of Vegetable and Fruit Consumption with Age-Related Cognitive Change," *Neurology* 67 (2006): 1370-6. Retrieved February 2008 from http://www.neurology.org/cgi/content/abstract/67/8/1370.
4. N. Z. Unlu et al., "Carotenoid Absorption from Salad and Salsa by Humans Is Enhanced by the Addition of Avocado or Avocado Oil," *Journal of Nutrition* 135, no. 3 (March 2005): 431-6. Retrieved February 2008 from http://jn.nutrition.org/cgi/content/abstract/135/3/431.
5. George Mateljan Foundation, "Avocado." Retrieved February 2008 from http://www.whfoods.org/genpage.php?tname=foodspice&dbid=5#healthbenefits.
6. George Mateljan Foundation, "Black Beans." Retrieved February 2008 from http://www.whfoods.com/genpage.php?tname=foodspice&dbid=2#foodspicename.
7. National Institute of Neurological Disorders and Stroke, "Folate Information Summary." Retrieved February 2008 from http://www.ninds.nih.gov/funding/research/parkinsonsweb/drug_summaries/folate.htm; George Mateljan Foundation, "Folate." Retrieved February 2008 from http://www.whfoods.org/genpage.php?tname=nutrient&dbid=63#function.
8. Mateljan Foundation, "Black Beans."
9. George Mateljan Foundation, "Cauliflower." Retrieved February 2008 from http://www.whfoods.org/genpage.php?tname=foodspice&dbid=13#healthbenefits.
10. Rebecca Wood, *The New Whole Foods Encyclopedia* (New York: Penguin, 1999), 63.
11. C. Galeone et al., "Onion and Garlic Use and Human Cancer," *American Journal of Clinical Nutrition* 84, no. 5 (November 2006): 1027-32; George Mateljan Foundation, "Garlic." Retrieved February 2008 from http://www.whfoods.org/genpage.php?tname=foodspice&dbid=60#foodspicename.
12. Mateljan Foundation, "Garlic."
13. Ibid.
14. George Mateljan Foundation, "Potatoes." Retrieved February 2008 from http://www.whfoods.org/genpage.php?tname=foodspice&dbid=48#safetyissues.
15. George Mateljan Foundation, "Soybeans." Retrieved February 2008 from http://www.whfoods.org/genpage.php?tname=foodspice&dbid=79#healthbenefits.

Chapter 16

1. George Mateljan Foundation, "Ginger." Retrieved February 2008 from http://www.whfoods.org/genpage.php?tname=foodspice&dbid=72#healthbenefits.

Chapter 17

1. Janet Raloff, "Reevaluating Eggs' Cholesterol Risks," Science News Online. Retrieved February 2008 from http://www.sciencenews.org/articles/20060506/food.asp.
2. Harvard School of Public Health, "Fats & Cholesterol." Retrieved February 2008 from http://www.hsph.harvard.edu/nutritionsource/fats.html.

Chapter 20

1. Rebecca Wood, *The New Whole Foods Encyclopedia* (New York: Penguin, 1999), 21.

Chapter 25

1. Mayo Foundation for Medical Education and Research, "Water: How Much Should You Drink Every Day?" April 23, 2006. Retrieved February 2008 from http://www.mayoclinic.com/health/water/NU00283#.
2. Mayo Foundation for Medical Education and Research, "Caffeine: How Much Is Too Much?" March 8, 2007. Retrieved February 2008 from http://www.mayoclinic.com/health/caffeine/NU00600#.
3. George Mateljan Foundation, "Green Tea: What Is a Safe Intake of Caffeine?" Retrieved February 2008 from http://www.whfoods.org/genpage.php?tname=foodspice&dbid=146#foodspicename.

Chapter 26

1. George Mateljan Foundation, "Spelt." Retrieved February 2008 from http://whfoods.org/genpage.php?tname=foodspice&dbid=143#descr.
2. Described on the box of quinoa produced by Quinoa Corporation, Gardena, CA.

Seasoning Glossary

1. George Mateljan Foundation, "Cinnamon." Retrieved February 2008 from http://www.whfoods.org/genpage.php?tname=foodspice&dbid=68#healthbenefits.

Gadgets, Measuring and More

1. The Pollution Information Site, scorecard, "Carcinogens." Retrieved February 2008 from http://www.scorecard.org/health-effects/chemicals.tcl?short_hazard_name=cancer&all_p=t.
2. C. Garcia-Viguera, "Phenolic Compound Contents in Edible Parts of Broccoli Inflorescences after Domestic Cooking," *Journal of the Science of Food and Agriculture* 83, no. 14 (October 15, 2003).
3. Interview with Andrew Weil, *Oprah Winfrey Show*, ABC, April 21, 2000.

Cook's Glossary

Al dente: describes cooked pasta and/or vegetables that are slightly firm
Baste: to brush, drizzle or spoon pan drippings, vegetable oil or other liquid over food during the cooking process to keep food moist and/or add flavor
Beat: to vigorously stir a mixture until smooth by hand or with mixer
Blanch: to partially cook in simmering water or over steam. After steaming, transfer food to cold water to stop the cooking process. Blanching is used to prepare some vegetables for use in stir-fry and salads or for freezing.
Blend: to combine ingredients creating a smooth mixture
Broil: to cook foods by placing them just a few inches over or under heat source
Butterfly: to cut meat (e.g., thick pork chop, chicken breast) in the center of the thickness without cutting all the way through to other side so it can be spread open (resembling butterfly wings) for faster cooking or for stuffing
Caramelize: to sauté a vegetable (e.g., onion) in small amount of oil long enough to break down the sugar in the food, producing a browner vegetable with a sweeter taste
Carryover-Cook: to allow retained heat, steam, hot water, etc., to cook (or continue cooking) a food when the food is no longer on the hot burner (pp. 38 and 107)
Chill: to cool quickly by immersing in cold water or placing in the refrigerator
Chop: to cut foods into small pieces (approximately ¼ to ½ inch)
"Chop & Drop": a method to sauté vegetables and/or meat in oil that generally speeds up the cooking process (see p. 34 for more explanation)
Coat: to use a food (e.g., a seasoning mixture) to cover another food
Core: to remove the center of a fruit or vegetable
Cube: to cut foods into small cubes (approximately ½ to 1 inch)
Crimp: to press two pieces of dough together along the edges (e.g., double-crusted pie)
Cut in: to mix fat (butter or oil) into flour with fork, knife or pastry blender/cutter
Dash: a sprinkle, such as that achieved by gently shaking a seasoning bottle
Deglaze: to remove the browned and flavorful drippings of cooked food (e.g., meat, caramelized onions) by adding liquid to the pan and stirring while briefly heating
Dice: to cut foods into cubes (approximately ¼ inch)
Drippings: the particles and juices from cooking meats and/or vegetables
Drizzle: to pour a thin stream of liquid over food
Fillet: a boneless piece of meat, fish or poultry; to remove such a piece for cooking
Fold: to gently combine ingredients without stirring
Flute: to make a decorative pattern (e.g., wavy edge on pie crust)

Fuse: to allow one flavor to integrate into another, usually over low heat (e.g., garlic flavor fused into olive oil)
Garnish: to decorate finished dish with attractive, edible ingredient
Glaze: to drizzle a liquid-like mixture on a food for the purpose of giving it a glossy appearance or adding taste (e.g., sweet taste to cinnamon rolls)
Grate: to finely shred by rubbing on a grater or microplane or using a food processor
Grill: to cook food such as steaks, hamburgers, fish and chicken on an outdoor or countertop grill or in a grill pan
Julienne: to cut (e.g., meats, cheeses, vegetables) in long thin strips
Knead: to press and stretch dough using your hands in a "fold toward, push away, quarter turn" action to work flour into dough and/or make dough smooth and elastic. Bread machines and mixers with dough hooks do this, but occasionally one might choose to knead in a little more flour when shaping dinner rolls, breadsticks or cinnamon rolls and making rolled biscuits (p.183).
Lightly Steam: to briefly cook foods in a small amount of simmering water to set color and allow to become slightly tender (as in blanching)
Marinate: to allow food to sit in seasoned liquid, allowing it to "marry" (blend) flavors and/or tenderize
Marry: to allow flavors to blend together
Mince: to finely chop foods (e.g., mincing garlic, p. 60)
Parbake: to partially bake, as with a pizza crust
Pinch: a small measure that can be held between your thumb and index finger
Poach: to cook by covering food in simmering liquid (e.g., fish, poultry, eggs)
Prick: to use a fork to make holes in food before baking (e.g., pizza crusts)
Proof: (1) to bring dough to the proper lightness by allowing the dough to rise; (2) to dissolve yeast in lukewarm water until bubbles form, confirming the yeast is active
Pull (meat off bones): removing cooked meat from bone in a pulling fashion
Puree: to make a food into a smooth mixture by pressing through a sieve or using a food processor or blender
Ribbon-Cut: to make ribbon-like pieces of vegetables and herbs (e.g., basil, spinach, chard, kale, collards, lettuce). First, if desired, remove center rib (e.g., kale, collard, sometimes chard). Then pile up leaves, tightly roll lengthwise and slice crosswise to make the ribbon-like pieces.
Roast: to cook in oven
Roux: a mixture of flour and fat that is cooked for one minute to enhance the nutty flavor of the flour while removing the starchy taste. The next step is to add a liquid and cook to thicken sauce or gravy.
Sauté: to cook briefly in a small amount of fat over medium heat, stirring regularly
Scald: to heat just below boiling (e.g., milk for pudding); milk steams and tiny bubbles appear at edge of pan

Season: to use spices and seasonings to flavor food
Sear: to seal in meat juices by browning meat on all sides using high heat
Set: to allow food to sit. Serves two purposes: (1) it allows batter (e.g., pancakes) or other food products (e.g., egg dishes) to set up; and (2) it allows meat juices to run back through the meat so that they do not run out when the meat is cut (keeps meat moist).
Shred: to cut food into long, thin pieces
Simmer: to cook foods at a gentle bubble
Sprinkle: to measure a small amount of food by shaking
Steam: to cook foods in small amount of simmering water in saucepan
Stir-fry: to sauté over medium heat while stirring constantly
Toss: to combine ingredients gently
Well: an indentation in a mixture of dry ingredients. Liquid ingredients are then placed in the well, allowing for more even distribution.
Whisk: to quickly stir ingredients with a fork or whisk to make a smooth, airy mixture
Zest: to grate the outer peel of a citrus fruit using a microplane (p. 222)

Nutrition Terms:

Phytonutrients are nutrients found in plants that are believed to promote human health. For example, flavonoids and carotonoids are specific groups of phytonutrients that, among other things, reduce the risk of many cancers, increase eye health and promote a healthy immune system. The rich supply of phytonutrients is a huge part of what makes vegetables and fruits so beneficial to our health.

Oxalates, purines and goitrogens are three naturally occurring substances in many vegetables that may be a concern for some people with specific health conditions. The vast majority of people do not need to be concerned. See our websites (p. 242) for more information.

Fiber Guide

Food Source	Serving Size	Fiber (grams)*	Food Source	Serving Size	Fiber (grams)*
Acorn sq, ck, mashed	½ cup	3.2	Grapes, raw	½ cup	0.7
Almonds, whole	¼ cup	4.2	Green beans, cooked	½ cup	2
Apple, raw with skin	medium	3.3	Kale, cooked	½ cup	1.3
Apricots, dried	4 count	2	Lettuce, romaine	1½ cups	1.8
Artichoke, globe, ck	large	4.5	Oatmeal, cooked	1 cup	4
Asparagus, cooked	1 cup	2.9	Orange, navel	medium	3.1
Banana	medium	3.1	Pasta, whole wheat	1 oz. dry	3
Barley, pearled, ck	½ cup	3	Peach	medium	2.3
Beans, black, cooked	½ cup	6	Peanut butter	2 Tbsp.	3
Beans, garbanzo, ck	½ cup	5	Pear, fresh	medium	5.1
Beans, red, cooked	½ cup	5	Peas, edible pods, ck	½ cup	2.5
Beets, cooked	½ cup	1.9	Peas, green, cooked	½ cup	4.4
Blackberries, fresh	½ cup	3.8	Pepper, bell, raw	1 cup	1.6
Blueberries, frozen	½ cup	2.5	Plum	1 count	0.9
Bread, 100% wh wheat	1 slice	3	Popcorn, popped	1 cup	1.2
Broccoli, cooked	½ cup	2.9	Potato, baked with skin	medium	4.4
Butternut sq, ck, mash	½ cup	2.9	Prune juice	½ cup	1.3
Cabbage, raw, chop	½ cup	1.1	Prunes	2 count	1.4
Cantaloupe, diced	½ cup	0.7	Pumpkin, canned	½ cup	3.6
Carrots, raw slices	½ cup	1.7	Raisins	¼ cup	2
Celery, raw	8-inch rib	1	Raspberries, fresh	½ cup	4
Chard, Swiss, cooked	½ cup	1.8	Rice, brown, cooked	½ cup	1.3
Collards, cooked	½ cup	2.7	Spinach, cooked	½ cup	3.5
Corn, wh kernel, frozen	½ cup	0.8	Strawberries, fr. sliced	½ cup	1.7
Dates	3 count	1.7	Sweet potato with peel	med. 5 oz	4.8
Edamame, shelled, ck	½ cup	3	Tomatoes, cherry	½ cup	0.9
Flour, whole wheat	1 Tbsp.	4	Zucchini squash, raw	1 cup	1.2

*as with all nutrients, fiber amounts vary

ck = cooked fr = fresh sq = squash wh = whole

Seasoning Glossary

Herbs

Herbs can be used fresh or dried. Generally, 1 teaspoon dried = 1 tablespoon fresh.

Selection: Select fresh herbs by looking for stems that are green and vibrant.

Storage: Once picked, **fresh herbs** do not last long. Store in refrigerator either in the crisper drawer (wrapped in a damp paper towel and placed in a plastic bag) or standing upright in a glass of water. Fresh herbs should be stored whole, as the best flavor is obtained when they are cut, chopped or torn right before using.

Most **dried herbs** and spices retain their strength of flavor for about a year if stored in an airtight container in a cool, dry place. (Do not store dried herbs and seasonings above or next to your stove.)

Washing: Before using fresh herbs, rinse herbs in cold water and shake dry. A salad spinner can be excellent for drying large quantities of herbs.

Drying: To dry fresh herbs, tie clean bunches together and hang upside down in a cool, dry place. When dry, crumble leaves in an airtight jar.

Growing and Freezing Fresh Herbs: Fresh herbs are easy to grow (even successfully in pots or flower boxes on a deck), and it is fun to cook with freshly picked herbs.

Basil: Basil adds a delightful sweetness to a variety of dishes. Fresh basil also add visual appeal, especially when ribbon-cut (p. 217). Best to add at the end of cooking time. A ¾ oz. package or bunch = 1 cup semi-packed leaves = ¾ cup ribbon-cut strips.

Freezing Fresh Basil: Place desired amount of ribbon-cut fresh basil in a small dish. Cover with a small amount of water and freeze. After frozen, thaw enough to remove from dish. Place iced blocks of basil in freezer bags. Keep frozen; add directly to recipes such as spaghetti sauce and soups whenever needed.

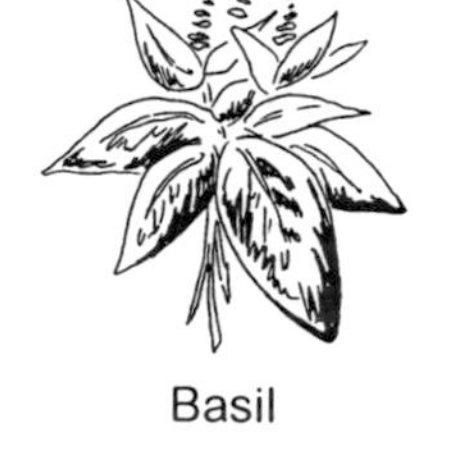

Basil

Chives: With garlic and onion varieties, fresh chives add great taste and visual appeal as a garnish to many soups, potatoes and egg dishes. The best flavor is obtained from chives when they are snipped with scissors rather than cut with a knife or torn.

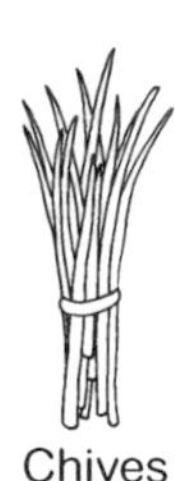

Chives

Cilantro: Often used in Mexican cooking, cilantro has a distinctive taste and should be used sparingly until taste preference is determined. There is a significant difference in taste between fresh and dried cilantro.

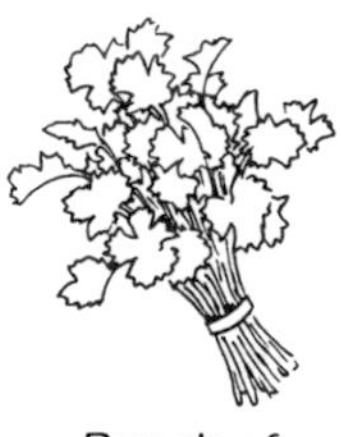

Bunch of Cilantro

Dill: Fresh or dried, dill offers a subtle flavor that enhances fish and chicken recipes and is great when added to salads. It has its best flavor when added toward the end of cooking time.

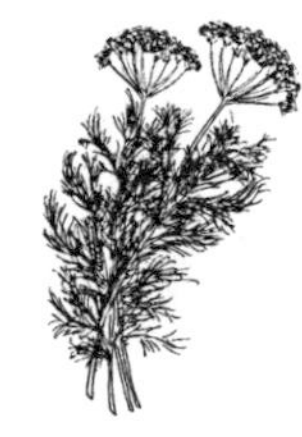
Dill with Seed Pod

Oregano: The flavor of oregano is strong and almost peppery, adding a kick to stews, sauces and meat. Try sprinkling fresh oregano on pizza or garlic bread.

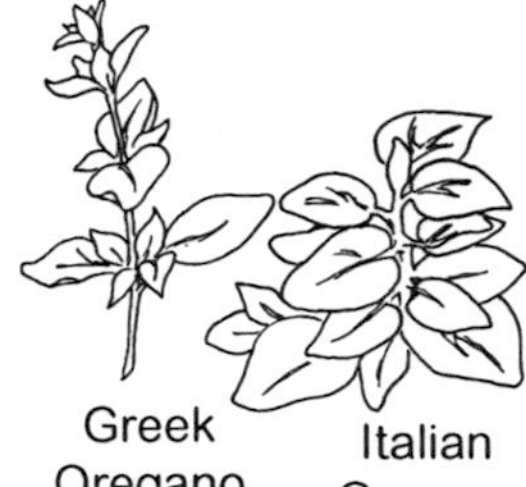
Greek Oregano   Italian Oregano

Parsley: A beautiful garnish, parsley can liven up almost any dish. Flat-leaf parsley (sometimes referred to as Italian parsley) is best when used in cooking. Curly parsley makes a dramatic but edible garnish.

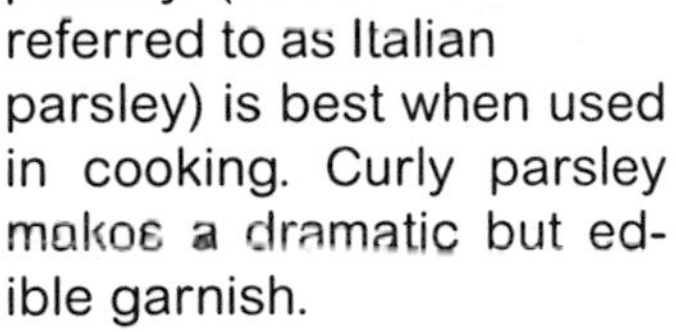

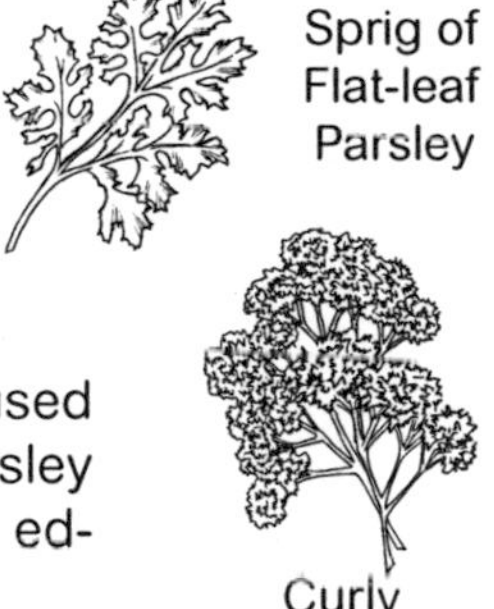
Sprig of Flat-leaf Parsley

Curly Parsley

Rosemary: Strong in flavor and aroma, rosemary is great for meats, lamb and pork. Dried, it can have a bit of a twiggy texture. Fresh sprigs can be placed in a soup or on a roasting piece of meat. For best flavor, release the oils by crushing some of the leaves as they are added to the dish being prepared. The branches of rosemary can be used as skewers for grilling.

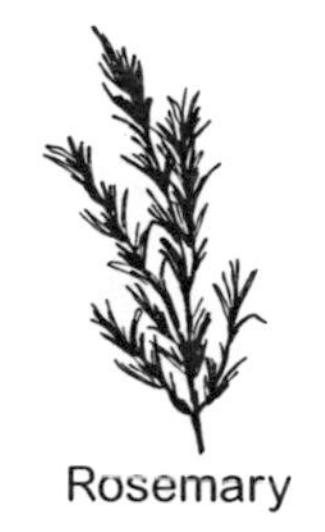
Rosemary

Sage: Easily used fresh or dried, sage adds a distinctive flavor to meats and soups. For best flavor, crush and rub between thumb and finger to release oils when adding to food.

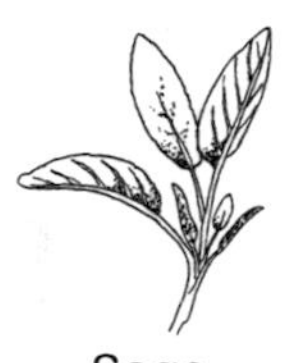
Sage

Thyme: Pungent, fresh thyme is good to use in soups and on roasted vegetables. Use sparingly until taste preference is determined.

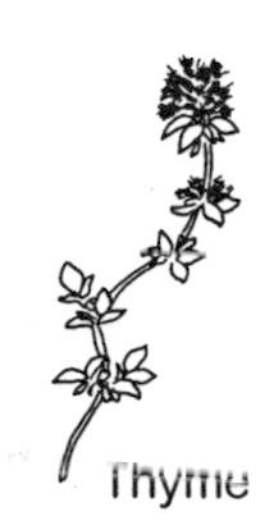
Thyme

Spices

Chili Powder: Companies use a variety of ingredients to make chili powder. Even the chilies used vary in color and heat. So experiment to find one that you like. (Many chili powders are high in salt; we prefer chili powders without salt added.)

Cinnamon: Used often in Middle Eastern cooking, cinnamon surprisingly enhances a variety of dishes. While the ground form is most common, cinnamon sticks are available and can be added to a simmering pot of beans or a warm beverage. The health properties of cinnamon are numerous. One of the most notable is its ability to lessen the impact of a high carbohydrate dish on blood sugar levels.[1] This makes it a great choice for seasoning oatmeal, toast or rice pudding.

Cloves: Complementing cinnamon and nutmeg, cloves are often used in the United States to flavor desserts, though elsewhere in the world they are used to season a variety of meat dishes. Along with garlic and chili powder, they help to give Worcestershire sauce its depth of flavor. Enjoy experimenting, but use in small amounts as it is strong in both aroma and taste.

Cumin: Cumin's slightly smoky flavor complements chili powder well. Generally a 1:2 ratio (cumin: chili powder) should be used unless you are using hot peppers, in which case you should use more cumin..

Garlic – see pages 60–61.

Nutmeg: Freshly grated nutmeg enhances many foods, especially cooked green vegetables (e.g., kale, collards, green beans, chard), winter squashes and sweet potatoes. Often adding more freshly grated nutmeg reduces the need for more salt (e.g., Pumpkin Pie Smoothie, Pumpkin Soup, Fall Harvest Stews and Southern-Style Shepherd's Pie). In baking, it is a nice complement to cinnamon.

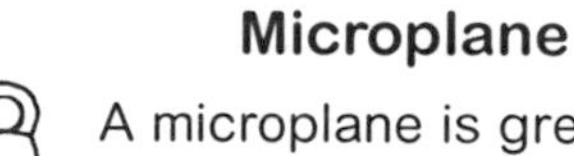

Microplane

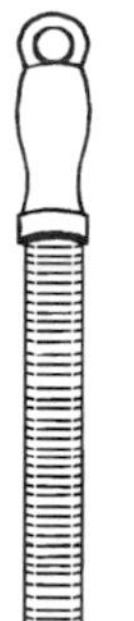

A microplane is great for grating fresh nutmeg, citrus peel, fresh Parmesan cheese and a little onion. There are many different designs, so choose one that finely grates and is comfortable to use without cutting your fingers.

A Few Seasoning Blends and a Word about Salt

There are many seasoning blends available and you can have fun creating your own. Three purchased blends that we use often and refer to in our recipes are:

Mama Garlic, by Frontier Herb, is our favorite seasoned garlic salt. It is a blend of sea salt, garlic, lemon peel, onion, parsley and black pepper.

Garlic 'n' Herb seasoning, by Simply Organic is a salt-free blend of sesame seeds, garlic, pepper, lemon peel, onion and parsley. It is Sondra's favorite on Roasted Asparagus, 20-Minute Stir-Fry Dinner (featured on the front cover) and other foods.

Hickory Barbeque, by Frontier Herbs is a salt-free blend of chili peppers, garlic, onion, paprika, hickory smoke, black pepper, cumin, nutmeg and cayenne. It is delicious on Seared Tofu.

Salt: Salt is used all over the world to enhance flavors and preserve food. It is necessary for the proper functioning of living cells, but too much can be harmful. (See chapter four for more information.)

Types of Salt

Table salt generally refers to salt that has been dried at high temperatures. This causes the salt to lose most of its trace nutrients. Iodine quickly dissipates from kiln-dried salt, so it is "attached" through a chemical process resulting in what is referred to as "iodized salt."

Sea salt generally refers to unrefined salt that has been mined directly from the ocean or from ancient ocean deposits deep within the earth (unaffected by modern pollution). Since it is dried in the sun, it retains the important trace elements of ocean salt, including iodine. It has a full flavor with no metallic aftertaste. Smaller amounts of sea salt usually provide more flavor than larger amounts of table salt.

Trace Elements

Sea Salt: typically 90% sodium and 10% trace elements

Table Salt: typically 98% sodium and up to 2% additives (usually synthetic versions of trace elements added by a chemical process)

Sweetener Glossary

Agave Nectar: a sweetener extracted from the pineapple-shaped core of the blue agave, a cactus-like plant native to Mexico.

Applesauce: adds moisture as well as a natural sweet flavor. Applesauce can be used to replace some fat as well as sugar. Do not overmix. Because applesauce is acidic, add about ¼ teaspoon of baking soda to the recipe to smooth its flavor.

Basil: has a mildly sweet flavor and can increase the sweetness of foods such as sauces, pilafs and meat dishes.

Brown Rice Syrup: an opaque golden liquid with a consistency similar to honey. It has a pleasant, lightly sweet taste and is excellent to use when only a touch of sweetness is needed. (To use brown rice syrup in recipes calling for sugar, replace 1 cup of sugar with ¾ cup brown rice syrup and reduce liquid by 2 to 4 tablespoons.)

Fruit: Many fruits can be added to baked goods, yogurts, salads and meats to increase their sweetness and add a rich and refreshing flavor. Remember that a little bit of sugar can help enhance the flavor of the fruit, maximizing the effect of the fruit, while still reducing the overall sugar by a significant amount.

Fruit Juice and Fruit Juice Concentrate: adds flavor as well as sweetness. Use only 100% juice. Do not overmix batters; add about ¼ teaspoon of baking soda to smooth the flavor.

Honey: a commonly used natural sweetener. Because honey is sweeter than sugar, not as much honey is needed in recipes. (Replace 1 cup of sugar with ⅔ cup of honey, reduce liquid by ¼ cup and consider adding ¼ teaspoon baking soda.) Darker honeys have a much stronger, more distinctive flavor and contain higher levels of minerals.

We recommend choosing local honey. Most local honey will be minimally processed to remove contaminates. Since the processing can destroy some natural enzymes and nutrients, we encourage you to learn the processing techniques used for your local honey. Absolutely choose honey that is labeled "undiluted," because some marketed honey is diluted with corn syrup.

Due to its ability to absorb and retain moisture, honey has a "keeping" quality that retards the drying out that occurs in baked goods. The flavor of baked goods made with honey is often better the day after baking. Because using honey as a sweetener will add an additional flavor factor to the end product, it is better to use a lighter, more mildly flavored honey when baking.

Almost all honey naturally crystallizes over time. It is easy to liquefy honey by placing the container in a pan of warm water (not hot) until the crystals disappear. This process does not affect the taste or purity of the honey.

Measuring Hint

When measuring syrup-style sweeteners such as honey, maple syrup and agave nectar, measure oil before the syrup to coat the measuring utensil. If the recipe does not call for oil, use water on the measuring utensil or "oil" the spoon with a dab of oil.

Maple Granules and Maple Syrup: Maple granules are a dehydrated form of 100% pure maple syrup. They are a great addition to crumb toppings on coffee cakes and muffins, often offering a more appealing flavor than regular sugar. Maple syrup, a concentrate of maple tree sap, has long been used as a mainstay natural food sweetener. When selecting a maple syrup, look for one that is labeled "100% pure," since many maple syrup products contain corn syrup or other fillers.

Spices and Herbs: Often, spices and herbs offer flavors that may not be sweet but are appealing to the taste buds in place of sweetness. For instance, cinnamon, nutmeg and cloves in a spice cake add to the richness of the cake and allow you to cut back on the amount of sweetener used without compromising flavor. A little bit of sugar along with the spices can help to carry the flavor of the spices throughout baked goods, maximizing their effectiveness.

Vegetables: Though not commonly considered in this category, some vegetables add sweetness to a variety of dishes. Both carrots and beets are high in natural sugars and add a nice dimension to baked goods, casseroles and sauces when pureed, grated, diced or sliced.

Gadgets, Measuring and More

Having the correct equipment is by far one of the best ways to save time in the kitchen. Within the recipes, we have highlighted a few equipment tips in the sidebars. While these are not required, they are helpful. For some gadgets and equipment, we have recommend brands listed on our websites (see p. 242).

Following the listing of handy gadgets and equipment, you will find a page on measuring tips and a page on healthy products to reduce cancer risks.

Suggested list of helpful equipment and gadgets:

- **Bench Knife** (p. 195)
- **Blender** and **Immersion Blender** (p. 122)
- **Bread Machine and/or Stand Mixer with Beaters and Dough Hooks:** Helpful to prepare yeasted breads (e.g., pizza crusts, cinnamon rolls, dinner rolls, pretzels). Stand mixer is handy for protein bars and cakes.
- **Broth/Fat Separator** (p. 157)
- **Chef Knife** (p. 60)
- **Colander:** Used to drain many things, including soaking water off dry beans.
- **Cutting Boards:** Used for many food preparation purposes (e.g., chopping vegetables, slicing meat, rolling dough [cinnamon rolls]). An easy-clean, smooth-surface style is good for chopping vegetables. A smooth-surfaced, flexible style is nice for dough preparation. See page 35 for sanitation notes.
- **Dippers:** Great for dipping drop biscuits and cookies (pp. 182 and 197).
- **Enclosed Manual Chopper** (p. 131)
- **Food Processor/Chopper:** Come in many sizes with many features. See pages 124, 154 and 162. A small chopper style is great for "shredding" cheese, grinding meat (p. 160) and chopping dried fruit (p. 187).
- **Food Scales:** Handy when you desire accurate measurements; saves time when measuring portions of canned products (see p. 206).
- **Kitchen (Meat) Thermometer** (p. 99)
- **Kitchen Spritzer** (p. 144)
- **Measuring Supplies:**
  (1) Dry-measuring cups (1/4, 1/3, 1/2 and 1 cup).
  (2) Clear liquid measures (1-cup and 2-cup and a ¼-cup measure mentioned on p. 182) that nest inside each other and have easy-to-read markings (see graphics on p. 227). The angled style allows for easier reading. Also a 4-cup and/or 8-cup batter

bowl are handy for measuring large amounts and double as mixing bowls.
(3) Measuring spoons (1 tablespoon, 1 teaspoon, 1/2 teaspoon, 1/4 teaspoon and 1/8 teaspoon). We prefer long-handled (approximately 5 inches in length).

- **Mesh Strainer** (fine): Useful for rinsing grains (e.g., quinoa, rice, barley) and straining meat broth.
- **Microplane** (p. 222).
- **Mixing and Cooking Utensils:** Mixing bowls, heat-resistant rubber spatulas/ spoonulas, whisk, metal spatulas, tongs, pastry brush, rolling pin (p. 110), vegetable peeler.
- **Pastry Blender** (p. 202)
- **Pizza Stone** (p. 169)
- **Potato Masher** (p. 135)
- **Salad Spinner** (p. 68)
- **Slow Cookers** (p. 126)
- **Vegetable Brush:** To scrub the skins of vegetables and fruit.

We recommend the following cookware. See page 228 for the healthy "whys."

- **Cast-Iron Cookware:** a **Griddle** for pancakes, etc., a **Skillet** for stir-fries, simple meats (cooked without sauces) and oven-roasted vegetables; and a **Grill Pan** for grilling steaks, hamburgers, fish and chicken
- **Glass Bakeware** (without nonstick coating), including an 8-inch square dish, 9x13-inch dish and variety of sizes of covered casseroles dishes
- **Stainless Steel Bakeware** (without nonstick coating), including baking (cookie) sheets and jelly roll pan (baking sheet with ½ inch sides)
- **Stainless Steel Cookware** (without nonstick coating), especially skillets, saucepans and larger pots for soups, all with lids
- **Stainless Steel Steamer Pan** and/or **Steamer Basket** (p. 38)
- **Toaster-Convection Oven:** Both of us enjoy using a countertop convection oven on a regular basis (pp. 160 and 228).

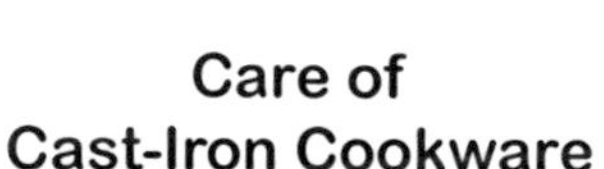

Care of Cast-Iron Cookware

To protect cast-iron cookware, heat it slowly, beginning with a cold burner or oven. Do not place cold cookware on preheated burner or in preheated oven.

Most manufacturers recommend not washing cast iron. However, we wash cooled pieces quickly (not soaking) with a mild nonchemical soap, then rinse and dry immediately.

Do not cook tomato products in cast iron.

Cast-iron cookware may be purchased preseasoned. As it is used, it becomes more seasoned, allowing for less oil to be needed

See more tips on page 39.

Measuring Guidelines

Measuring Dry Ingredients (e.g., flour, baking powder, seasonings)

1. Use dry measuring cups or measuring spoons.
   a. Fill the measure a little overfull with the dry ingredient, especially on backside (side nearest handle).
   b. Using a table knife, move the straight edge across top of the measure to level off the ingredient.

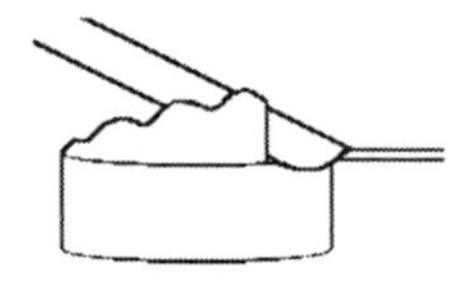

Measuring
Dry Ingredients

2. Salt and seasonings often do not need to be measured as accurately. Simply shake spoon gently over food container to level ingredient.
3. Sometimes very small amounts are measured by a pinch, shake, sprinkle or dash.

Measuring Liquid Ingredients (e.g., water, juice, syrup, oil, broth)

1. Use a clear liquid measuring cup that has markings to indicate the fractional divisions of the measure.
   Using the **side-view-style** liquid measure:
   a. Place measure on a level table or counter.
   b. Bend down so your eyes are level with measure lines.
   c. Liquids are measured at the bottom of the meniscus (the saucer-like depression along the top edge of the liquid). Add liquid gradually until the meniscus is lined up with desired mark on liquid measure.

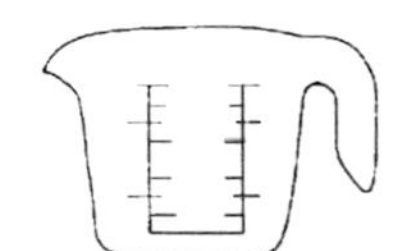

Measuring
Liquid Ingredients
with Side-View-Style
Measure

   Using the **angled-style** liquid measure:
   a. Place measure on a level table or counter.
   b. Look down from the top to read measurements as you add liquids into measure.

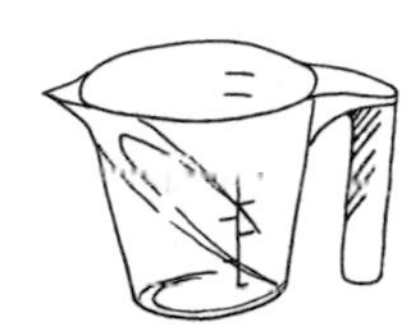

Liquid Measure
Angled-Style

2. Measure small amounts of liquid ingredients with measuring spoons. However, this is not very accurate. A one-fourth clear angled-style measure is handy (p. 182).

Measuring Equivalents

4 cups	=	2 pints or 1 quart or $^1/_4$ gallon	1 Tbsp.	=	3 tsp.
1 cup	=	16 Tbsp. ($^1/_2$ pint)	$^1/_2$ Tbsp.	=	$1^1/_2$ tsp.
$^7/_8$ cup	=	14 Tbsp. (1 cup – 2 Tbsp.)	$^7/_8$ tsp.	=	$^1/_2$ tsp + $^1/_4$ tsp. + $^1/_8$ tsp.
$^1/_2$ cup	=	8 Tbsp.	$^3/_4$ tsp.	=	$^1/_2$ tsp, + $^1/_4$ tsp
$^1/_3$ cup	=	$5^1/_3$ Tbsp (5 Tbsp. + 1 tsp.)	$^5/_8$ tsp.	=	$^1/_2$ tsp. + $^1/_8$ tsp.
$^1/_4$ cup	=	4 Tbsp.	$^3/_8$ tsp.	=	$^1/_4$ tsp. + $^1/_8$ tsp.
$^1/_8$ cup	=	2 Tbsp.	$^1/_8$ tsp.	=	one-half of a $^1/_4$ tsp.

Reducing Cancer Risks

In addition to the herbicides, pesticides and fungicides discussed in chapter eleven, chemicals such as chlorine, dioxins and formaldehyde can be found in our homes, in our air, water and food and even in our cookware. These chemicals can weaken our immune system and are often carcinogenic;[1] that is, over time, they can increase our risk of developing cancer. This section looks at some of the things we can do to reduce the chemicals in our kitchens and retain nutrient values in our foods. The strategies are in alphabetical order. Just like with other pieces of the healthy puzzle, an effective way to make changes is to start with the strategies and materials that are easiest to use, prioritizing based on convenience, time, money and personal preference.

Cookware: To reduce the toxic load, gradually replace aluminum, copper (copper bottomed is okay) and nonstick coated cookware (formaldehyde based) with stainless steel, preseasoned cast iron, high-quality enamel baked and/or glass bake and cookware. (As you use cast iron, it will continue to season more. When well seasoned, its surface becomes almost nonstick, requiring less oil. See page 226 for our recommended pieces and how to care of cast-iron cookware.)

Food Storage Wraps and Paper Products: Use unbleached parchment paper and muffin liners to reduce dioxin exposure. Avoid having aluminum foil directly touch food, since aluminum toxicity leads to forms of dementia (if you choose to use the foil on occasion, place the shiny side toward the food).

Household Cleaners: The fragrances and chemicals breathed in from a variety of chemical-based cleansers (e.g., laundry, dish, multipurpose, disinfectants, air sanitizers) are a source of indoor air pollution. Instead, use fully biodegradable, natural, plant-based cleaners (see our websites, p. 242, for an excellent resource).

Toaster Oven versus Microwave: We recommend using a toaster oven over microwaves since microwaves can drastically reduce the levels of valuable nutrients from foods. Studies show that 90 percent of antioxidants are destroyed in microwave-cooked foods.[2] If you use a microwave, do not use plastic dishes or plastic wraps to cover foods when cooking, since the microwaves cause the dioxins from the plastics to leach into the food.[3]

Water: It is important to drink water throughout the day. However, our drinking water supply often contains high levels of mercury and chemical runoff from pesticides and herbicides used on farms and homeowners' lawns. Consider installing a water filter to purify your drinking water. If you desire to freeze plastic water bottles, first remove a bit of the water. This allows room for the freezing water to expand without stretching the plastic. The process of the plastic expanding releases dioxins.

Healthier Choices Shopping Guide

This glossary is designed to guide you in determining the quality of a food product. Listed first are some key nutrient levels to keep in mind (see chapter two for more details) and a list of keywords or phrases to look for and to avoid. Following that is a list of food products we use in our recipes, along with specific things to look for or avoid. For some we have included the brand we used in our nutritional analysis. By no means does this cover all acceptable brands; we have not been paid to support any particular company. The brands are available at natural food stores and major chain grocery stores.

Nutrient quantities to consider:

- Calories: These factor into your total caloric intake and are an individual determination (see p. 4).
- Fat: It is the quantity of saturated and trans fats that really counts. Trans fats should be zero and saturated fats should be kept below two or three grams for most items.
- Cholesterol: This may not be too critical, but go with your doctor's guidelines.
- Sodium: Since the overall goal is to consume fewer than 2,300 milligrams per day, a good target is to stay under 600 milligrams per meal. This leaves 500 milligrams for snacks and beverages. If you are purchasing prepared foods, consider the amount you will be eating and the sodium levels in the foods you will be eating with it. Suggested sodium levels for broths can be found on page 119; for beans, see page 123; and for tomatoes, see pages 119 and 137.
- Fiber: Whenever you can, get more than two or three grams per serving.

The majority of key words to look for are:

- Whole-grain
- Nitrite-free
- Non-GMO
- No trans fats
- No antibiotics or growth hormones used

The majority of key words to consider avoiding are:

- Corn syrup
- High-fructose corn syrup
- Saturated fats
- Hydrogenated or partially hydrogenated oils
- Artificial flavorings (imitation)
- Additives (e.g., MSG)
- Food Dyes (e.g., "Yellow No. 5," "Red 40," "Blue No. 1"); caramel flavoring/coloring
- Preservatives (e.g., BHA, BHT, TBHQ, sodium benzoate, nitrites, sulfites). The preservatives may be listed as "antioxidants" because they prevent the fats in foods from "oxidizing," or becoming rancid (spoiling).

See our websites (p. 242) for more information.

Food Item: (Brand) **P:** key words to look for when **P**urchasing; **A:** key words to **A**void. 365 refers to Whole Foods brand

All-Purpose Gluten-Free Baking Flour: (Bob's Red Mill)

Aminos, liquid: (Bragg's) ... this is a great substitute for soy sauce

Apple Cider Vinegar: (Braggs) **P:** raw

Applesauce: (Santa Cruz) **P:** 100%, unsweetened; **A:** corn syrup

Baking Powder: (Rumford) **P:** aluminum-free

Beans, canned: (Eden and 365 brands used in our testing and nutritional analysis; Westbrae Natural is a good brand, but they have more sugar and are higher in sodium than we prefer) **A:** corn syrup, high sodium (p. 123), high sugar

Blue Corn Chips: (Garden of Eatin, Bearitos; p. 143) **A:** high sodium

Bread/Buns: (Rudi's, Food for Life) **P:** highest whole-grain flours possible and/or Ezekiel (made from sprouted grains); **A:** corn syrup, high sugars, bleached flour

Bread Crumbs: (p. 98)

Broth – Beef, Chicken, Vegetable and low-sodium broths: (365, Imagine, Pacific) **P:** p. 119; **A:** corn syrup, MSG and other preservatives, artificial flavorings

Brown Rice Crispy Cereal: (Erewhon, Nature Path and EnviroKidz for cocoa flavored) **P:** brown rice, low sweetener; **A:** corn syrup, enriched white rice, preservatives

Cooking Spray: use Kitchen Spritzer (p. 144); **A:** preservatives, contains oils not designed for temperature the oil is being used for (p. 10)

Cornmeal: P: non-GMO

Cornstarch: (Rapunzel) **P:** non-GMO

Crackers: (Back to Nature, Barbara's Bakery) **P:** 100% whole grain or blend, low sodium if possible; **A:** corn syrup, hydrogenated oil, trans fat, preservatives

Cream Cheese: (Neufchâtel, p. 42) **A:** artificial flavorings, artificial colorings

Creamy Potato Leek Soup: (Imagine) **A:** additives, sweeteners, high sodium if possible

Dip: (p. 42)

English Muffins: (p. 191)

Extracts: (Flavorganics, Simply Organic) **A:** imitation flavorings, corn syrup

Flatbread: (p. 191)

Flax Oil: (Spectrum Essentials) **P:** dark bottles, cold-pressed, unrefined

Fruit, dried: (Made in Nature is gluten free, Woodstock) **P:** 100% fruit (try to find apple juice-sweetened dried cranberries); **A:** sulfites, articifial sweeteners

Fruit, frozen: (Cascadian Farms, Woodstock Farms, Wyman's, SnoPac) **P:** frozen when fresh; **A:** sweeteners, preservatives

Graham Crackers (crumbs): (New Morning) **P:** at least some whole-grain flours used, low sugars; **A:** preservatives, corn syrup,

Ham: (Beeler's, Applegate Farms) **P:** free of nitrates, nitrites, antibiotics and steroids; **A:** artificial colorings, MSG

Juices: P: unsweetened, 100% juice; **A:** sweeteners, additives, corn syrup

Ketchup: (Westbrae, Annie's Naturals) **P:** lowest sugar and sodium possible; **A:** high-fructose corn syrup, corn syrup, high sodium, high sugar

Luncheon Meats: (Applegate Farms) **P:** free of nitrates, nitrites, antibiotics, steroids and growth hormones; **A:** artificial colorings, MSG

Maple Syrup: (Spring Tree, Grade A) **P:** pure, 100%; **A:** corn syrup, artificial flavorings

Margarine: P: with flax oil if possible (do not use margarine with flax oil for baking); **A:** trans fats, preservatives, food colorings

Mayo: (Spectrum Naturals, Vegenaise) **P:** with flax oil and raw apple cider vinegar if possible; **A:** hydrogenated fat, sugar, corn syrup, preservatives

"Milks": low-fat cow milk (prefer organic), unsweetened soy (Silk), unsweetened almond (Pacific), sweetened almond (Pacific), unsweetened rice (Imagine Rice Dream)

Mustard, Dijon-style: (Natural Value, Westbrae Natural) **A:** preservatives, sugars, high sodium

Nuts: P: raw or at least unsalted; **A:** sodium, sugars

Oils: (pp. 10–11) **P:** specific oil for intended purpose

Olive Oil: (Bionaturae) **P:** dark bottles, extra virgin, cold-pressed; **A:** refined

Pasta: (p. 137) **P:** 100% whole grain or whole-grain blend; **A:** all refined flour

Peanut & Nut Butters: (East Wind) **P:** unsweetened, low sodium; **A:** corn syrup, high-fructose corn syrup, dextrose, hydrogenated vegetable oil, high sodium

Polynesian Sauce: (San-J) **P:** sweetened with honey; **A:** high-fructose corn syrup

Pretzels: (Newman's Own Organics – we enjoy spelt pretzels); **A:** corn syrup, hydrogenated oils, artificial flavorings and preservatives

Salad Dressing: (Seeds of Change; Cardini, Nasoya, Organic Ville) **P:** see pp. 44, 70, 97 and 99 for easy low-sodium recipes; **A:** high sodium, fat free as they usually have high sugar and/or corn syrup, preservatives (e.g., potassium sorbate, calcium disodium, EDTA, propylene glycol alginate, sulfates, phosphoric acid, polysorbate 60)

Salsa: (pp. 91 and 153) **A:** high sodium, high sugars, preservatives

Salt, real (Redmond)

Sausage (Fully Cooked Links and Ground): (Applegate Farms, Beeler's, Trader Joe's) **P:** free of nitrates, nitrites, antibiotics and steroids; consider chicken/turkey sausage (Applegate Farms was used in our testing and nutritional analysis for fully cooked links; we grind the links for ground chicken sausage in a couple of recipes); chose as low sodium as possible **A:** artificial colorings, MSG

Seasoned Garlic Salt (p. 222)

Seasonings/Herbs: (Simply Organic, Frontier)

Soy Sauce: most soy sauces are 700–1000+ milligrams of sodium per tablespoon; we use Bragg's liquid aminos in place of soy sauce

Soy Protein Isolate, unsweetened: (Shaklee; see our websites on p. 242) **P:** determine that the processing does not destroy isoflavones

Sugar: (Wholesome Organic Sweeteners, Organic Florida Crystals, 365)

Tomato Products: (Bionaturae, 365, some Muir Glen) **A:** high sodium (pp. 119 & 137)

Tortillas, soft whole-grain: (p. 191)

Tortilla Chips: (Garden of Eatin, Bearitos; p. 143); **A:** high sodium

Vegetables, frozen: (Woodstock Farms, Cascadian Farms, 365) **P:** frozen when fresh, low or no salt added; **A:** preservatives, high sodium added, high calorie sauces

Vegetables, frozen mixes: (Cascadian Farms) Chinese-Style Stir-Fry, Thai-Style Stir-Fry, Gardener's

Wine: (Frey red table wine) **P:** no sulfites added; **A:** sulfites

Worcestershire Sauce: (Annie's Naturals) **P:** raw apple cider vinegar, non-GMO cornstarch; **A:** high sugar, high sodium, additives

Topic and Recipe Index

15-Minute Pumpkin Soup, 84
20-Minute Stir-Fry, 61
abbreviations, 34
absorption (see nutrients, sugars)
acid reflux, 16, 166, 223
acorn squash, 19, 82, 219
  recipes using, 82, 160
Acorn Squash & Sausage Bake, 82
Acorn Squash with Pork Chops, 160
activity level, 4, 172
acupuncture, 31
additives, 7, 229
agave nectar, 223
al dente pasta, 137
allicin, 55, 61
all-purpose flour, 21
almonds, 21, 219
altitude, 172
aluminum, 205, 228
Alzheimer's disease, 48
amino acids, 18
aminos (liquid), 139, 148, 230
antibiotics, 28, 29, 60, 72, 229
antifungal, 72
anti-inflammatory, 60, 63, 72, 74, 96
antioxidants, 28, 48, 52, 53, 55, 59, 76, 96, 107, 120, 172, 186, 228, 229
antiviral, 60, 72
apple, 219
Apple Crisp Pie, 204
Apple Crisp, 203
applesauce, 223
apriocts, 219
arthritis (aiding), 60, 63, 67
artichoke, 19, 43, 219
artichoke hearts, recipes using, 95
artificial colors and flavorings, 7, 42, 70, 92, 229
artificial sweeteners, 7, 17, 112, 173
arugula, 44
  recipes using, 44, 45, 93, 95, 109, 170
Arugula Pesto Salad Dressing, 44
Asian Salmon Salad, 96–97
asparagus, 19, 46, 219
  recipes using, 39, 46, 95, 111, 118, 127, 148
asthma (easing), 84
avocado, 19, 47
  recipes using, 47, 95
Baby Bok Choy & Leeks, 51
bacteria, 76
bacterial infections (fighting), (see antibiotic)
Baked Sweet Potato, 88
bakeware, 226
Baking Mix, 181
  recipes using, 182, 183, 184, 185, 197, 206
baking powder, 175
baking soda, 7
Balsamic Vinaigrette Salad Dressing, 70
banana, 19, 219
barley, 21, 27, 180, 219
  recipes using, 121, 180
Barley Casserole, 180
Basic Rice, 176
basil, 220
  recipes using fresh, 63, 81, 93, 95, 136, 170, 179, 223
Basil Quinoa Pilaf, 179
Bean Salsa, 91
Bean-Corn Salsa, 91
beans (canned), 48, 123
beans, 20, 48–49, 219
  recipes using, 49, 81, 91, 94, 100, 122, 123, 129, 132, 138, 139, 149
Beef Barley Soup, 121
Beef Teriyaki 148–149
beef, nutritional value, 19
beef, purchasing, 18, 29
beef
  recipes using chunks (cooked), 94, 118
  recipes using ground (lean), 87, 100, 125, 134, 138, 146, 155, 170
  recipes using roasts, 156
  recipes using round steak, 121, 132, 136, 148
  recipes using sirloin steak, 132
  recipes using stew meat, 132
beet, 19, 50
beet, recipes using, 50, 64, 95, 102
Beet Salad, 102
bench knife, 195
betacryptoxanthis, 86
beverages, 172–173
BHA, 229
BHT, 229
Biscuit Mix, 182
Black Bean Dip, 149
Black Bean Soup, 123
blackberries, 19, 219
blood glucose (sugar) levels, 14, 24–25, 30, 48, 66, 67, 84, 88, 89, 186, 221
blood pressure, 5, 12, 13, 18, 22, 23, 25, 30, 47, 89
blue corn, 58
blueberries, 19, 185, 219
Blueberry Muffins, 187
blueberry syrup (see pancake syup)
bodyweight, 16, 22, 25, 30, 166
bodywork therapies, 31
bok choy, 51
  recipes using, 51, 108, 109
bone health, 48, 56, 62, 89
Bran Muffins, 186–187
bran, 21, 174
bread, 101, 219
bread machine, 161, 191, 225

Bread with Olive Oil, 191
breading, safety tip, 99
breads and grains, 174–195
Broadsticks, 193
breakfast and brunch, 103–115
Breakfast Pizza, 110–111
Breakfast Squares, 108
breastfeeding (needs), 6, 172, 178
breathing exercises, 30, 31
broccoli, 19, 52, 147, 219
recipes using, 52, 95, 118, 119, 147, 152, 163
Broccoli & Red Pepper, 52
broth-fat separator, 157
broths (purchased), 118, 119
brown rice syrup, 223
brown rice, 21
butter, 9, 11
butternut squash, 19, 83, 219
recipes using, 83, 128, 129, 209
cabbage, 19, 53, 219
recipes using, 53, 95, 109, 118, 126, 150, 156, 157, 180
Cabbage-Fish Bake, 150–151
Cabbage Patch Soup, 126
caffeine, 173
cakes, 200
calcium, 12
calcium (foods high in), 43, 48, 50, 51, 52, 57, 71, 84, 178
calories, 4, 5, 8, 14, 17, 173, 229
cancer, 7, 10, 12
cancer-prevention, 52, 53, 60, 63, 64, 65, 68, 72, 86, 90, 150, 228
Candy Fries, 88
canned fruits and vegetables, 29
cantaloupe, 19, 219
caramel coloring/flavoring, 229
Caramelized Onion Dinner, 72–73
Caramelized Onions, 72
Caramelized Soups, 124–127
carbohydrates, 5, 7, 25
carcinogenic, 7, 228
care packages, 112
carotenoids (foods high in), 47, 54, 86, 90, 218
carrots, 19, 54, 120, 219
recipes using, 39, 51, 54, 78, 90, 95, 118, 119, 120, 121, 126, 127, 128, 129, 132, 134, 136, 148, 150, 152, 154, 157, 160, 163, 179, 200
cast-iron cookware, 10, 226
celery, 55, 219
recipes using, 43, 74, 75, 79, 87, 95, 113, 118, 121, 125, 134, 157, 177, 162, 163
celiac disease, 26–27, 33
cell development, growth and repair, 8, 18, 31, 48
cereals, 104, 174
chard, 56, 219
recipes using, 56, 64, 95, 109, 178
Chard & Potato Bake, 56
Cheese Biscuit Mix, 183
Cheeseburger Soup, 125
chef's knife, 60
chemical residues, 37, 76
chemicals, 7, 28, 29, 37, 228
chemicals (removing from body), 15, 72
cherries, 19
chicken, nutritonal value, 19
chicken, purchasing, 18, 29
chicken
recipes using chunks (cooked), 94, 118, 130, 133
recipes using chunks (raw boneless), 56, 57, 61, 72, 81, 98, 111, 118, 119, 120, 127, 128, 130, 132, 133, 145, 147, 153
recipes using pieces (bone-in), 99, 144, 157
recipes using whole, 157
Chicken Broccoli Mac 'n' Cheese, 147
Chicken Cabbage Delight, 157
Chicken Vegetable Bake, 133
Chicken-Vegetable Spread, 160
children (also see Little Chefs), xii, 13, 14–15, 25
Chili Meat Loaf Patties, 155
chili powder, 221
chili, 130–133
chiropractic care, 31
chives, 220
recipes using fresh, 108, 109, 119
chlorine, 228
Chocolate Chip Cookies, 197
Chocolate Chip Crispy Granola Bars, 112–113
cholesterol, 5, 8, 9, 14, 22, 23, 25, 43, 48, 63, 67, 72, 89, 120, 186
Chop & Drop (definition), 34
Chunky Garden Spaghetti Dinner, 136–137
cilantro, 220
recipes using fresh, 81, 91, 93, 95, 109
cinnamon rolls, 194–195
cinnamon, 221
cinnamon blend, 158
circulation, 31, 48, 50
Citrus Vinaigrette Salad Dressing, 97
cleaners, 228
cloves, 221
Cocoa Frosting, 207
coffee cakes, 184–185
colander, 225
Collard Wraps, 57
collards, 19, 57, 219
colorings, natural, 199
community supported agriculture (CSA), 29
complete protein, 18, 178
complex carbohydrates, 174
concentration (inability), 7, 103
condiments, 10, 92–93
Confetti Dip, 42
congestion (easing), 74
constipation (relief of), 50
cookies, 85, 197–199
cooking oil (see oil)
cooking spray, 144
cooking utensils, 226
cookware, 10, 226, 228
copper, 228
Corn on the Cob, 58
corn syrup, 16, 17, 42, 58, 70, 92, 118, 143, 171, 173, 208, 223, 229
corn, 19, 27, 58, 219
recipes using, 58, 81, 95, 111, 118, 119, 130, 138, 139
cornmeal, 21
recipes using, 138

crackers, 121, 174
Cranberry-Pecan Muffins, 187
Cream Cheese Frosting, 207
cream cheese, 42
creamy soups (purchased), 118
Crescents, 193
crisps, 202, 203
croutons, 190
crucifers, 53, 208
crusts, freezing, 168
crusts, purchased, 168, 205
cumin, 222
cupcakes, 200, 206
cutting boards, 35, 225
dates, 219
defense molecules (in plants), 28
degermed grains, 174
dementia, 48
depression, 7, 173
desserts, 85, 164, 165, 196–209
diabetes, 5, 14, 16, 22, 24–25, 66, 89, 175
diet drinks, 173
digestion, 8, 14, 15, 16, 18, 30, 31, 68, 73
Dijon Salad Dressing, 99
dill, 221
  recipes using fresh, 95, 152, 157
dinner rolls, 192–193
dinosaurs, 150
dioxins, 228
dipper, 182
diverticulitis, 14
dizziness, 172
Do-Ahead Day, 142
Do-Ahead Quick-Fix Meals, 141–142
Dramamine, 96
Easy Baked Fish, 151
Easy Guacamole, 47
edamame (soy) beans, 20, 219
  recipes using, 94, 101, 118
eggs, 19, 29, 44, 107
  recipes using, 59,78, 89, 94, 95, 99, 102, 107, 108, 109, 110, 111, 114, 115, 138, 139, 160, 165, 184, 185, 186, 187, 189, 200, 206
empty calories, 5
enclosed chopper, 131
energy, 5, 8, 30, 31, 48, 89
English Muffin Pizza, 170
enzymes, 48
essential amino acids, 18, 178
essential fatty acids (see fats)
ethylene gas, 55
exercise, 24, 30
eye health, 56, 64, 65, 68, 120, 218
Fall Harvest Stew, 128
Fall Harvest Vegan Stew, 129
Family Fun Nights, 167–171
Fancy Hamburgers, 146
Fancy Scrambled Eggs, 109
fat, 5, 7, 8-11, 22, 23, 25, 29, 103, 104, 229
  essential fatty acids, 5, 22, 174
  healthy fats, 5, 8-11, 47, 104, 192
  hydrogenated oils, 9, 42, 92, 229
  "low-fat" foods, 17
  lowering consumption, 9
  oleic acid, 47
  omega-3 fatty acids, 8, 57, 82, 84
  saturated fats, 5, 7, 9, 10, 11, 18, 22, 23, 229
  trans fats, 5, 9, 10, 11, 22, 23, 143, 161, 168, 182, 229
  unsaturated fats, 5, 8, 9, 11, 107
fatigue, 26, 172
fennel, 19, 59, 153
  recipes using, 59, 150, 152, 180
Fennel & Mashed Potatoes, 59
fetal development, 48
fiber, 5, 7, 14–15, 22, 23, 25, 52, 229
  benefits of, 14
  amounts needed, 5, 14
  foods high in, 43, 46, 48, 56, 57, 59, 62, 63, 66, 68, 71, 74, 91, 176, 180
  increasing, 42, 161, 196
  insoluble fiber, 14
  soluble fiber, 14
fish, 9, 18, 19, 97
  recipes using, 94, 95, 150, 151, 152
flavonoids, 79, 218
flavorings, artificial, 7
flaxseed meal, 21
  recipes using, 15, 78, 79, 105, 106, 112, 144, 115, 188, 189
flaxseed oil, 9, 10, 11
  recipes using, 43, 52, 61, 64, 101, 192
flours, 175
  all-purpose, 21, 175
  brown rice, 177
  helpful hint, 168
  spelt, 21, 175
  white whole wheat, 21, 175, 219
  whole wheat pastry, 21, 175
  whole wheat, 21, 174-5
folate (foods high in), 43, 47, 48, 53, 58, 59, 107
folate, 47, 48, 58
food dyes, 229
food processor/chopper, 124, 225
food scales, 206, 225
formaldehydes, 228
free radicals, 10, 11, 49
free range, 18, 19, 29
fresh produce, 28, 29
friendly flora, 15
frostings, 207
frozen fruits and vegetables, 29, 41
Frozen Yogurt, 196
Fruit Pancake Syrup, 188
fruit, 17, 29, 116, 196, 223
Fruit-Gazed Sweet Potatoes, 164
Fruity Crispy Granola Bars, 112–113
fungicides, 228
Garlic 'n' Herb Seasoning, 222
Garlic Bread, 136
Garlic Butter, 183
garlic, 55, 60–61
  exposure to air, 61
  recipes using fresh, 44, 59, 61, 63, 64, 72, 75, 79, 81, 87, 90, 91, 100, 101, 109, 118, 121, 122, 123, 128, 129, 130, 134, 138, 139, 152, 170
  impact of cooking on nutrients, 61
gastritis (aiding), 60
genetically-modified (GMO) foods, 28

GERD (see acid reflux)
germ (of grain), 174
gifts, 112
ginger, recipes using fresh, 96
Gingerbread Cookies, 198–199
glass bakeware, 226
Glazed Carrots, 54
glucosinolates, 218
glutathione (foods high in), 46, 150
gluten (sensitivity to), 26–27
gluten, 26–27, 190
Gluten-Free Chocolate Chips Cookies, 197
Gluten-Free Crisp Topping, 202
Gluten-Free Flour Mix, 27
gluten-free foods, 27, 33, 115, 176
Gluten-Free Granola Bars, 112–113
Gluten-Free Protein Bars, 115
glycemic-index (of pasta), 137
GMO (see non-GMO)
goitrogens, 218
grain biscuits, 182-183
grains (see whole grains, flours, oat, quinoa, rice, spelt and wheat)
Granola Bars, 112–113
Granola, 208
grapefruit, 19
grapes, 219
grass fed, 18, 19, 29
Green Bean Basil Salad, 63
green beans, 19, 62–63, 219
  recipes using, 45, 62, 63, 83, 118, 121, 128, 126, 132, 134, 152, 180
green onions (scallions), 73
  recipes using, 109
Green tea, 172-173
Greens & Onions (sautéed and simmered), 64
greens, 64
  recipes using, 56, 57, 64, 65
grill pan, 226
Grilled Chicken Kale-Carrot Soup, 120
Grilled Chicken Rubs, 145
Grilled Pork Rubs, 145
groats, 186
growth hormones, 28, 29, 229
Hamburger Buns, 193
Hamburger Pizza, 170
Hamburger Soup, 125
hamburgers, 146
Ham-Leek-Asparagus Breakfast Pizza, 111
Hard-Cooked Egg, 107
headaches, 26, 103, 172, 175
healthier eating (definition), xi, 1
healthy fats (see fats)
heart disease (risk), 5, 12, 22–23, 47
heart disease, 22–23, 25
heart health, 22–23, 25, 47, 48, 49, 56, 59, 60, 62, 64, 68, 74, 89, 90, 107, 120, 186
heartburn, 166
Hearty Chicken Noodle Soup, 127
Hearty Chicken Rice Soup, 127
Hearty Homemade Bread for Bread Machines, 190
Hearty Meat & Veggie Chili, 132–133
herbal teas, 172
Herbed Noodles, 157, 158
herbicides, 28, 228
herbs + spices, 10, 17, 220–222
  dried herbs, 220
  drying herbs, 220
  growing herbs, 220
  fresh herbs, 220
  freezing herbs, 220
  washing herbs, 200
Hickory Barbeque, 158, 222
High Fiber Oat Spice Pancakes, 188–189
high-fructose corn syrup (see corn syrup)
high-heat oil, 10
hoisin sauce, 97
Holiday Dinner Makeover, 161–165
holidays, 112, 161
honey, 223
Honey-Applesauce Bran Muffins, 186–187
hormone production and regulation, 8, 18, 31
hot peppers (see peppers)
household cleaners, 228
hydrogenated oils (see oils)
hypoglycemia, 66
ice cream (selecting), 208
ice cream maker, 208
ice cube trays (using), 43
immersion blender, 122
immune system, 15, 31, 37, 63, 186, 218, 228
in season, 28, 209
indoor air pollution, 228
infertility, 173
inflammation reduction (see anti-inflammatory)
inflammation, 26
insulin, 24
intestinal health, 48, 89
iodine, 222
iron (foods high in), 46, 48, 50, 62, 74, 74, 79, 84, 178
Italian Meat Loaf Patties, 155
joint pain, 26
juice, 17, 105, 172, 223
Kale & Potato Bake, 65
kale, 19, 65, 120, 219
  recipes using, 51, 64, 65, 95, 120, 121, 129, 130
Kid-Friendly Granola Bars
kidney disease (risk), 12, 25
kitchen spritzer, 144
kohlrabi, 66, 95
lamb, recipes using ground, 134
leeks, 19, 67
  recipes using, 51, 53, 95, 109, 118, 126, 180
legumes, 20
Lemon-Butter Sauce, 43
lettuce and salad greens, 68–69, 219
  recipes using, 69, 95, 96, 98, 100, 153
liquid aminos (see aminos)
Little Chefs (also see children), 41, 55, 77, 79, 99, 112, 113, 120, 131, 167, 176, 181, 193, 199, 204, 209
liver health, 43, 50, 68
local food, 28, 29, 41
Low Sugar Cinnamon Rolls, 194–195
low-heat oil, 10
lunches (school, work), 112, 116–117, 131
lutein (foods high in), 47, 107, 120
lycopene, 90, 91
lysine, 178

macaroni and cheese, 147
macular degeneration, 120
magnesium (foods high in), 43, 48, 50, 56
magnesium, 48, 49
Mama Garlic, 222
maple granules, 224
maple syrup (see also pancake syrup), 224
marathon, 153
margarine, 11, 192
marinade safety, 148
Marinara Sauce, 90
massage, 31
Meal-in-a-Salad, 94–95
measuring, 34
  angled-style measure, 182
  dry ingredients, 227
  equivalents, 227
  liquid ingredients, 227
  sticky liquids, 224
  supplies, 225
meat thermometer, 99
meatloaf patties, 154, 155
medium-heat oil, 10
mercury, 228
mesh strainer, 226
metabolism (speeding up), 166
microplane, 222
microwave, 61, 228
migraine (see headache)
minerals, 6, 7, 23
mini food processor, 154, 162
Mixed Vegetables, 163
mixing utensils, 226
monosodium glutamate (MSG), 7, 42, 118, 143, 229
mood swings, 7
mother's milk, 178
motion sickness, 96
MSG (see monosodium glutamate)
muffin liners, 228
muffins, 186–187
muscle pain, 26
muscle relaxation, 48
muscle weakness, 172
Mushroom Hamburgers, 146
napa cabbage, 53
National Academy of Sciences, 178
National Cancer Institutes, 150
natural sweeteners, 17
nectarine, 19
nervous system function, 31
neurological disorders, 48, 173
nitrates/nitrites, 29, 143, 229
no-heat oil, 10
non-GMO foods, 29, 229
nonstick cookware, 228
nutmeg, 222
  recipes using freshly grated, 44, 65, 83, 84, 93, 106, 128, 129, 134
nutrient absorption and utilization, 8, 31
nutrient dense (definition), xi
nutrient depletion, 28, 29, 36
nutrients (definition), 4
nutrition facts panel, 4
nutritional analysis of recipes (description), 6-7
nutritional value of food, 31
nuts and seeds, 9, 117
  recipes using, 38, 62, 69, 78, 80, 85, 93, 94, 95, 97, 98, 105, 112, 114, 115, 117, 125, 160, 164, 165, 177, 179, 184, 185, 187, 189, 194, 196, 197, 201, 209
oat, 21, 27, 186, 219
  recipes using, 112, 114, 154, 186, 188, 194, 202, 208
oat bran, 21
  recipes using, 186, 187, 188, 202
Oat Bran Muffins, 186–187
Oat Crisp Topping, 202
Oatmeal Cookies, 197
oil (cooking), 10
  butter/margarine, 11
  coconut, 11
  cold-pressed, 11
  expeller-pressed, 11
  flaxseed, 11
  high-heat, 10
  high-oleic, 11
  "light," 11
  low-heat, 10
  medium-heat, 10
  oxidation of, 11
  plastics (exposure to), 11
  rancid, 11
  refined/unrefined, 11
  smoke point of, 10
  storing, 11
  use, 9, 10
  virgin/extra-virgin, 11
  toasted, 11
okra, 71
oleic acid (see fats)
olive oil, 10, 11
  recipes using, 44, 45, 49, 61, 63, 70, 93, 97, 99, 136, 191
Omega Butter, 192
Onion Hamburgers, 146
onions, 19, 72–73
  recipes using, 39, 45, 50, 56, 58, 59, 61, 64, 65, 72, 74, 75, 78, 80, 81, 82, 83, 84, 87, 89, 90, 91, 95, 100, 101, 102, 108, 109, 110, 111, 118, 119, 120, 121, 122, 123, 126, 127, 128, 129, 130, 132, 133, 134, 136, 138, 139, 146, 147, 148, 152, 154, 155, 157, 160, 162, 170, 179, 180
orange, 219
oregano, 221
  recipes using fresh, 170
organic foods, 28, 29
osteoporosis, 12, 48
Oven Fries, 76
Oven-Fried Chicken Chunks, 144
Oven-Fried Chicken, 144
Overnight Blueberry Coffee Cake, 184
oxalates, 218
oxidation, 10, 11
oxygen, 48
pain reduction, 31, 74
pak choi (see bok choy)
pancake syrup, 102, 103, 188
pancakes, 188–189
Pan-Fried Okra, 71
paper products, 228
paprika, 45
parchment paper, 228
Parkinson's disease, 48
parsley, 221
  recipes using fresh, 81, 86, 87, 91, 93, 95, 109, 121, 152, 162
pasta tips, 137, 174
pasta (whole wheat), 219
pastry blender, 202
pattypan squash, recipes using, 61, 62, 80, 81, 152
pecans, 21
peach, 19, 219

Peach or Mango-Blueberry Crisp, 203
peanut butter, 219
Peanut Butter Frosting, 207
pear, 219
Peas & Celery Salad, 74
peas, 19, 74, 219
  recipes using, 74, 94, 118, 134
Pecan Crusted Chicken Salad, 98
Pecan Pie, 165
peel, 37, 54, 76, 83, 94, 129, 204, 209
Pepper-Corn Chili Soup, 130–131
peppers, hot (chili), 74–75, 138
  recipes using, 100, 108, 130, 132, 138, 139, 149
peppers, sweet bell, 19, 75, 219
  recipes using, 39, 45, 52, 58, 61, 72, 75, 78, 81, 87, 90, 95, 108, 109, 128, 130, 132, 136, 146, 157, 160, 170, 177, 179, 180
pesticides, 28, 29, 228
Pesto, 93
phosphorous (foods high in), 50, 84, 178
physical activity, 4, 23
phytonutrients, 218
pies, 164-165, 204
pilaf mixes (boxed), 177
pilafs, 177, 179
pineapple (crushed), recipe using, 153
Pizza Crust, 168–169
pizza stones, 169
pizza, 149, 167–170
plastics, 228
plum, 219
polished grains, 174
popcorn, 58, 171, 219
pork
  recipes using chops, 83, 145, 153, 160, 177
  recipes using chunks (cooked), 94, 118
  recipes using ground, 134
  recipes using ham, 65, 89, 94, 108, 109, 111, 113, 193
  recipes using roasts, 128, 132, 156
portions, 25, 166, 173, 196
potassium (foods high in), 43, 46, 47, 48, 59, 66, 84
potassium, 47, 48, 71
potato, 19, 76, 219
  recipes using, 21, 39, 45, 56, 59, 65, 76, 95, 118, 126, 156, 157
potato masher, 135
potato salad, 45
potlucks, 94, 181
poultry (see chicken, turkey)
poultry mix, recipes using, 162
prayer, 30
pregnancy needs, 6, 172, 178
prepared food meals, 143
preservatives, 7, 29, 42, 92, 229
produce (see fruit, vegetables)
protein (see also vegetable proteins), 6, 7, 18–21, 25, 48, 104, 107, 174, 178, 196
Protein Bars, 114
protein combining, 18
prunes and juice, 219
pumpkin, 19, 29, 84–85, 219
  recipes using, 84, 85, 106, 165, 188, 189, 201, 202
Pumpkin Cake, 206
Pumpkin Cheesecake, 201
Pumpkin Cookies, 85
Pumpkin Cupcakes, 206
Pumpkin Deluxe Pancakes, 189
Pumpkin Pancakes, 188–189
Pumpkin Pie Smoothie, 106
Pumpkin Pie, 165
pureeing vegetables (see vegetables)
purines, 218
Quick Basic Soup, 119–120
Quick Easy Hummus, 48
Quick-Fix Meals, 140–158
Quick-Fix Prepared Food Meals, 143
quinoa, 21, 27, 178–179
  recipes using, 75, 154, 179
Quinoa Pilaf, 179
raisins, 219
raspberry, 19, 219
refrigerated dough, 168, 182, 192, 194
rice (brown), 21, 27, 176–177 219
  recipes using, 57, 75, 78, 176, 177
rice flour (brown), recipes using, 58, 84, 85, 89, 132, 134, 144, 147, 150, 152, 162, 177
Rice 'n' Fruit, 105
rice pilaf, 163
Roasted Asparagus, 46
Roasted Beets with Greens, 50
Roasted Butternut Squash, 83
Roasted Potato Salad, 45
Roasted Rice Pilaf Dinner, 177
Roasted Vegetables, 39
roasts (see beef and pork)
rosemary, 221
  recipes using fresh, 75, 157, 162
roux (making), 176
Rum-Pecan Sugar Cookies, 197
rutin (foods high in), 46
safe internal temperatures, 35
safe refrigerated storage time, 35
sage, 221
  recipes using fresh, 157, 162
salad dressings, 10, 44, 47, 70, 97, 99, 153
salad greens, 68–69
salad spinner, 68
salads, 45, 69, 74, 92–100, 153
Salmon & Pasta, 152–153
salmonella poisoning, 107
Salsa Chicken Salad, 153
Salsa Pork Salad, 153
Salsa, 91
salt (see also sodium), 137, 221, 222
sanitation tips, 35
saturated fats (see fat)
Saucy Apple Pie, 204
sausage, recipes using, 83, 108, 109, 110, 126, 127, 170, 180
Sausage-Pepper Breakfast Pizza, 110
Sausage-Pepper Pizza, 170
Sausage-Pepper-Onion Mix, 110

Sautéed Cabbage, 53
Sautéed Chard with Balsamic Grilled Chicken, 56
Sautéed Green Beans with Almonds, 62
scallions (see green onions)
Scalloped Corn, 58
Scarborough Fair Turkey Breast, 162–163
sea salt, 222
Seared Tofu, 158
Seasoned Croutons, 190
Seasoned Nuts, 117
Seasoned Spaghetti Squash, 86
Seasoned Squash Dinner, 81
Seasoned Squash Side, 80
seeds (see nuts and seeds)
selenium, 180
serving size, 6, 25, 196
shallots, 73
  recipes using, 95, 109, 147, 148
Shaped Sugar Cookies, 199
Shepherd's Pie Make-Over, 134
shopping list hints, 141
Shortcake Mix, 182
Shortcake, 196
shortening, 11, 184
Side Salad, 69
Simmered Beets and Greens, 50
Simple Choices for –
  blood glucose, 25
  breakfast, 103–105
  diabetes, prevent or delay, 25
  fats, 9
  fiber, 15
  healthier eating, 1
  heart health, 22, 23
  sodium, 13
  sugar, 17
  treats, 196
  vegetable (increasing), 40
Simple Pizza Sauce, 169
skillet, 226
sleep, 30, 31
Slow Cooker Beef Roast, 156
Slow Cooker Black Bean Soup, 122
Slow Cooker Chicken and Veggies, 157
Slow Cooker Chowder, 119
Slow Cooker Pork Roast, 156
Slow Cooker Quick-Fix Meal, 140
slow cooker, recipes using, 119, 121, 122, 124, 125, 126, 127, 128, 133, 153, 156, 157, 162, 180
slow cooker tips, 126
smoke point (oil), 10
Smoothies, 106
snacks, 112, 166, 171
sodium, 5, 6, 7, 12-13, 23, 29, 48, 49, 56, 70, 92, 119, 123, 137, 173, 221, 222, 229
sodium benzoate, 229
soups (purchased), 118, 119
soups, 84, 118–127, 130–133, 157
Southern-Style Shepherd's Pie, 134–135
Southwestern Casserole, 138–139
Southwestern Chicken Breakfast Pizza, 111
Southwestern Hamburgers, 146
soy (see soy beans, soy protein isolate and tofu)
Soy Deluxe Pancakes, 189
soy protein isolate, 20, 89
  recipes using, 78, 85, 89, 106, 114, 115
spaghetti squash, 19, 86–87
  recipes using, 86, 87
Spaghetti Dinner Night, 136–137
Spaghetti Squash Casserole, 87
sparkling apple cider, 161
spelt, 21, 27, 175
spelt flour, 21, 175
  recipes using, 85, 114, 138, 168, 187, 189, 192, 194, 205, 208
Spelt Oat Bran Muffins, 187
Spice "Muffin" Cake, 200
Spiced Sweet Potatoes, 164
Spicy Flatbread Pizza, 149
Spicy Southwestern Bean Breakfast Pizza, 111
spinach, 19, 41, 79, 219
  recipes using, 44, 64, 79, 93, 95, 101, 108, 109, 118, 126, 127, 128, 129, 130, 132, 138, 139, 156, 170, 171
Spinach Dip, 79
Spinach-Red Potato, 135
Spinach-Sweet Potato, 135
squash (see summer squash and winter squash)
Squash Apple Bake, 209
stainless steel bakeware/cookware, 226
stand mixer, 225
Start-to-Finish Quick-Fix Meals, 140
Steamed Asparagus, 46
Steamed Broccoli, 52
Steamed Vegetables, 38
steroids, 29
stews, 128–129
Stir & Press Pie Crust, 205
Stir-Fry Vegetables, 38
stomach upset, 96
storage
  oils, 11
  raw and cooked foods, 25
  wraps, 228
strawberries, 185, 219
Strawberry-Rhubarb Crisp, 202
stress in plants, 28
stress reduction, 30, 31
stress, 173
stroke (risk), 12, 23, 25, 68
Stuffed Crescent, 193
stuffed peppers, 75
sugar (see also blood sugar and natural sweeteners), 5-6, 7, 14, 16-17, 25
  absorption of, 14, 25
  added, 29
  consumption of, 5-6 14, 16-17, 25
Sugar Cookies, 197, 199
sugar highs, 14
sulfites, 229
summer squash, 19, 80–81
  recipes using, 61, 80, 81, 95, 118, 136, 152, 157, 158, 170
sunlight, 30
supplements, 31
sweet corn, 58
sweet potato, 19, 88, 164, 219
  recipes using, 88, 89, 134, 156, 164
Sweet Potato Cakes, 89
sweeteners (see sugar, natural sweeteners), 17
Swiss chard (see chard)

symbols, 32
synthetic products (see also artificial and chemicals), 7
syrup (see brown rice, corn, pancake)
table salt, 222
Taco Pizza, 170
Taco Salad, 101
Tacos, 100
taste buds, 13, 36, 54, 125, 174, 181, 196
tea, 172–3
temperatures, cooking, 35
Tex-Mex Soup, 125
thermometer (food), 35
thickening agent, 176
thirst, 172
thyme, 221
  recipes using fresh, 75, 76, 162
toaster-convection oven, 160, 226, 228
tofu, 20
  recipes using, 81, 83, 94, 118, 158
Tofu Sandwich, 158
tomatoes, 19, 29, 90–91, 119, 137, 219, 226
  recipes using, 47, 63, 72, 81, 87, 91, 95, 100, 101, 108, 109, 111, 119, 128, 130, 132, 136, 146, 155, 169, 170
Topped Baked Potato, 21
Tortilla Wrap, 153, 160
Trail Mix, 117
trans fats (see fat)
transitions, xii, 30–31, 174–5, 184, 190, 196
travel meals, 112, 116–117, 131
triglycerides, 5
Turkey Loaf Patties, 154
turkey, purchasing, 18, 19, 29
turkey
  recipes using breast halves (raw, boneless), 162
  recipes using chunks (cooked), 75, 94, 118, 130
  recipes using chunks/strips (raw), 72, 118, 130
  recipes using ground, 100, 136, 138, 154
  recipes using leg/thigh, 157
Tuscan-style tomatoes, 137
ulcers (prevention), 74
unsaturated fats (see fat)
utensils, 226
Vanilla Frosting, 207
vascular disease, 9
vegan diet, 18
vegetables, 18, 19, 25, 29, 36–91, 116, 224
vegetable brush, 226
vegetable peeler, 40, 55
Vegetable Pizza, 170
vegetable proteins, 18–21, 48
vegetables (descriptions and tips), 36–91
vegetables (pureeing), 40, 137
vegetarian diet, 18, 33
Vegetarian Southwestern Casserole, 139
Vegetarian Spread, 160
Vegetarian Tacos, 91
Veggie Burgers, 78
Venison Teriyaki, 148–149
venison, 19
  recipes using ground, 146, 155
  recipes using round steak/chops, 132, 148
viral infections (fighting) (see antiviral)
vitamin A (foods high in), 46, 50, 51, 54, 62, 65, 82, 86, 107
vitamin A, 63
vitamin B (foods high in), 46, 50, 74, 84, 107, 176, 178
vitamin C (foods high in), 43, 46, 51, 62, 75, 147
vitamin C, 37, 50, 63, 74
vitamin D (foods high in), 84, 107
vitamin E (foods high in), 46, 107, 178
vitamin E, 174
vitamin K (foods high in), 46, 54, 62, 65
vitamins, 6, 7, 23
walnuts (English), 21
water, 171, 172, 228
water bottles, 228
watercress, recipes using, 93
watermelon, 19
weight (see bodyweight)
weight gain (preventing), 60
wheat, 27, 175 (see also flours)
  duram, 175
  germ, 21
  gluten, 26-27, 175, 190
  hard, 175
  red, 175
  sensitivity, 175
  soft, 175
  spring, 175
  white, 21, 175
  winter, 175
  whole, 21
Wheat Bran Muffins, 186–187
wheat bran, recipes using, 186,
wheat flours, recipes using, 85, 114, 138, 144, 168, 181, 182, 183, 184, 185, 186, 188, 189, 190, 192, 194, 197, 198, 199, 200, 205, 206, 208, 229
wheat germ, recipes using, 15, 103, 105, 106, 208
Whipped Cream, 165
white cabbage, 51
whole foods, 28-29, 171, 173
Whole-Grain Dinner Rolls, 192–193
Whole Grain Heart-Healthy Blueberry Coffee Cake, 185
whole grains, 21, 23, 25, 29, 167, 174
Wilted Spinach Salad, 101
winter squash, recipes using, 82, 83, 84, 85, 86, 87, 106, 128, 129, 160, 165, 188, 189, 201, 202, 209
xanthan gum, 70
xanthan gum, recipes using, 70, 97
yams, 88
yeast overgrowth, 16
yeast, 175
yoga, 31
Yogurt, Fruit & Nuts, 105
zeaxanthin, 107, 120
zinc (foods high in), 46, 56, 84
zucchini squash, 80, 219
  recipes using, 80, 109, 121, 152, 163

Our Synergism in Action

The Making of a Cookbook

We first met while participating in a food buying club, and our early conversations centered on food choices and options for meeting the nutritional needs of our families. We shared food from a CSA (Community Supported Agriculture, see p. 29) and compared notes on recipes. It is no surprise, then, that one of the fruits of our friendship is a cookbook. But our relationship – and this book – is so much more.

As we have worked and laughed and dreamed together over the last few years, we have marveled at God's amazing design in bringing us together. From a human standpoint, there is little reason why our lives should have intersected. And yet, because of our knowing and caring for one another, our lives have been enriched beyond measure.

And yes, our cooking has changed because of the influence of each other. Many of our favorite recipes are ones that we created together. Few recipes are "only Sondra's" or "only Dorie's." For example, Sondra's original recipe for Black Bean Soup was made in a pressure cooker. Dorie didn't have a pressure cooker, so a slow-cooker version was born. But the beans used were dry beans, and though it was easy to set them out to soak overnight, Dorie was at a point in her life when she often couldn't think about what to cook for dinner until just before it was time to eat – let alone get her act together the night before! And so she created a stovetop version using canned beans.

We've enjoyed laughing at our mistakes (like the time baking soda ended up in the cupcakes instead of salt!) and celebrating our discoveries (like the time we created our favorite blueberry and walnut salad by just chatting about possibilities while testing salad dressings). But so much more than our cooking has changed. Both intentionally and without trying, we have encouraged each other spiritually, physically, mentally and emotionally. This cookbook is a reflection of how God has intertwined our lives.

Our friends and family are an integral part of this book because they are an integral part of our lives. As we poured ourselves into this book, they supported us, prayed for us and tested our food. (Sometimes over and over again!) Their differing preferences led to many of the variations offered in the recipes. Looking at the front cover of the book is like looking at a patchwork quilt of memories. Dorie's small group ate that exact bowl of dip; Sondra's friends at church ate those biscuits; Dorie's son Justin ate that hamburger after operating the camera lights for us; and we devoured those pancakes, starved after a morning of work. Man, were they good!

We truly wrote this book from the trenches. During the three-plus years that we worked on this project, we encountered sickness, major life changes and family emergencies. We put plans on hold, ate on the run and regrouped more times than we dreamed imaginable. And we cooked with children very much present. We still laugh about Dorie's inability to accurately test the timing of a recipe because there are always interruptions at her house. But even the interruptions have shaped this book – we want others who cook with interruptions to have easier, healthier ways to do so and still keep their sanity!

And children are a major reason we want to share this book with you. This current generation of children may be the first in modern history to have a life expectancy shorter than that of their parents. As we provide healthy options for our children, we are able to teach them how to make good choices. This happens as we do these things ourselves. It isn't easy. The fact that it's taken us two years longer than expected to complete this cookbook is evidence of that! But the fact that the cookbook is in your hands is also evidence that it can be done – not because of our ability but because of God's grace.

We have no question that God uses the circumstances in our lives for His glory, and we know that this book — a patchwork of our lives — is His. We hope that He will use it in your life and that He will be glorified by the work of our hands, minds and hearts.

Contact Us

We would love to hear from you – your stories, your experiences, your variations and your recipes. We would be happy to look at recipes with you (working toward making them healthier, finding alternative ingredients, etc.). We also welcome your questions, answering what we can and brainstorming solutions with you. The best way to contact us is via our websites:

www.Transitions2BetterLiving.com
www.SimpleChoices4HealthierEating.com

About the Authors

Sondra Lewis has a bachelor of science degree, and has taken graduate studies, in family and consumer science. Prior to authoring cookbooks, she was an educator and an assistant manager in college food service. Lewis enjoys healthy cooking to maintain health and manage allergies. She lives with her husband in Coralville, IA.

Dorie Fink has taught elementary school and enjoys free-lance editing and speaking. Supporting family members with health challenges propelled her into the world of food preparation and nutrition. She lives with her husband and their two sons in Eau Claire, WI.

Lewis and Fink share a love of cooking, gardening, learning and educating. They also enjoy sharing recipes and produce from their local CSAs and farmer's markets. Between them, Lewis and Fink have nearly twenty-five years of healthy cooking experience.

Printed in the United States
119400LV00002B/127-166/P

9 780964 34628